CARLAT PUBLISHING

HOSPITAL PSYCHIATRY FACT BOOK

FIRST EDITION

Victoria Hendrick, MD

Editor-in-Chief, *The Carlat Hospital Psychiatry Report*

Clinical Professor, David Geffen School of Medicine at UCLA

Director of Inpatient Psychiatry, Olive View–UCLA Medical Center, Los Angeles, CA

Daniel J. Carlat, MD

Publisher, *The Carlat Report* newsletters and books

Associate Clinical Professor, Tufts University School of Medicine, Boston, MA

Published by Carlat Publishing, LLC

PO Box 626, Newburyport, MA 01950

CARLAT PUBLISHING

Hospital Psychiatry Fact Book

FIRST EDITION

Published by Carlat Publishing, LLC
PO Box 626, Newburyport, MA 01950

Publisher and Editor-in-Chief: Daniel J. Carlat, MD
Deputy Editor: Talia Puzantian, PharmD, BCPP
Senior Editor: Ilana Fogelson

This CME/CE activity is intended for psychiatrists, psychiatric nurses, psychologists, and other health care professionals with an interest in mental health. The Carlat CME Institute is accredited by the Accreditation Council for Continuing Medical Education to provide continuing medical education for physicians. Carlat CME Institute maintains responsibility for this program and its content. Carlat CME Institute designates this enduring material educational activity for a maximum of fourteen (14) *AMA PRA Category 1 Credits*™. Physicians or psychologists should claim credit commensurate only with the extent of their participation in the activity. The American Board of Psychiatry and Neurology has reviewed the *Hospital Psychiatry Fact Book* and has approved this program as part of a comprehensive Self-Assessment and CME Program, which is mandated by ABMS as a necessary component of maintenance of certification. CME tests must be taken online at www.thecarlatreport.com/cme (for ABPN SA course subscribers).

To order, visit www.thecarlatreport.com
or call (866) 348-9279

2 3 4 5 6 7 8 9 10

ISBN #:
Print: 979-8-9893264-2-6
eBook: 979-8-9893264-3-3

PRINTED IN THE UNITED STATES OF AMERICA

Table of Contents

Introduction **7**

Working in Multidisciplinary Teams **9**

Nurses: Key Responsibilities and Communication Tips 10
Social Workers & Case Managers: Collaboration Strategies 12
Occupational and Recreation Therapists: Roles in Recovery 13
Psychiatric Technicians: Safety and Patient Engagement 14
Pharmacists: Supporting Medication Management 15
Working with the Hospital Pharmacy 16

Patient Assessment and Documentation **17**

How to Conduct a Psychiatric Emergency Department Evaluation 18
Psychiatric Admission Notes: Structure and Key Elements 20
How to Document Daily Progress Notes 25
Discharge Summaries: Essential Components for Continuity of Care 26
Techniques for the Psychiatric Interview 28
The Psychiatric Review of Symptoms 29
Mental Status Examination: Key Components and Interpretation 32

Physical Examination in Psychiatry **35**

How to Conduct the Physical Exam 36
How to Perform the Neurological Exam 37

Legal and Ethical Considerations **39**

Informed Consent: Legal and Practical Aspects 40
Commitment Hearings: Testimony and Procedures 41
Health Care Proxy and Power of Attorney 42
Involuntary Medications: Guidelines and Considerations 43
How to Evaluate Capacity to Make Decisions 44
Confidentiality and Release of Patient Information 45

Health Care Administration and Compliance **47**

Medicare and Medicaid: Overview and Billing 48
Utilization Review (UR) and Compliance 50
Coding and Billing Protocols 52
The Joint Commission and Psychiatric Hospitals 54
Quality Measures in Psychiatric Care 55

Hospital Safety Protocols **57**

How to Use Precaution Orders 58
Managing Sexual Activity Incidents on the Inpatient Unit 59
Workplace Violence Prevention and Safety 60
Minimizing PTSD from Workplace Trauma 61
Reportable Events: Documentation and Compliance 62

Agitation Management **63**

How to Verbally De-Escalate an Aggressive Patient 64

How to Medicate an Agitated Patient. 66
How to Minimize Use of Restraints 67
Physical Restraints and Seclusion: Guidelines and Safety 68

Suicide and Self-Injurious Behaviors 71
How to Identify and Respond to Self-Injurious Behaviors 72
Medical Management of Self-Injurious Behaviors 73
Assessing Suicide Risk 74
Creating a Patient Safety Plan 76
Protocols Following a Patient Suicide. 77
How to Manage Deliberate Foreign Body Ingestion 78

Danger to Others 79
Assessing and Managing Homicide Risk 80
Handling Tarasoff Obligations. 81

COMMON PSYCHIATRIC CONDITIONS

Anxiety Disorders 83
Screening for Common Anxiety Disorders 84
Obsessive-Compulsive Disorder (OCD) 85
Panic Disorder. 86
Trauma-Related Disorders 87
How to Manage Anxiety with Nonaddictive Medications 89
Choosing and Managing Benzodiazepines. 90

Bipolar Disorder 92
Bipolar Disorder Diagnostic Interview 93
How to Medicate Manic Episodes 94
How to Treat Bipolar Depression 96

Depressive Disorders 97
Differential Diagnosis of Depressive Disorders 98
How to Diagnose Major Depressive Disorder. 99
Depression with Psychotic Features 100
How to Choose Medications for Major Depressive Disorder. 101
Prolonged Grief Disorder 102
Electroconvulsive Therapy (ECT) 103
Transcranial Magnetic Stimulation (TMS) 105

Developmental and Intellectual Disabilities 106
Intellectual Disabilities: Management in Inpatient Psychiatry 107
ADHD in Adults 108
Autism Spectrum Disorder 109

Eating Disorders 110
Anorexia Nervosa. 111
Forced Refeeding in Anorexia Nervosa 113
Bulimia Nervosa 114

Insomnia 115
Sleep Disturbances in Inpatient Psychiatry. 116
Insomnia: Medication Management 117

Neurocognitive Disorders **118**
Major Neurocognitive Disorder: Evaluation 119
Major Neurocognitive Disorder: Medication Treatment 121
How to Identify and Manage Confusion and Delirium 122
Behavioral and Psychological Symptoms of Dementia 123
Traumatic Brain Injury 124

Personality Disorders **126**
Overview of Personality Disorders 127
Borderline Personality Disorder 128

Schizophrenia and Other Psychotic Disorders **130**
Interviewing Patients with Psychosis 131
DSM-5 Diagnosis for Psychotic Disorders 132
Schizophrenia: Assessment and Management 133
Medication Strategies for Schizophrenia 135
Schizoaffective Disorder: Diagnosis and Treatment 136
Delusional Disorder 137
Brief Psychotic Disorder 138
Antipsychotic Comparison: Quick Reference 139
Clozapine: Guidelines for Use and Monitoring 142
Long-Acting Injectable Antipsychotics 143
Discontinuing and Switching Antipsychotics 147

Substance Use Disorders **148**
Managing Alcohol Withdrawal 149
Managing Opioid Withdrawal 150
Treatment of Stimulant Use Disorders 151
Wernicke's Encephalopathy 153

Less Common Syndromes **154**
Catatonia 155
Dissociative Identity Disorder 156
Factitious Disorder 157
Functional Neurological Disorder 158

Psychotherapy on the Inpatient Unit **159**
Introduction to Inpatient Psychotherapy 160
Motivational Interviewing Techniques 161
Cognitive Behavioral Therapy Techniques 162
Supportive Therapy in the Inpatient Setting 163
Group Programs 164
Psychotherapy for Psychotic Disorders 166
Relaxation and Deep Breathing Exercises 167
Anger Management Techniques 168
Sample Behavior Management Plan 169
Establishing a Token Economy 170

Medication Side Effects **171**
Discussing and Managing Medication Side Effects 172
Metabolic Syndrome 173
Akathisia 174
Bruxism 175

Constipation ... 176
Diarrhea ... 177
Dry Mouth (Xerostomia) ... 178
Dystonia ... 179
Excessive Sweating (Hyperhidrosis) ... 180
Fatigue ... 181
Hyperprolactinemia ... 182
Nausea ... 183
Neuroleptic Malignant Syndrome ... 184
Orthostatic Hypotension ... 185
Parkinsonism ... 186
QT Interval Prolongation ... 187
Serotonin Syndrome ... 189
Sexual Dysfunction ... 190
Sialorrhea (Hypersalivation) ... 191
Tardive Dyskinesia ... 192
Tremor ... 193
Weight Gain ... 194

Diagnostic and Monitoring Tools ... 195

Which Diagnostic Labs Should You Order? ... 196
Complete Blood Count ... 198
Basic Metabolic Panel ... 201
Kidney Function Testing ... 203
Liver Function Tests ... 204
Urinalysis ... 205
Therapeutic Drug Monitoring ... 206
Urine Drug Screening ... 207
Neuroimaging in Psychiatry ... 209
Pharmacogenetic Testing ... 210
ECG in Inpatient Psychiatry ... 211

Prescribing and Medication Management ... 213

Clinically Significant Drug Interactions ... 214
Recommended Labs for Psychiatric Medications ... 216
Prescribing Psychiatric Medications in Kidney Impairment ... 218
Prescribing Psychiatric Medications in Liver Impairment ... 219
Routine Medications for Common Patient Needs ... 221

Managing Comorbid Medical Conditions ... 223

Abnormal Lipid Levels ... 224
Abdominal Pain ... 226
Acute Stroke Symptoms ... 227
Anti-NMDA Receptor Encephalitis ... 228
Chest Pain in Psychiatric Settings ... 229
Chronic Obstructive Pulmonary Disease (COPD) ... 231
CPR Guidelines for Inpatient Psychiatry ... 233
Diabetes ... 235
Gastroesophageal Reflux Disease (GERD) ... 237
Headaches ... 238
HIV ... 240
Huntington's Disease ... 242
Hypertension ... 243

Hyponatremia 245
Lice and Scabies 246
Pain Management 247
Parkinson's Disease 248
Poststroke Psychiatric Symptoms 250
Psychogenic Polydipsia: Diagnosis and Treatment 252
Seizure Disorders 253
Sexually Transmitted Diseases 255
Swollen Feet, Ankles, and Calves 256
Syphilis 258
Systemic Lupus Erythematosus 259
Thyroid Disease 260
Upper Respiratory Infections 262
Urinary Tract Infections 263
Viral Hepatitis 264

Specific Populations 265

Management of Agitation in Children and Adolescents in Hospital Settings 266
Management of Suicidality and Self-Harm in Children and Adolescents 268
Working with Pregnant Patients 269
Treatment of Bipolar Disorder in Pregnant and Postpartum Women 271
Depression in Pregnancy: Diagnosis and Treatment 273
How to Recognize and Treat Postpartum Depression 274
Postpartum Psychosis: Diagnosis and Treatment 275
Use of Psychiatric Medications in Breastfeeding Patients 276
Cross-Cultural Issues on the Inpatient Psychiatric Unit 280
Providing Gender-Affirming Care to LGBTQIA+ Patients in Hospital Units 281

Appendices 283

Appendix A: National Mental Health Resources 284
Appendix B: SMART Goals and Interventions in Psychiatric Care 286
Appendix C: Clinical Scales 288

Index 289

List of Tables

Table 1: Suicide Risk and Protective Factors 75
Table 2: Comparative Table of Benzodiazepines 91
Table 3: Long-Acting Injectable Antipsychotics 144
Table 4: QTc Interval Classification for Adults 187
Table 5: Top QT-Prolonging Non-Psychotropic Meds 187
Table 6: Risk of QT Prolongation with Psychiatric Medications 188
Table 7: Recommended Diagnostic Tests 197
Table 8: Elements of a Urinalysis: Quick Reference Chart 205
Table 9: Urine Drug Screening 208
Table 10: Pharmacogenetic Recommendations from the FDA 210
Table 11: Most Common Clinically Significant Drug Interactions in Psychiatry 215
Table 12: Recommended Laboratory Tests for Psychiatric Medications 216
Table 13: Illustrative Insulin Sliding Scale Protocol 236
Table 14: Distinguishing Antipsychotic-Induced Parkinsonism from PD 248
Table 15: ED Dosing Recommendations for Children and Adolescents 267
Table 16: Psychiatric Medications in Pregnancy and Lactation 277
Table 17: Commonly Used Clinical Scales 288

Introduction

Inpatient psychiatric care in the United States faces many challenges, from a shortage of beds and psychiatrists to the pressures of managed care. These obstacles can make the system feel overwhelming. As an inpatient psychiatrist, you'll encounter demanding workloads and patients eager for discharge. Hospital administrators will require meticulous documentation and completion of numerous forms. And yet, there is nothing as endlessly fascinating and rewarding as working in a psychiatric inpatient unit. You have a front row seat to the human drama, and the "actors" reach out to hoist you onto the stage—because you are the key player in resolving all manner of crises.

This book was born of our delights and frustrations working in several inpatient units over our careers. Its purpose is to help you get your work done efficiently. We'll cover everything from reviewing old charts and handling administrative tasks to navigating forensic issues and managing psychiatric emergencies. Our advice derives from a combination of sources, including our own experiences, interviews with highly experienced unit staff, and the scientific literature (though oddly enough, there's not much published on how to do inpatient psychiatry). While there are already some good inpatient psychiatry textbooks around, most of them are comprehensive textbooks of psychiatric practice rather than truly useful manuals—so we wrote our own.

To complement what we've covered in this book, we've also put together a variety of online resources at www.thecarlatreport.com/inpatient. These include more in-depth coverage of daily inpatient routines, interview techniques, and patient management strategies, plus practical tools like downloadable scales and patient handouts. We hope these will help you navigate the complexities of inpatient psychiatry with even more confidence.

Enjoy the book, but more importantly, enjoy the work.

Victoria Hendrick, MD
Daniel J. Carlat, MD

Working in Multidisciplinary Teams

Nurses: Key Responsibilities and Communication Tips

Nurses are arguably the most important staff members in a psychiatric hospital. They not only administer the medical and psychiatric care prescribed by health care providers, but also act as your eyes and ears on the unit, promptly identifying and alerting you to any new issues. It's important to understand how nurses work, because the more in sync you are with them, the more effectively and efficiently you can manage your responsibilities.

Training

There are two primary types of nurses: registered nurses (RNs) and licensed practical nurses (LPNs)/licensed vocational nurses (LVNs). RNs must have at least an associate degree in nursing, which usually takes two to three years, depending on the program. Some RNs also pursue a bachelor's degree in nursing (BSN), which is increasingly becoming a requirement in hospitals. LPNs (or LVNs, as they are called in California and Texas), on the other hand, can get a certificate after only one year of training. To a casual observer (ie, you) it will be hard to tell the difference between an RN and an LPN/LVN. While more extensive training is desirable, in reality nursing competence is related more to the degree of experience on a psychiatric unit.

Duties

- *Medication administration:* Nurses deliver medications in various forms (eg, pills, nebulizers, patches, injections).
- *Psychotherapy and counseling:* Nurses often provide emotional support and crisis intervention for patients who are agitated or distressed, and they decide when to administer PRNs.
- *Behavioral management:* Nurses oversee behavioral plans to monitor and manage patient safety, including restraints if necessary. The actual work of things like 15-minute checks is generally done by psychiatric technicians (see the "Psychiatric Technicians: Safety and Patient Engagement" fact sheet in this section).
- *Medical symptom evaluation and management:* Nurses obtain vital signs and fingerstick glucoses; manage constipation, nausea, and pain; provide wound care; and so on.
- *Self-care assistance:* Nurses aid patients with activities of daily living like bathing and dressing.

Roles

Nurses may assume different roles during a shift:

- *Charge nurse:* There is often a designated "charge nurse" who is involved in reviewing admissions and escalating clinical issues as needed following the hospital's chain of command.
- *Patient assignments:* Specific patients are assigned to nurses for personalized care.
- *Admissions/discharges:* Some nurses specialize in managing patient admissions and discharges.
- *Medication:* Nurses may each be responsible for their assigned patients' medication administration, or there may be a dedicated nurse (a "med nurse") who handles all the medication dispensing.
- *Vital signs:* Vitals are usually done once a day in the morning. Knowing who is responsible for vitals each day is useful, as this nurse can address questions about abnormalities and perform rechecks upon request. (Sometimes psychiatric technicians will also do vitals.)

Staffing Ratios and Patient Acuity

You'll notice that staffing may vary from day to day. While there are no specific national guidelines for the ratio of nurses and other staff to patients, the nurse-to-patient ratio in psychiatric units is usually in the range of 1:4 to 1:6 (although the ratio changes during the night shift due to lower activity levels and patient needs, potentially reaching 1:8 or higher). Clearly, more staff are needed when the unit is full. Even at a given census level, the intensity of patients will vary. The intensity of the patient mix is termed "acuity," and you'll often hear this mentioned when the charge nurse is deciding whether they can take a new admission: "We're too acute right now for this kind of patient." There are various acuity rating scales, but here is a typical breakdown:

- *Low acuity:* Patients who are ready for discharge.
- *Medium acuity:* Patients in need of treatment who are cooperative with their treatment plan.
- *Higher acuity:* Patients who are highly symptomatic, such as those who are manic, actively responding to delusions and hallucinations, or suicidal. They are usually on at least 15-minute checks.
- *Highest acuity:* Patients at highest risk for suicide or violence. They may be on constant observation and may be at risk for needing to be physically or chemically restrained.

Collaborating Effectively with Nurses

- At the beginning of the day, make sure you know each nurse by name and their specific roles—especially who is assigned to your patients. Knowing team members' names is critical for effective teamwork throughout medicine. For example, in Atul Gawande's *The Checklist Manifesto*, he points out that knowing names in the operating room decreases surgery complication rates by 35%. The better you know your co-workers, the easier it is to communicate with them, and patient care benefits as a result.

- Read nursing assessments. Nurses write brief shift notes that describe the patient's symptoms and behaviors over each eight-hour shift. These will give you valuable insights into a patient's condition and response to treatment.
- Determine which nurses are the most competent. Like doctors, nurses vary in their skill and competence. It may seem obvious, but unless you spend some time talking to the nurses you work with, you may not recognize these variations in clinical prowess. This is important because the best nurses will give you the best advice, and you should get in the habit of consulting them on difficult patients. (Often the most competent nurse will be the charge nurse.)
- When asking nurses about patients, rather than simply asking, "How is the patient doing?" ask for specifics: "How do you think the medications are working for Mr. Jones? How many hours of sleep did he get last night?"
- Since nurses are on the front line of dealing with complaints, agitation, and suicidal ideation, they often have astute insights to help you deal with these problems. Ask them what they think will help address these issues.

Social Workers & Case Managers: Collaboration Strategies

Social workers are key players on the inpatient psych unit, and working well with them can make your job a lot easier. They bring a wealth of expertise, especially in addressing the social and psychological aspects of treatment, and they excel at coordinating services that support patients during and after their hospital stay. While social workers often handle discharge planning, larger units may also include case managers specifically for this task.

Training

Social workers must complete a master's degree in social work (MSW), and many go on to become psychotherapists, typically obtaining a Licensed Clinical Social Worker (LCSW) designation, which requires about two years of post-master's clinical experience. Social workers are well versed in many of the clinical areas familiar to psychiatrists, except with more emphasis on psychosocial treatments. They also become highly knowledgeable about public assistance programs like Medicaid, Social Security disability, and various human service agencies to aid the indigent.

Case managers typically hold degrees in social work, nursing, or a related field, often with specialized training in mental health. Many have a background as LCSWs or RNs with additional certifications in case management.

Duties

Like you, social workers and case managers see their assigned patients daily (or nearly every day) and write a note. Their schedule will be similar to yours, so it's often helpful for you and the social worker to see patients together. Their responsibilities can include:

- *Psychosocial assessments:* Evaluating all new patients.
- *Family and caregiver liaison:* Contacting family members and outside caregivers for additional insights and to address issues during the hospitalization.
- *Discharge planning:* Coordinating outpatient services, referrals, and appointments.
- *Utilization review:* Securing authorization for extended inpatient care from insurance companies. Some hospitals have dedicated utilization review staff.
- *Resource connection:* Case managers connect patients with community resources, including social services, support groups, and financial assistance programs.

Collaborating Effectively with Social Workers & Case Managers

- *Communicate*: A common complaint from social workers is that the psychiatrist comes in, writes a bunch of orders, and then leaves. Often the patients are not told about the medication changes, and then the social worker bears the brunt of the patient's questions or complaints. Before leaving the hospital, always check in with the social worker to discuss any new orders.
- *Be involved in family meetings*: While social workers often lead family meetings, families often have questions for the doctors, like about medication choices and side effects. They also often want to find out why the patient is not being discharged. The social worker can rarely provide answers to all these questions, so it's helpful for you to at least make a brief appearance in these meetings.
- *Assist with forms*: Coordinate on filling out forms that require extensive clinical information, like applications for guardianship/conservatorship and follow-ups with the department of mental health. Doctors often hate dealing with forms and delegate them to social workers, who then must struggle through the clinical portions—which doctors could complete more easily.

Occupational and Recreation Therapists: Roles in Recovery

Occupational therapists (OTs) play a pivotal role in inpatient treatment settings. While the term "occupational therapy" might initially seem puzzling, its roots are deeply intertwined with the history of psychiatric treatment. In the era before modern psychiatric care, wards primarily served as containment facilities, offering basic necessities but little in terms of holistic treatment. The revolution arrived in the form of occupational therapy, founded on the belief that mental illnesses arose from imbalances between work and leisure. The Johns Hopkins Department of Psychiatry was among the early pioneers of this approach, creating a "habit training" program where patients engaged in activities like basket weaving and bookbinding to restore balance. Over time, occupational therapy expanded beyond psychiatry, offering patients across medical fields a pathway to reengage in meaningful life activities after illness.

Recreation therapists are vital to the holistic care of patients on the psychiatric unit, using therapeutic activities to enhance mental and emotional well-being. Their work focuses on improving patients' physical, social, and cognitive functioning through structured recreational activities. Understanding their role and collaborating effectively can significantly enhance patient recovery and engagement in the therapeutic process.

Training

OTs are required to complete a master's degree in occupational therapy, which includes coursework in medical and psychological sciences, as well as at least 24 weeks of fieldwork. Graduates must pass the National Board for Certification in Occupational Therapy (NBCOT) exam and obtain state licensure.

Recreation therapists typically hold a bachelor's or master's degree in recreational therapy or a related field and are often certified as Certified Therapeutic Recreation Specialists (CTRS). Their training includes work in therapeutic techniques, psychology, and physical health, letting them design and implement activities that promote overall well-being.

Duties

OTs focus on bridging the gap between symptomatic relief and functional improvement in daily life. While psychiatrists and nurses alleviate symptoms through medications and therapy, OTs help patients apply these psychological gains to real-world situations.

Key duties of an OT include:

- Conducting initial assessments and creating personalized treatment plans related to activities of daily living (ADLs), social skills, work skills, and money management skills.
- Conducting more specific assessments as necessary, such as fall risk and cognitive functioning evaluations.
- Facilitating therapeutic groups, from goal setting and life skills to art, music, and substance abuse therapy.
- Assessing patients' readiness for discharge and providing insights into the level of care needed post-discharge.

Duties of recreation therapists include:

- *Activity planning:* Recreation therapists develop individualized and group activities that promote physical health, social interaction, and mental stimulation.
- *Skill development:* Through therapeutic activities, they help patients build coping skills, improve self-esteem, and manage stress.
- *Behavioral activation:* They use activities to engage patients in meaningful experiences, reducing symptoms of depression and anxiety.
- *Progress assessment:* Recreation therapists monitor and assess patients' participation and progress, adjusting interventions as necessary to meet therapeutic goals.

Collaborating Effectively with Occupational Therapists

Understanding the work of an OT can greatly enhance your collaborative efforts. Here are some strategies:

- *Attend OT-run groups:* This will familiarize you with group activities—the primary source of psychosocial treatment on units—and provide insight into your patients' progress.
- *Review OT documentation:* OTs record their activities, initial evaluations, and patient participation in the medical chart. Reviewing these can offer valuable information for your treatment plans.
- *Understand ADLs:* OTs assess both basic and instrumental ADLs. Basic ADLs include walking, feeding, dressing, grooming, toileting, bathing, and transferring. Instrumental ADLs are more complex tasks required for independent living, such as managing finances, transportation, shopping, meal preparation, housecleaning, home maintenance, communication management, and medication management.

Collaborating Effectively with Recreation Therapists

- *Participate in care planning:* Include recreation therapists in treatment team meetings to ensure their activities support the patient's therapeutic goals.
- *Encourage patient participation:* Reinforce the importance of recreational activities as part of the patient's overall treatment, motivating patients to engage in these interventions.
- *Provide feedback:* Share observations about how patients respond to recreational activities and collaborate on adjusting interventions to better meet patients' needs.

Psychiatric Technicians: Safety and Patient Engagement

Psychiatric technicians, also known as mental health aides or specialists, are unsung but vital members of the mental health care team.

Training

Requirements for psych techs vary widely from state to state. Some states require only a high school diploma, whereas others require specific psych tech licensure. The American Association of Psychiatric Technicians is the main organization offering certifications, and there are four certificate levels, corresponding with increasing training requirements. The lowest, Level 1, requires a high school diploma or GED, while the highest, Level 4, requires a bachelor's degree in the mental health field plus at least three years of experience in a mental health setting.

Duties

To the uninitiated psychiatrist, psych techs may appear to be random staff members milling around. When we were new to inpatient work, we didn't know if they were nurses, custodians, or security staff. In some ways, psych techs are all these things, plus therapists. Duties include:

- Observing patients throughout their shifts and documenting their observations.
- Monitoring patient safety, such as doing 15-minute checks.
- Helping with activities of daily living, including dressing, toileting, and eating.
- Participating in restraints.
- Escorting patients off the unit, such as for outdoor breaks or for 12-step meetings.
- At higher levels of training, taking vital signs, writing shift notes, and running therapeutic groups (eg, coping skills or mindfulness).
- Providing emotional support and counseling.

Collaborating Effectively with Psych Techs

Get to know the psych techs who are working with your patients—don't underestimate them as "low level" staff. Many are actively pursuing further education in nursing, medicine, or related fields and choose to work in this setting for both experience and financial reasons. Make a point of asking psych techs about their impressions of your patients. They bring a unique perspective, often spending significant time engaging in casual conversations with patients, and can provide insights beyond clinical symptoms.

Pharmacists: Supporting Medication Management

Pharmacists play a critical role in managing medication safety and efficacy and identifying potential drug interactions. You'll collaborate closely with them to ensure optimal pharmacological care for patients.

Training

Most pharmacists hold a Doctor of Pharmacy (Pharm.D) degree, typically earned after four years of postcollege education. Some pharmacists enter the field through six-year programs that begin after high school. Additionally, pharmacists can pursue specialization as Board Certified Psychiatric Pharmacists (BCPPs) through a variety of pathways, culminating in a board certification examination.

Duties

- Managing the in-hospital pharmacy, including creating formularies, helping to develop clinical guidelines, purchasing medications, and dispensing medications as they are ordered on the units.
- Reviewing medication orders, clarifying unclear orders, and discussing potential issues with physicians.
- In some settings, clinical psychiatric pharmacists participate in patient rounds and act as psychopharmacological consultants. They may provide medication-related education to medical, nursing, and other professional staff and conduct medication education groups for patients.

Common Issues and Interactions

Pharmacists frequently need to clarify orders when there are discrepancies in dosages or potential drug interactions that could be harmful. They may recommend dosing adjustments or alternative medications, based on hepatic or renal function, or for patients who are pregnant or who have medical comorbidities. They also assist in optimizing nonpsychiatric medication regimens (eg, for infections or diabetes).

Formulary and Nonformulary Requests

- The formulary—a list of approved medications—is determined by a hospital committee, which is usually called the P&T (Pharmacy and Therapeutics) committee or the formulary committee. This committee includes pharmacists, physicians, and nurses. It makes decisions by balancing patient care with budget considerations.
- You can request a list of all formulary drugs from the pharmacy.
- If a drug is not on the formulary, you can request that it be added. Call the pharmacy and ask them what the protocol is for making that request. Alternatively, a pharmacist may also provide a suitable therapeutic substitution.

How Pharmacists Can Help You

Get to know your hospital's pharmacists and communicate with them frequently. They can assist you with:

- Checking availability of and procuring new medications.
- Advising on dosing and titration schedules.
- Managing transitions, like from oral antipsychotics to injectables.
- Providing guidance on drug-drug interactions.
- Gathering patient medication history either from the patient or through available records, including the state's prescription drug monitoring program (PDMP): https://www.pdmpassist.org/
- Coordinating "meds to beds" programs at some hospitals, in which discharge meds are delivered to the bedside before patients are discharged, with the pharmacist providing medication counseling and education.

Working with the Hospital Pharmacy

The process from when you order a medication in an electronic health record (EHR) to when it arrives at the nursing station is complex and involves multiple steps. Understanding this process, including medication reconciliation, can help you ensure more efficient care and minimize delays in medication administration.

The Medication Order Process

1. *Order entry:* Once you order a medication through the EHR, the order is electronically transmitted to the pharmacy. This system reduces errors related to handwriting and immediately alerts pharmacists to new orders.
2. *Pharmacist review:* The pharmacist receives the order and reviews it for any potential issues, such as drug interactions, allergies, or dosing errors.
3. *Medication preparation:* After approval, the pharmacy staff prepares the medication. This might involve measuring the correct dose, compounding drugs if necessary, and labeling the medication.
4. *Dispensing:* The prepared medication is then dispensed, typically into a secure cart that is transported to the nursing station. Controlled substances often require additional verification steps.

Medication Reconciliation Explained

Medication reconciliation is a safety process in which health care providers compare a patient's medication orders to all the medications that the patient has been taking. This is to avoid medication errors such as omissions, duplications, dosing errors, or drug interactions. Pharmacists play a key role in this process by:

- Verifying the accuracy of medication lists at admission, transfer, and discharge.
- Ensuring that any medication changes are intentional and documented.
- Consulting with psychiatrists and nurses to clarify any discrepancies.

Common Delays and How to Mitigate Them

Delays in getting medications to the nursing station can be caused by:

- The need for thorough review and preparation, especially for high-risk medications.
- The physical distance between the pharmacy and patient care area.
- Waiting for approval of controlled substances.
- Limited pharmacy staffing, particularly during off hours.

Strategies to Make the Medication Process as Seamless as Possible

- Enter orders into the EHR as early as possible, especially for medications known to require extra processing time.
- Participate in medication reconciliation by providing accurate and complete medication histories.
- Educate yourself on formulary options and choose first-line medications that are readily available in the hospital pharmacy.
- Communicate directly with pharmacists when prescribing complex or unusual medication regimens.

Patient Assessment and Documentation

How to Conduct a Psychiatric Emergency Department Evaluation

Evaluating new patients in the psychiatric emergency department (ED) can be demanding and high-pressure. You will likely be dealing with multiple patients simultaneously, all needing evaluations or attention for agitation, suicidality, or other urgent concerns. Here's a guide to help you navigate the process effectively.

Safety Assessment

- Quickly assess if the patient poses a risk to themselves or others. Check for weapons or harmful objects. If the patient is agitated, ensure you have adequate support from security or other staff.
- Make sure the environment is safe. Remove potential hazards, and if necessary, place the patient in a safe room.

Rapid Physical and Mental Status Exam (MSE)

- Ensure nurses have obtained vital signs. Abnormal vitals can indicate common medical issues masquerading as psychiatric symptoms, like substance intoxication/withdrawal.
- Perform a brief physical exam to check for signs of medical conditions that could affect mental status, like head trauma, infections, dehydration, or neurological deficits.
- Complete an MSE to assess appearance, behavior, speech, mood, affect, thought process, thought content, cognition, insight, and judgment.

Obtain a Comprehensive History

Chief complaint and history of present illness

- Understand why the patient is here today. What event or symptom brought them in?
- When did the symptoms start? How have they progressed?

Psychiatric history

- Previous diagnoses, hospitalizations, treatments, and response to treatments.
- History of alcohol or drug use.
- Family history of psychiatric diagnoses.

Legal history

- Find out if there's a history of arrests or other encounters with the law.

Medical history

- Medical conditions, current and past.
- Current medications, as well as any recent changes or noncompliance issues.
- Any known allergies.
- Obtain a review of systems to identify symptoms that may contribute to the psychiatric presentation. Cover the major systems (general health, cardiovascular, respiratory, gastrointestinal, genitourinary, musculoskeletal, neurological, skin).

Suicide and Violence Risk Assessment

- Ask direct questions about thoughts of self-harm, plans, and means.
- Similarly, inquire about any thoughts of harming others.
- Watch for risk factors, like previous attempts, family history, substance abuse, and recent stressors.
- Your electronic health record likely includes a suicide risk assessment template that you will need to complete before you wrap up your note.

Collateral Information

- If the patient consents, contact family members or friends for additional information, especially if the patient's account is unclear or inconsistent.
- Don't disclose information without the patient's consent, but if family or friends reach out to you, you are free to listen to what they have to say.
- Review previous medical records if available.

Laboratory and Diagnostic Tests

- Obtain a urine drug screen.
- Order other relevant labs (eg, complete blood count, complete metabolic panel, thyroid function tests) based on the patient's presentation and medical history.
- For patients of reproductive age, obtain a urine pregnancy test if applicable.

Prescription Drug Monitoring Program (PDMP) Check

- Before finalizing your assessment and plan, check the patient's use of controlled substances through your state's PDMP. This will help you identify any potential misuse of controlled substances, doctor shopping, or overprescription, which could contribute to the patient's current psychiatric presentation.
- In California, this is known as the Controlled Substance Utilization Review and Evaluation System (CURES). Other states have their own systems, such as MassPAT in Massachusetts, the Illinois Prescription Monitoring Program (ILPMP), KASPER in Kentucky, and PMP Aware in Texas.

Differential Diagnosis and Treatment Planning

- Based on history and MSE, narrow down potential psychiatric diagnoses.
- Consider medical causes for new-onset psychiatric symptoms:
  - Substance intoxication/withdrawal—a common reason patients show up in psychiatric EDs.
  - Medication side effects like from anticholinergics (causing delirium), corticosteroids and stimulants (causing psychosis or mania), or antidepressants (causing serotonin syndrome).
  - Thyroid disorders: Hyperthyroidism or hypothyroidism can cause anxiety, depression, or psychosis.
  - Neurological conditions: Seizure disorders, traumatic brain injury, or encephalopathy can lead to confusion, mood changes, or psychosis.
  - Autoimmune conditions: Such as systemic lupus erythematosus, which can cause psychosis, depression, or cognitive dysfunction.
  - Infections: Such as meningitis or encephalitis. Even urinary tract infections can cause altered mental status, especially in elderly individuals.
  - Electrolyte imbalances: Hyponatremia or hypercalcemia, which can lead to confusion or psychosis.

Immediate Management

- Patients are often brought to the ED by police or psychiatric mobile response teams, already on involuntary holds, and you will need to decide whether to keep the hold. Talk to the staff who brought the patient to understand what happened and read the involuntary hold paperwork.
- If the patient is in acute distress, stabilize with medications as necessary (eg, benzodiazepines for agitation, antipsychotics for psychosis).
- Determine if the patient needs to be admitted for further observation and treatment or if they can be safely discharged with outpatient follow-up.
- For patients who need inpatient admission: Consider starting treatment in the psych ED, especially in cases where the patient won't be able to transfer to the inpatient unit immediately.
- If you initiate psychiatric medications, provide information to the patient about their diagnosis and the medication you'll be prescribing, including risks, side effects, and alternatives. Patients will often be unwilling or unable to discuss treatment, but have them sign the informed consent for medications if they're willing.
- For patients stable enough to be discharged, provide resources for outpatient follow-up. Prescribe discharge medications in a quantity sufficient for the follow-up appointment, to encourage attending the appointment.
- If you identify urgent medical issues, obtain a medical consultation for management and clearance before admitting or discharging the patient.

Document Your Assessment, Differential Diagnosis, and Plan

- Make sure your documentation includes assessments of decision-making capacity and any involuntary hold criteria if applicable.
- If you speak to collateral contacts, include a brief synopsis of the information they shared with you, along with their names and contact information.
- Depending on your state, you may need to perform a firearms advisement, informing the patient that their right to buy a weapon is nullified for a certain period (usually for five years).

Psychiatric Admission Notes: Structure and Key Elements

Admission notes are meant to serve as a succinct summary of why the patient is hospitalized, their mental status, the diagnosis, and your initial treatment plan. Current electronic health record software often spits out admission notes that are excessively long and are often ignored. To the extent that you have control over your admission notes, try to keep the narrative sections concise and to the point. They should generally be no longer than 1,000 words.

To help with this, we've provided a comprehensive template. It includes structured fields and suggested language to guide your admission documentation, as well as placeholders for specific data and descriptions that you can customize for each patient. The goal is to standardize the documentation process, making it easier for you to capture all necessary information thoroughly and concisely.

Patient Name

Preferred Language

Date of Admission

Chief Complaint

Exact quote from patient of why they believe they are here.

Identifying Information

"[Patient name] is a [age]-year-old [race] [gender] with a history of [diagnoses], admitted from the [ED/medical unit/xxx facility] for assessment and treatment of [xxx]."

Admission Legal Status

Typical broad options include "voluntary" and "involuntary," but each state has specific legal designations.

History of Present Illness

How and when patient got to the hospital

"On [date], the patient [self-presented/was brought in by xxx] after 911 was called by [person]."

Reason/precipitant

Describe events, symptoms, and behaviors leading to the patient's presentation.

ED report

Include observations and assessments by ED staff, as well as reports by family, friends, police, or EMTs.

Life stressors

Describe any significant life stressors contributing to the current situation.

Example

"On June 24, 2024, the patient was brought in by ambulance after 911 was called by a neighbor. The patient had been experiencing increasing paranoia and hallucinations, which culminated in aggressive behavior toward a family member. ED staff noted the patient was agitated and disoriented upon arrival. The patient's family reported a history of schizophrenia with recent noncompliance with medication. EMTs observed the patient making incoherent statements and displaying aggressive behavior during transport. Recent job loss and the death of a close relative have been significant stressors for the patient."

Past Psychiatric History

Prior psychiatric admissions

List dates of previous admissions, names of facilities, lengths of stay, and reasons for each admission. Example format: "[Date] at [facility name], [length of stay], for [reason]."

Medication history

List all psychiatric medications the patient has tried in the past, including dosages and durations. Include any adverse effects experienced with each medication.

Safety risks and incidents

- If there is no history, state, "Patient denied any history of suicide attempts or violent acts."
- If there is a history, describe each suicide or homicide attempt, each act of violence, and each other relevant safety issue.
- Access to firearms:
  - "Patient denied access to firearms."
  - "Patient endorsed access to firearms, including [type and location]."

Trauma history

Describe any significant traumatic events the patient has experienced, including the nature of the trauma and the patient's age at the time of the trauma.

Family Psychiatric History

Describe family history of clinical mental illness, substance use issues, and suicides, if any.

Social History

Residence

- Current living conditions:
  - "Homeless [on street/in shelter]."
  - "Lives in a group home."
  - "Owns or rents home."
  - "Lives with [family/partner/friends]."

Family

Family composition and history: Describe family structure (eg, "Only child," "Youngest of three siblings"). Include significant events like deaths, divorces, or notable family dynamics. Mention if the patient was adopted or raised in foster care.

Relationships

- Marital status: Single, married, divorced, widowed.
- Children: Number of children, if any. Describe relationship with children (eg, "Estranged," "Close contact," "Children live with patient").
- Other significant relationships: Detail any other significant romantic partnerships, friendships, or community ties.

Education

- Educational background: List highest level of education achieved (eg, "High school diploma," "College degree in [subject]").
- Learning challenges: Describe any diagnosed learning disabilities or difficulties faced during schooling.

Employment/income source

- Current employment status:
  - "Employed as [job title, eg, 'construction worker']."
  - "Unemployed, previously worked as [previous job]."
- Income source: "Collects SSI/SSDI due to [diagnosis, eg, 'chronic mental health condition']."

Military history

- Service record:
  - "Patient denied military history."
  - "Served from [start date] to [end date] in [branch of military, eg, 'US Army']."
- Discharge status: Honorable/nonhonorable discharge. If applicable, describe reasons for discharge.

Collateral Contact Information

Does patient consent to contacting their collaterals? (Y/N)

Legal History

- Arrests: List any instances of arrest, including dates and charges.
- Convictions: Detail any criminal convictions, including dates and nature of the offenses.
- Incarcerations: Note periods of incarceration and facilities involved.
- Probation/parole: Specify any terms of probation or parole, including the supervising agency, duration, and conditions.
- Outstanding warrants: Mention any existing warrants.
- Court dates: List upcoming or recent court appearances and the nature of the proceedings.
- Restraining orders: Detail any restraining orders issued, including the parties involved and the reasons.
- Involvement with Department of Children and Family Services (DCFS): Describe if applicable.

Substance Use History

- "Patient [denied/endorsed] current or prior tobacco, drug, or significant alcohol use."
- If endorsed, describe substance history, including first and most recent use, withdrawal complications, drug rehabilitation treatments, and programs.

Outpatient Providers

- "Prescriber: [Name, phone number, address]."
- "Psychotherapist: [Name, phone number, address]."
- "PCP: [Name, phone number, address]."
- "Others: [Name, role, phone number, address]."

Past Medical History

- "Unremarkable."
- "Remarkable for [list of current/past pathologies, surgeries, injuries]."

Outpatient Medications

List current medications, both psychiatric and nonpsychiatric. Include dosages and frequencies.

Allergies/Reactions

- "[No known allergies/NKA]."
- "[List of allergies and reactions]."

Review of Systems

- General: Fevers, chills, or sweats? Weight change?
- Respiratory: Shortness of breath, cough, or sore throat?
- Cardio: Chest pain or palpitations?
- GI: Nausea, vomiting, diarrhea, constipation, or heartburn?
- Genitourinary: Dysuria or urgency?
- Gynecological: Menses: Regular/irregular? Cramping? Intermenstrual or postmenopausal bleeding? Vaginal discharge?
- Musculoskeletal: Joint or muscle pain? Reduced range of motion?
- Skin: Easy bruising or bleeding? Rashes?
- Neurological: Headache, weakness, tremor, or dizziness? Vision changes?

Physical Examination

- "Hospitalist consulted to perform a standard physical examination upon admission; refer to hospitalist progress note for details."

If the psychiatric clinician does the physical and the patient has typical findings, you can use the following template (and see the related fact sheet in the Physical Examination in Psychiatry section for more details):

- General
- Head, eyes, ears, nose, and throat (HEENT)
- Neck
- Cardiovascular
- Respiratory
- Abdomen
- Extremities
- Skin
- Musculoskeletal
- Neurological

Laboratory Data

- Routine admission labs: List specific routine admission labs.
- Urine drug screen: List results or state results are pending.
- Pregnancy test: List results or state results are pending.

Mental Status Exam

Example statements are presented with spaced slashes for ease of reading. Brackets indicate places to provide additional information if applicable.

Appearance

- Clothing: Hospital gown / Casually dressed in own attire / Disheveled.
- Grooming: Groomed / Unkempt.
- Nutritional status: Well-nourished / Undernourished / Obese.
- Age appearance: Appears [older than / younger than] chronological age.

Behavior
- General: Calm / Psychomotor agitation (PMA) / Psychomotor retardation (PMR).
- Specific actions: Pacing / Catatonic / Disorganized / Bizarre gestures / [Other details].
- Eye contact: Appropriate / Intermittent / Poor / Intense.

Speech
- Rate: Normal / Rapid / Pressured / Paucity of speech / Mute.
- Rhythm: Regular / Irregular.
- Volume: Normal / Soft / Loud.
- Prosody: Normal / Monotone / Variable.
- Latency: Spontaneous / Prolonged.
- Articulation: Clear / Slurred / Dysarthric.

Mood
- Self-report: "[Exact patient quote]."

Affect
- Type: Mood-congruent / Euthymic / Flat / Blunted / Irritable / Dysthymic / Anxious / Angry / Expansive.
- Range: Full / Restricted / No range / Labile.

Thought process
- Goal-directed / Organized and linear / Disorganized / Circumstantial / Tangential / Loose associations / Flight of ideas / Thought blocking.

Thought content
- Delusions / Paranoia / Grandiosity / Ruminations / Obsessions or perseverations / Paucity of expressed thought / [Other: Describe remarkable content] / Suicidal ideation [Patient denied / Passive / Active with plan / Active without plan] / Homicidal ideation [Patient denied / Generalized / Active toward [target]].

Perceptions
- Patient denied / Auditory hallucinations [with / without] commands / Visual / Tactile.
- Response to internal stimuli (RTIS): Observed / Not observed.

Orientation
- Awareness: Alert and oriented x4 (to name, date, location, and reason for hospitalization).
- Deficits: [Describe any deficits if present.]

Attention and concentration
- Normal / Distracted / Impaired.
- [Able / Unable] to name calendar months backward for a year.

Memory
- Intact / Impaired (short term or long term).
- Tests:
  - [Able / Unable] to register three pairs of words. [Describe any problem.]
  - [Able / Unable] to recall all three pairs one minute later.

Knowledge
- [Able / Unable] to name the current and previous four presidents.

Insight
- [Reasonable / Limited / Poor] regarding understanding the nature and severity of [mental illness] and need for treatment.

Judgment
- [Reasonable / Limited / Poor] regarding seeking and accepting help and regarding safety.

Reliability as a reporter
- Strong / Limited / Poor or inconsistent.

Admission Diagnoses

List as appropriate.

Assessment

[Patient name] is a [age]-year-old [race] [gender] with a history of [diagnoses, drug use], admitted for assessment and treatment of [describe primary reason for admission]. [Brief summary of patient info and brief evidence for the admitting diagnoses.] Due to the presentation, patient requires hospital level of care for safety and stabilization, evaluation of medications, and exploration of aftercare options.

Initial Treatment Plan

Psych

- "Admit to [facility] for comprehensive psychiatric assessment and treatment."
- "Continue medication: [Name of medication / Dose / Frequency]."
- "Initiate medication: [Name / Dose / Frequency] to treat [condition] (eg, 'lithium 600 mg BID to treat bipolar disorder, manic episode')."
- "Initiate PRN medications: [Name / Dose / Frequency] (eg, 'diphenhydramine 50 mg every 6 hours PRN extrapyramidal symptoms; lorazepam 2 mg every 6 hours PRN anxiety')."
- "Behavioral checks: [Indicate frequency and type, eg, Q30 minutes for moderate-risk behaviors / Q15 minutes for high-risk behaviors such as suicidal ideation or aggression / 1:1 observation for imminent-risk behaviors]."
- Reach out to community-based providers, if any.
- Encourage patient participation in therapeutic groups and milieu activities.

Medical

- List specific medical interventions or monitoring required.
- List additional medical needs or considerations (eg, PRN meds for pain, heartburn, constipation, nicotine cravings).

Labs

- Urine drug screen.
- Admission labs.
- Pregnancy test when indicated.

Diet

Specify diet type.

Vitals

"Monitor vitals [frequency, eg, 'every shift']."

Legal

Hold details:

- Start and end time/date.
- Hold criteria: Danger to self / Danger to others / Gravely disabled.

Disposition

"Plan for disposition: [Mention tentative discharge plan, eg, to home, back to facility when stable, to be determined]."

How to Document Daily Progress Notes

Progress notes should be succinct, readable notes that summarize your patient's progress over the last 24 hours (or whatever interval your hospital requires). Your hospital has likely adopted electronic health record software that uses templates, leading to reams of excessive data. This makes the progress notes unreadable and relatively useless for efficiently tracking patient progress—but all hope is not lost. In this fact sheet, we recommend the tried-and-true SOAP note (Subjective, Objective, Assessment, Plan) format. Alternatively, you can use the increasingly common APSO note (Assessment, Plan, Subjective, Objective) format that places the most important sections at the beginning.

Progress Note Format

Patient name:

Date of birth:

Medical record #:

Date of visit:

Subjective

This section covers how the patient is doing on the unit, plus their interval history (any relevant clinical information obtained since the last progress note).

- Status of target symptoms (eg, main symptoms leading to hospitalization).
  - It's helpful to include a representative quote from your interview that illustrates how the patient is presenting to you. Eg: "I don't need to take medications—I am a god." "The medication's working, but it makes me sleepy. Can I take it all at bedtime?" "I'm super bored here; can I just leave today?"
- Any significant events occurring over the last 24 hours (eg, restraints, medication refusals, conflicts with staff).
- Status of activities of daily living (eg, sleep, eating, hygiene, visibility in milieu).
- Group attendance.
- Information recently obtained from contact with collaterals, such as outpatient providers or family members.

Objective

- Formal mental status exam
- Labs of note
- Vital signs

Assessment

- DSM-5 diagnoses: Include all DSM-5 diagnoses, not just the main one requiring inpatient hospitalization (eg, schizophrenia, paranoid type; methamphetamine use disorder; antisocial personality disorder).
- Medical diagnoses
  - Comorbid medical diagnoses (eg, diabetes, hypertension) are common among psychiatric patients.
  - Make a note indicating whether diagnoses are stable or require attention (eg, consultation with endocrinology service to adjust medications for diabetes).
- Assessment of whether patient is improving
  - If symptoms are not improving, comment on why (eg, awaiting response to a new medication trial, medication dose is too low, side effects interfering with response, diagnosis is in doubt).
  - Explain why your patient needs continued hospitalization and provide details. Examples: Don't just say the patient is suicidal; instead, say the patient has a plan to overdose on pills if discharged. Don't just say the patient doesn't have a safe aftercare plan in place; instead, say the patient's discharge plan is not reasonable because they intend to move into their parents' home despite the parents having a restraining order against the patient.

Do not simply type the admission diagnosis without some comment on whether the problem is improving.

Plan

- Medication plan
  - List all active psychiatric meds that the patient is taking, including dosage, and PRNs if patient has required them.
    - Specify which meds are to be started, continued, discontinued, increased in dose, or decreased in dose.
    - If you are making med changes, the reasons for the changes should be clear based on your assessment above; if they aren't, add a few words in the plan to clarify your thinking.
  - List nonpsychiatric meds the patient is taking for medical reasons (eg, diabetes).
- Legal status
  - Mention the start and end dates of the psychiatric hold.
  - If there's an order for involuntary medications, include start and end dates.
  - If the patient's legal status is in flux (eg, awaiting a commitment hearing), provide relevant updates.
- Discharge plan: Comment on whether there is a plan for disposition/discharge.

Make sure the plan relates directly to your assessment. For example, if you said the diagnosis was in doubt, then you should add something to your plan to do more assessment (such as asking another attending for a second opinion or initiating contact with the outpatient provider for more information).

Discharge Summaries: Essential Components for Continuity of Care

The discharge summary serves as a detailed and comprehensive review of a patient's hospital stay, treatment received, and plans for outpatient care or follow-up. Electronic health record software often can automatically create discharge summaries from existing data in the patient's record. While this saves time, it generally results in excessively long discharge summaries that are difficult for clinicians to read quickly. This fact sheet outlines what we consider best practices for writing discharge summaries for psychiatric inpatients. The goal is to create a concise document that *you* would want to read to quickly learn about a new patient that you are admitting.

Basic Demographics

- Patient name.
- Date of birth.
- Medical record #.
- Date of admission.
- Date of discharge.

Discharge Diagnoses

Place this at the beginning of the summary to give readers quick context.

Identifying Information

Provide a snapshot of the patient's demographics, including age, marital status, ethnicity, gender, work status, and primary diagnosis at admission.

Chief Complaint at Admission

Summarize the patient's initial presenting issues/pathology.

History of Present Illness and Past Psychiatric History

You can typically copy and paste this information from your initial admission evaluation. You get extra credit if you edit and improve this section based on information you have learned over the course of the hospitalization.

Hospital Course

This section is the essence of the discharge summary, since it will help future providers understand how they can most effectively approach and help the patient in the event of another admission. Provide a comprehensive review of the patient's hospital stay, including changes in mental and physical health status and treatments provided. Highlight any significant events or complications during the stay. The course should start with the state of the patient at admission and cover progress or changes until discharge.

- How long was the admission (clue for probable length of the next admission)?
- Was the patient cooperative with treatment?
- What was the time course of response to medications?
- Were any PRNs especially effective?
- Were any medications clearly ineffective?
- Was the patient an active participant, going to groups and interacting with staff and peers?
- Or were they reluctant, staying in their room and resisting significant contact with anyone?
- Were there any behavioral events, such as the need for restraints?
- Were there any legal hiccups, such as signing a three-day notice and triggering a commitment hearing?
- Were family or friends involved in treatment?

Medication Changes Made During Admission

You could argue that this repeats some of the information from the preceding Hospital Course section and from the Discharge Medications section later in the summary, but it is helpful to detail all medication changes in one place.

Mental Status on Discharge

The discharge mental status should be clearly improved from admission. Carefully document the patient's level of suicidality, homicidality, and/or impulsivity—all of which should be stable and consistent with safe discharge.

Consultations

List any consultations from other medical specialists or mental health professionals during the hospital stay. Include their recommendations and how the recommendations were incorporated into the treatment plan.

Laboratory Data

Include any significant laboratory or test results obtained during the hospital stay. Highlight any changes or developments from the time of admission.

Discharge Diagnoses

List the final diagnoses at the time of discharge, according to DSM-5 criteria. While this may seem redundant given that you have started the summary with the discharge diagnoses, it is helpful to repeat this information here since many providers will ignore most of the summary and skip right to the end. Include medical diagnoses also.

Discharge Medications

Detail all medications the patient will continue to take after discharge. Include dosages and administration schedule.

Discharge Plan

- Disposition: Where the patient will go from the hospital and how they will get there.
- Aftercare: Detail the follow-up plan, including any scheduled appointments with mental health professionals or medical practitioners. Include dates, times, and contact information if possible.

Techniques for the Psychiatric Interview

To conduct an efficient psychiatric interview, you'll need to develop key interviewing skills to gather valid information in a time-effective way. This fact sheet outlines some major techniques experienced clinicians rely on.

Validity Techniques

These techniques help elicit valid information about sensitive topics.

- *Normalization*
  - *Normal reaction to experiences:* "With all the stress you've been under, I wonder if you've been drinking more."
  - *You've seen other patients react that way:* "I've talked to a number of patients who've said they get so depressed that they have strange experiences like hearing voices."
- *Symptom expectation*
  - "What sorts of drugs do you normally use when you're drinking?"
  - "What have you done to harm yourself in the past?"
- *Symptom exaggeration*
  - "How many nips of vodka do you have per day? 10? 15?"
  - "How many times each day do you think about suicide?"
- *Reduction of guilt:* "Have you ever been in situations where fights occurred and you were affected?"
- *Using familiar language:* "Do you get high?" instead of "Do you smoke marijuana?"
- *Changing topics sensitively*
  - *Smooth transition:* "Speaking of anxiety, have you noticed that you've had panic attacks?"
  - *Referred transition:* "Earlier, you mentioned..."
  - *Introduced transition:* "Now I'd like to switch gears and ask about..."

Content Enhancement

These techniques are helpful for patients who need encouragement to provide more information (eg, people who have negative symptoms of mental illness or are withdrawn, shy, reluctant to reveal information, etc).

- *Open-ended questions:* "What kinds of symptoms do you have when you are depressed?"
- *Gentle commands:* "Tell me what kinds of symptoms you've had."
- *Continuation techniques*
  - *Expressions:* "Go on." "Uh huh." "Really?" "Continue with what you were saying about..."
  - *Repeating the last few words*
    - Patient: "I usually just sit around the house." Psychiatrist: "You sit around the house and...?"
    - Patient: "I watch TV or talk to my roommate." Psychiatrist: "You talk to your roommate about...?"
  - *Enhancing recall*
    - *Anchoring questions to memorable events*
      - "Do you recall what you were doing around high school graduation? Were you depressed? Drinking a lot?"
      - Birthdays, graduations, accidents, illnesses, major purchases, public events (eg, 9/11, Jan 6 Capitol attack)
    - *Tagging questions with examples (multiple-choice questions)*
      - List possible antidepressant medications

Content Control (Redirection)

These techniques help for patients who are so expressive, talkative, or tangential that you cannot obtain relevant information. They also help for patients who are manic or have racing thoughts due to anxiety.

- *Closed-ended and multiple-choice questions*
  - Eg, rather than "How have you been sleeping?" try:
    - *Yes or no:* "Have you been sleeping normally?"
    - *Numerical answers:* "How many hours do you sleep?"
    - *Multiple choice:* "Have you been sleeping more than normal, less than normal, or a normal amount?"
- *Gentle interruptions (redirecting)*
    - *Empathic interruption:* "I can tell that's been a tough situation. Have you been drinking more to cope?"
    - *Delaying interruption:* "I can see this situation has been difficult, and I'd like to talk about that a bit later. Right now I need to ask you about some of your signs of depression..."
    - *Educating interruption:* "I'm sorry, but I need to interrupt because we have a lot of ground to cover..."

This fact sheet is derived from Daniel Carlat's The Psychiatric Interview *(5th ed., Wolters Kluwer, 2023).*

The Psychiatric Review of Symptoms

The psychiatric review of symptoms is an important though often neglected part of the initial psychiatric evaluation. This fact sheet provides a framework to help you screen for the major psychiatric disorders that your patient may have. It starts with a mnemonic that will help you recall all the major categories of disorders, followed by brief reminders of the diagnostic criteria. It's helpful to have this at your side when doing your interviews, though with practice you'll eventually memorize most of the information.

Overall Mnemonic for Each Major Category of DSM Diagnoses

Depressed **P**atients **S**ound **A**nxious, **S**o **C**laim **P**sychiatrists

- **D**epression and other mood disorders (including bipolar disorder).
- **P**sychotic disorders.
- **S**ubstance use disorders.
- **A**nxiety disorders (includes panic disorder, generalized anxiety disorder, obsessive-compulsive disorder, PTSD).
- **S**omatic disorders (includes eating disorders, somatic symptom disorder).
- **C**ognitive disorders (includes ADHD, dementia).
- **P**ersonality disorders.

Specific Disorders

Major depression

- *Screening question:* "Are you depressed? Have you felt depressed pretty much every day over the past two weeks?"
- *DSM criteria:* **SIGECAPS** (four out of the following eight, plus depressed mood or anhedonia, for at least two weeks.):
  - **S**leep disorder (either increased or decreased sleep).
  - **I**nterest deficit (anhedonia).
  - **G**uilt (worthlessness, hopelessness, regret).
  - **E**nergy deficit.
  - **C**oncentration deficit.
  - **A**ppetite disorder (either decreased or increased appetite).
  - **P**sychomotor retardation or agitation.
  - **S**uicidality.

Manic episode

- *Screening question:* "Has there been a time of several days when your mood felt great and you slept only two or three hours a night, or even less, but still had a lot of energy?"
- *DSM criteria:* **DIGFAST** (elevated mood with three of these seven, or irritable mood with four of these seven, for one week):
  - **D**istractibility.
  - **I**ndiscretion (DSM-5-TR's "excessive involvement in pleasurable activities").
  - **G**randiosity.
  - **F**light of ideas.
  - **A**ctivity increase.
  - **S**leep deficit (decreased need for sleep).
  - **T**alkativeness (pressured speech).

Psychotic disorders

- *Screening question:* "Have you had any strange or odd experiences lately that you can't explain, like seeing or hearing things that aren't there?"
- *DSM criteria:* **D**elusions **H**asten **S**chizophrenic's **B**ad **N**ews (requires two symptoms for one month, plus five months of prodromal or residual symptoms; one or more of the three core symptoms—delusions, hallucinations, speech disorganization—must be present):
  - **D**elusions.
  - **H**allucinations.
  - **S**peech/thought disorganization.
  - **B**ehavior disorganization.
  - **N**egative symptoms.

Substance use disorder

- *Screening question:* "Do you enjoy a drink or getting high now and then?"

Patient Assessment and Documentation

- *DSM criteria:* **T**empted **W**ith **C**ocaine (must meet at least two of the following 11 criteria):
  - **T**olerance (ie, a need for increasing amounts of a substance to achieve intoxication).
  - **W**ithdrawal syndrome.
  - Loss of **C**ontrol of substance use (nine criteria follow):
    - More substance ingested than the patient intended.
    - Unsuccessful attempts to cut down.
    - Much time spent in activities related to obtaining or recovering from the effects of the substance.
    - Craving the substance.
    - Substance use continued despite significant problems caused by its use.
    - Important social, occupational, or recreational activities given up or reduced because of substance use.
    - Failure to fulfill major role obligations at work, school, or home.
    - Persistent social and interpersonal problems caused by substance use.
    - Recurrent substance use in situations in which it is physically hazardous.

Panic disorder

- *Screening question:* "Have you ever had a panic or anxiety attack? A panic attack is a sudden rush of fear and nervousness in which your heart pounds, you get short of breath, and you're afraid you're going to lose control or even die. Has that ever happened to you?"
- *DSM criteria:* Recurrent panic attacks plus one month or more of worrying about the next attack.
  - Heart, breathlessness, fear (must have at least four of the following 13 symptoms):
    - Heart cluster: Palpitations, chest pain, nausea.
    - Breathlessness cluster: Shortness of breath, choking sensation, dizziness, paresthesia, hot/cold waves.
    - Fear cluster: Fear of dying, fear of going crazy, sweating, shaking, derealization/depersonalization.

Agoraphobia

- *Screening question:* "Have you started to avoid things because of your panic attacks? Do you have problems with crowds? Buses or subways? Restaurants? Bridges? Driving places?"
- *DSM criteria:* Anxiety about (and avoidance of) places or situations from which escape might be difficult or embarrassing.

Generalized anxiety disorder

- *Screening question:* "Are you a worrier? What do you worry about?"
- *DSM criteria:* Excessive worry for at least six months, plus three of the following six symptoms:
  - **M**acbeth **F**rets **C**onstantly **R**egarding **I**llicit **S**ins:
    - **M**uscle tension.
    - **F**atigue.
    - **C**oncentration difficulty.
    - **R**estlessness or feeling on edge.
    - **I**rritability.
    - **S**leep disturbance.

Social anxiety disorder

- *Screening question:* "Are you uncomfortable in social situations?"
- *DSM criteria:* Panic or near-panic attack in social situations.
  - "Do you get to the point of having a panic attack?"
  - "Is this anxiety so intolerable that you would go out of your way to avoid any social situations?"

PTSD

- *Screening question:* "Do you have posttraumatic stress disorder, which means having memories or dreams of a terrible experience, like being attacked by someone or surviving a natural disaster?"
- *DSM criteria:* **R**emembers **A**trocious **N**uclear **A**ttacks (person has all four of the following, lasting at least one month):
  - **R**emembers: The traumatic event is persistently **R**eexperienced via memories, dreams, flashbacks, or intense distress when the person is exposed to events that are symbolic of the original event.
  - **A**trocious: Stimuli associated with the event are persistently **A**voided (eg, avoiding certain activities or thoughts, amnesia for the event).
  - **N**uclear: The person experiences **N**egative cognitions and feelings (eg, negative beliefs about oneself or the world, inability to have positive emotions, diminished interest in various activities, a sense of foreshortened future).
  - **A**ttacks: Increased **A**rousal occurs: Sleep disturbance, irritability, difficulty concentrating, hypervigilance, exaggerated startle response.

Anorexia nervosa

- *Screening question:* "Have you ever had an eating disorder, such as anorexia or bulimia?"
- *DSM criteria:* **W**eight **F**ear **B**others anorexics (all three criteria required):
  - **W**eight significantly low.
  - Intense **F**ear of gaining weight or becoming fat.
  - Distorted **B**ody image.

Bulimia nervosa

- *Screening question:* "Have you ever felt like your eating was out of control? Do you have eating binges when you eat a larger amount of food than you should and feel like you can't stop eating?"
- *DSM criteria:* **B**ulimics **O**ver-**C**onsume **P**astries:
  - **B**inge eating episodes (at least once a week for three months).
  - **O**ut of control: Feeling of being out of control when binging.
  - **C**oncern with body shape and weight that is excessive.
  - **P**urging behaviors, such as self-induced vomiting; misuse of laxatives, diuretics, enemas, or other medications; fasting; or excessive exercise.

Somatic symptom disorder (formerly somatization disorder)

- *Screening question:* "Do you tend to worry a lot about your health?"
- *DSM criteria:*
  - Patient has one or more somatic symptoms (may or may not be medically documented as "real").
  - Overly focused on the symptoms, as defined by one or more of the following:
    - Excessive thoughts about the seriousness of the symptoms.
    - High levels of anxiety about the symptoms.
    - Too much time devoted to thinking about or responding to the symptoms.

ADHD

- *Screening question:* "When you were in elementary or junior high school, did you have problems with hyperactivity or paying attention in class?"
- *DSM criteria:* Children should eat their **OATM**eal to concentrate better in class:
  - **O**rganization problems (difficulty finishing tasks).
  - **A**ttention problems (difficulty concentrating).
  - **T**alking impulsively (impulsivity).
  - **M**ovement excess (hyperactivity).

Neurocognitive disorder (dementia)

- *Screening question:* "Have you noticed that your memory has been getting worse over the last year or two?"
- *DSM criteria:* **Memory LAPSE** (significant impairment in at least one of the six domains):
  - **M**emory.
  - **L**anguage.
  - **A**ttention (complex).
  - **P**erceptual-motor.
  - **S**ocial cognition.
  - **E**xecutive function.

This material is derived from Daniel Carlat's The Psychiatric Interview *(5th ed., Wolters Kluwer, 2023).*

Mental Status Examination: Key Components and Interpretation

The mental status examination (MSE) provides a structured way of observing and describing a patient's current mental state. Here we review the MSE's various components and typical descriptors. Be mindful of the patient's age, cultural background, language proficiency, and level of education when you perform the MSE. For instance, minimal speech in a non-English-speaking individual may reflect a language barrier rather than poverty of thought; beliefs that may initially appear delusional, like believing supernatural spirits communicate with and influence an individual, can be normal in certain cultures.

Appearance

- Gait; posture; grooming; dress; distinctive markings like tattoos, scars, or medical aids (eg, hearing aids).

Behavior

- Patient's behavior during the examination: Cooperative, agitated, restless, guarded (ie, hesitant or mistrustful).
- Eye contact: Consistent, intense, avoidant, minimal.
- Note unusual behaviors, such as pacing, grimacing, responding to internal stimuli (like hallucinations or delusions), or catatonic posturing (maintaining rigid, unusual postures for extended periods).

Psychomotor

- Movement patterns: Calm; restless; psychomotor retardation/agitation, tremors, tics.

Speech

- Rate: Normal, rapid, interruptible, pressured, prolonged speech latency (ie, delayed response before speaking).
- Quantity: Talkative, spontaneous, hypoverbal (minimal speech), hyperverbal (excessive speech), mute, paucity of speech (reduced quantity).
- Volume/tone: Soft, loud, monotone.
- Fluency/rhythm: Clear, good articulation, slurred, dysarthric.

Mood

- Patient's self-reported emotional state: Sad, happy, anxious, apathetic, irritable, angry.
- Alexithymia: Difficulty identifying/expressing emotions.

Affect

- Observed emotional expression: Appropriate, full range, cheerful, euphoric, sad, tearful, blunted, flat, constricted, withdrawn, demanding, hostile, agitated, expansive, labile, mood congruent/incongruent, indifferent, suspicious.

Thought Process

- Linear/logical (thoughts that are coherent and goal directed).
- Disorganized (thoughts that are difficult to follow, nonsensical).
- Circumstantial (excessive, unnecessary details before reaching the point).
- Tangential (replies to questions that deviate from the topic and do not circle back).
- Loosening of associations (a lack of logical connection between thoughts, jumping from one topic to another).
- Flight of ideas (rapid switching of topics with superficial connections).
- Perseveration (persistent repetition of the same idea in response to different questions).
- Thought blocking (abrupt interruption in the train of thought, leading to a sudden cessation of speech, after which the patient may not recall what they were talking about).
- Word salad (a severe form of disorganized speech that is essentially incoherent and incomprehensible, consisting of a random assortment of words).
- Concrete thinking (difficulty with abstract thinking, such as understanding metaphors).

Thought Content

- Suicidal/homicidal ideation and/or plan.
- Delusions: Paranoid, grandiose, somatic; nihilistic; of guilt/sin; delusions of reference (a belief that unrelated events are directly related to the patient, like a person speaking on TV is specifically sending messages to them).
- Overvalued ideas (strongly held beliefs that are neither delusional nor obsessional but are exaggerated in importance and are maintained despite evidence to the contrary).
- Preoccupations, ruminations, obsessions.
- Poverty of thought: Limited quantity and content of speech, not due to reduced intelligence.
- Echolalia: Repetition of another person's spoken words.
- Neologisms: Inventing new words that only have meaning to the patient.

- Clang associations: Speech guided by words' sound rather than their meaning, often rhyming.
- Thought insertion: Belief that thoughts that are not the patient's own are being inserted into their mind.
- Thought withdrawal: Belief that thoughts are being removed by an external force.
- Thought broadcasting: Belief that thoughts are being broadcasted or transmitted so that others can hear them.

Perception

- Hallucinations: Auditory, visual, olfactory, gustatory, tactile.

Insight/Judgment

- Patient's awareness of their condition and their decision-making ability.

Cognition

- Orientation: Awareness of time, place, person, and situation (eg, "oriented X 4").
- Consciousness/level of awareness (eg, alert, drowsy, stuporous).
- Memory: Immediate recall, recent (short term), remote (long term).
- Attention: Ability to focus/sustain attention: Digit span test, spell "world" backward, serial 7s.

Consider adding the Montreal Cognitive Assessment (MoCA) for further assessment.

Sample MSE for a Young Male Patient with Schizophrenia

- *Appearance:* Disheveled, malodorous, with unkempt hair and unwashed clothing; scar on left forearm.
- *Behavior:* Uncooperative, restless, muttering to himself.
- *Psychomotor:* Psychomotor agitation; patient is pacing and was seen shadow boxing earlier.
- *Speech:* Low volume; demonstrates paucity of speech.
- *Mood:* "I don't know, I just need to get out of here."
- *Affect:* Flat; patient shows little facial expression in response to conversation or environmental stimuli.
- *Thought process:* Disorganized, with loose associations, impoverished thought content, and evidence of thought blocking.
- *Thought content:* Describes paranoid delusions that a chip has been placed in his tooth to transmit messages to him and control his behavior.
- *Perception:* Endorses auditory hallucinations of voices that comment on his actions and command him to assume a boxing stance to defend himself from an unseen enemy.
- *Insight/judgment:* Insight and judgment are severely impaired, with poor decision making, such as refusing necessary medical treatment and neglecting personal hygiene.
- *Cognition:* Oriented to name and place only; unable to state the current month or year or reason for his admission to the hospital. Attention is impaired, as evidenced by his inability to follow simple instructions or engage in a coherent conversation. Memory assessment is difficult due to his disorganized thought process.

Physical Examination in Psychiatry

How to Conduct the Physical Exam

In many hospitals, medical hospitalists conduct screening physicals for all admissions. However, on occasion you may need to perform your own exams. The guidelines below are a quick refresher for those situations.

When to Perform a Physical Exam

Every new patient should receive an exam, especially if they haven't had a recent physical. Also, perform an exam to check for medication side effects, new physical symptoms (especially unexplained ones), signs of intoxication or withdrawal, or sudden/unexplained mental status changes.

Key Components of the Physical Exam

General observation

- *Appearance:* Hygiene, clothing appropriateness, signs of neglect.
- *Behavior:* Agitation, lethargy, unusual movements.
- *Vital signs:* Blood pressure, pulse, temperature, respiratory rate.

Head, ears, eyes, nose, and throat

- *Eyes:* Pupil size, reactivity, nystagmus, jaundice.
- *Mouth:* Oral hygiene, signs of nutritional deficiencies, tremor of the tongue.

Neck

- *Inspect:* For signs of thyroid enlargement.
- *Palpation:* For lymphadenopathy, thyroid enlargement or nodules.

Cardiovascular system

- *Heart:* Rate, rhythm, any murmurs or irregularities.

Respiratory system

- *Lungs:* Breath sounds, wheezing, rales, or rhonchi.

Abdominal exam

- *Inspection:* Distension, scars, striae.
- *Palpation:* Tenderness, masses, organomegaly, abdominal softness or firmness.

Skin

- *Observation:* Cyanosis, pallor, rashes, lesions, signs of infection or jaundice.

Extremities

- *Inspection:* Edema, cyanosis, clubbing of fingers, and joint abnormalities.

Neurological exam

- *Motor function:* Strength, tone, coordination.
- *Sensory exam:* Light touch, vibration, proprioception.
- *Cranial nerves:* Basic assessment for abnormalities.
- *Reflexes:* Patellar and Achilles reflexes.

Tips for Conducting the Exam

- *Explain the process:* Patients may be anxious; explaining what you're doing and why helps ease fears.
- *Be systematic:* Follow a consistent order to ensure nothing is missed.
- *Document findings:* Clear, concise documentation aids in ongoing patient care.
- *Use a chaperone:* Particularly for sensitive examinations.

Example of a Physical Exam on a Healthy Patient

- General: Appears stated age, dressed in hospital gown, disheveled hair, sitting up in bed; in no acute distress (NAD).
- Head, eyes, ears, nose, and throat (HEENT): Normocephalic/atraumatic (NCAT); pupils equal, round, and reactive to light (PERRL); extraocular muscles intact (EOMI); mucus membranes moist.
- Neck: Supple; no lymphadenopathy, thyromegaly, or masses.
- Cardiovascular: Regular rate and rhythm (RRR); normal S1/S2; no murmurs/rubs/gallops; no visible peripheral edema.
- Respiratory: Clear to auscultation bilaterally (CTAB); breathing unlabored on room air.
- Abdomen: Soft; nontender and nondistended (NTND); normal bowel sounds (NBS).
- Skin: Warm, dry, and intact; no rashes, lesions, or bruises.
- Extremities: Warm, well perfused (WWP); no cyanosis, clubbing, or edema (C/C/E).
- Neurological: Normal speech; muscle strength 5/5 in all extremities; sensation intact to light touch; gait steady; cranial nerves II–XII intact; deep tendon reflexes (DTRs) normal and symmetric in upper and lower extremities.

How to Perform the Neurological Exam

Occasionally, you'll need to assess neurological function in a patient on the psych unit, going beyond the routine physical exam that all new patients receive. In this fact sheet, we give you a brief refresher course on how to do the standard neurological exam.

Focused Neurological Exam Components

Cranial nerves

- *I (olfactory):* Briefly assess the sense of smell by asking the patient to identify common odors with each nostril separately.
- *II (optic):* Check visual acuity and visual fields. Inquire about any changes in vision.
- *III (oculomotor), IV (trochlear), VI (abducens):* Evaluate eye movements by having the patient follow your finger in an "H" pattern. Examine pupil reactions to light.
- *V (trigeminal):* Assess facial sensation by lightly touching the forehead, cheeks, and jaw.
- *VII (facial):* Evaluate facial symmetry by asking the patient to smile, frown, and close their eyes tightly.
- *VIII (vestibulocochlear):* Screen for hearing loss by whispering a word in each ear while masking the other.
- *IX (glossopharyngeal), X (vagus):* Check for palate elevation and gag reflex. Assess speech quality for hoarseness.
- *XI (accessory):* Evaluate shoulder-shrug and head-turn strength against resistance.
- *XII (hypoglossal):* Assess tongue protrusion for symmetry and strength.

Motor system

- Observe for involuntary movements, muscle wasting, or abnormal postures.
- Assess muscle tone and strength by asking the patient to push or pull against your hand with their arms and legs.

Reflexes

- Check biceps, triceps, and Achilles reflexes using a reflex hammer.
- Perform the Babinski test to check for pathological reflexes.

Sensory system

- Do a brief check for gross sensory deficits by asking about any areas of numbness and then testing light touch and pain with a pinprick in those areas.

Coordination

- Hold up a finger and ask the patient to touch their nose with their finger, then touch your finger, alternating rapidly.

Questions to Guide the Exam

- "Have you noticed any changes in your vision or hearing?"
- "Do you feel any weakness or numbness in your limbs?"
- "Have you experienced any problems with your balance or coordination?"

Special Considerations

- For patients on antipsychotics, pay attention to extrapyramidal symptoms such as tremors, rigidity, and involuntary movements.
- In patients with diagnoses like bipolar disorder or schizophrenia, assess for tardive dyskinesia and other movement disorders.

Legal and Ethical Considerations

Informed Consent: Legal and Practical Aspects

Informed consent is a cornerstone of ethical psychiatric practice. It's not just a formality—it's a dynamic process that ensures patients understand the nature of their treatment, the risks involved, and their alternatives. In psychiatry, where interventions can significantly impact a patient's autonomy and well-being, informed consent is particularly critical.

Key Elements of Informed Consent

1. *Capacity:* Before obtaining informed consent, you must assess whether the patient has the capacity to understand and appreciate the information provided. Capacity involves the ability to comprehend the situation, weigh the options, and make a reasoned decision. For patients with impaired capacity, you might need to involve a legal guardian or health care proxy.
2. *Disclosure:* You're responsible for providing comprehensive information about the proposed treatment. This includes:
    - *Diagnosis:* What condition is being treated?
    - *Nature and purpose of the proposed treatment:* What exactly will be done, and why?
    - *Risks and benefits:* What are the potential outcomes, both positive and negative?
    - *Alternatives:* Are there other treatment options available, and what are their respective risks and benefits?
    - *Consequences of refusal:* What might happen if the patient chooses not to undergo the treatment?
3. *Understanding:* It's crucial to ensure that the patient truly understands the information. This involves more than just reciting the facts—engage in a dialogue, ask questions, and encourage the patient to ask their own. If there are language barriers, consider using interpreters or written materials in the patient's preferred language. Also, be mindful of how cultural factors may influence a patient's understanding and decisions.
4. *Voluntariness:* Consent must be given freely, without any form of coercion or undue influence. In a psychiatric setting, where patients might feel pressured or may lack full autonomy, this can be a sensitive area. Always be mindful of the power dynamics and make sure the patient knows they have the right to refuse or withdraw consent at any time.
5. *Documentation:* While the process of informed consent is largely conversational, document it thoroughly in the patient's medical record. This includes notes on the patient's capacity, the information provided, their understanding, and the voluntariness of their consent.

Special Considerations in Psychiatry

- *Involuntary treatment:* In situations where a patient is deemed a danger to themselves or others, involuntary treatment might be necessary. Even in these cases, try to seek informed consent whenever possible, and explain the reasons for involuntary treatment and the patient's legal rights.
- *Emergency situations:* In emergencies where immediate treatment is required to prevent harm, you might not be able to complete the usual informed consent process. Document the emergency nature of the situation and any attempts to obtain consent or involve the patient in decision making.
- *Ongoing consent:* Informed consent is not a one-time event but an ongoing process. Treatment plans can evolve, and patients' circumstances or preferences may change. Revisit consent periodically, particularly when there are significant changes in treatment.

Commitment Hearings: Testimony and Procedures

Patients often arrive at psychiatric hospitals under involuntary commitment orders, typically initiated by police or psychiatric mobile response teams. Short holds (eg, 72 hours) don't get a judicial review, but if you extend the hold, you'll need to provide legal testimony to a hearing officer or judge. Here are some strategies for providing testimony. Procedures vary across jurisdictions, but the overarching goal is to balance individual safety and rights with preventing undue deprivation of liberty.

Key Points in Testifying

- Your primary role is to act as a fact witness, providing evidence on the patient's condition and the need for involuntary commitment.
- Base your testimony on your direct observations and clinical judgment. Third-party information, like nursing observations or family reports, might be considered hearsay and therefore inadmissible.
- Offer concrete examples of the patient's behavior or statements demonstrating that they pose a significant risk to themselves or others. Don't just vaguely say the patient is suicidal—mention the specific threats they've made (eg, overdosing on pills or jumping off a bridge).
- The legal system is designed to be adversarial. Expect your diagnostic conclusions and treatment decisions to be scrutinized and questioned. Maintain composure during cross-examination.
- There are no standardized definitions for "imminent harm" or "imminent risk"; those terms are subject to interpretation based on state statutes, case law, and individual judges. Familiarize yourself with how these terms are typically interpreted in your jurisdiction.

Understanding Commitment Hearings

- Hearings involve you, the patient, a hearing officer (eg, a judge), and the patients' rights advocate (and/or a lawyer) who represents the patient's interests. In some areas, an attorney will also be present to represent the hospital. Legal representation is mandatory in some places, while in others it's provided upon request. Some jurisdictions allow the inclusion of witnesses, like family members. Patients may choose not to contest their holds and might not attend, but the hearing will still proceed as scheduled.
- Hearings typically take place in the hospital or via teleconference.
- The structure of hearings varies depending on the jurisdiction. As you gain experience in your hospital, you will become familiar with the process local to your institution. If your hearings involve an attorney who represents the hospital, meet with them ahead of time to prepare. Typical hearings will include some variation of the following:
  - You will be sworn in.
  - Your credentials as an expert will be stipulated and the opposing attorney may question you about them.
  - You will be asked to read the legal hold documents and explain why the patient poses an imminent risk to themselves or others or cannot provide for their basic needs.
  - The attorney representing the hospital may ask you for several prearranged pieces of information that you should be prepared to provide. They include the patient's diagnosis, how you arrived at the diagnosis, the circumstances of the admission, the patient's current symptoms and behavior, and whether there is a safe and less restrictive alternative to inpatient admission.
    - Following your testimony, the patients' rights advocate or lawyer will typically challenge your claims and might argue that the patient is safe to be discharged and has a reasonable plan for self-care.
    - Finally, the patient will have an opportunity to speak.
    - The hearing officer will then decide whether to continue the hold, though they may keep you and the patient waiting for a day or two, depending on the judge.
  - In some states, if the hold is kept in place, patients have the right to appeal the decision through habeas corpus. There is usually a timeline (eg, two business days) for this second hearing. Appeal hearings tend to be more formal and take place in a courtroom. You'll be cross-examined by attorneys, including a public defender representing the patient and a district attorney supporting the hold, and a judge will preside over the hearing and make the final decision.

Post-Discharge Preparedness

- If the hearing officer or judge decides that the patient does not meet criteria for involuntary hospitalization due to a psychiatric disorder, you'll need to discharge the patient promptly, often within an hour of the decision. Be prepared for this possibility (eg, by having discharge medications already ordered).
- If you believe the patient would benefit from remaining in the hospital even though the hearing officer or judge has discontinued the hold, consider proposing voluntary admission. Should the patient decline, ensure a solid discharge plan is in place.

Health Care Proxy and Power of Attorney

Health care proxy (HCP) and power of attorney (POA) are types of advance directives, which are legal documents allowing individuals to designate someone else to make decisions on their behalf, particularly when they are incapacitated. Unlike conservatorships or guardianships, which are court-assigned, advance directives like an HCP or POA allow the individual to proactively choose a representative. This delegate is tasked with making decisions that align with the person's wishes and values, encompassing medical, legal, and occasionally financial matters. This fact sheet delves into these important legal tools.

HCP

An HCP is a legal document that allows an individual (the principal) to appoint someone else (the proxy or agent) to make health care decisions on the principal's behalf if the principal is unable to do so. This includes decisions about medical or psychiatric treatments, surgical procedures, and other health care services.

POA

A POA is a broader legal document that grants an agent the authority to make decisions on behalf of the principal, which may include financial, legal, and sometimes health decisions. POA types include:

- *General POA:* Gives broad powers but ceases to be effective if the principal becomes incapacitated.
- *Durable POA:* Remains in effect even if the principal becomes incapacitated.
- *Health care POA:* Specifically for health decisions, like an HCP. Sometimes referred to as "durable power of attorney for health care."

A POA has a couple of key differences from an HCP:

- An HCP is solely for health care decisions, while a POA can include various types of decisions, depending on its scope.
- An HCP becomes effective only when the principal is determined to be unable to make health care decisions.

Legal and Ethical Considerations

- HCP and POA laws vary by state. Familiarize yourself with the regulations and legal requirements in your jurisdiction.
  - Jurisdictions may have different legal and medical definitions of what constitutes incapacity and may have specific criteria for what mental or physical conditions qualify.
  - Some states require a single physician's determination, while others might need concurrence from multiple health care professionals. Some areas have broadened the scope of health care professionals who can make such determinations to include nurse practitioners.
- Upholding patient wishes vs proxy decisions:
  - You may encounter situations where the wishes of the proxy or agent conflict with your clinical judgment or the known preferences of the patient. For example, an HCP, who may be a family member, may insist on changing a medication due to perceived side effects they've read about, despite the patient's stable condition and your clinical assessment that the current medication is appropriate.
  - Try to resolve the disagreement through discussion, focusing on the patient's best interests and previously expressed wishes.
  - If the conflict persists, you may need to seek legal advice or consult with the hospital ethics committee.
- In the absence of a named HCP, the next of kin often steps in as the surrogate decision maker, with some states outlining a specific next-of-kin hierarchy (eg, first spouse, then child, etc). Work with your hospital's risk management department to ensure compliance with state laws and hospital policies when determining the appropriate surrogate decision maker.

Sample Scenario

Marcus, a 32-year-old male with severe bipolar disorder, experiences a manic episode characterized by psychosis and impaired judgment. Prior to this episode, he had appointed his sibling, Nancy, as his HCP via an advance health care directive. Upon Marcus' hospitalization, you conduct a comprehensive evaluation of his mental state. Recognizing Marcus' inability to make informed health decisions due to his current condition, the psychiatrist documents this assessment in Marcus' medical record, officially determining that Marcus is incapacitated. This documentation serves as the formal trigger to activate Nancy's role as the HCP, as outlined in the advance directive. Nancy, now officially acting as the HCP, engages with the medical team to align treatment decisions with her brother's known preferences and values. She is aware, for example, that to continue his hobby as a painter, Marcus would want to avoid any medication that might cause a hand tremor. Nancy meets regularly with the treating physicians to ensure Marcus' care remains focused on his best interests and prior wishes. After three weeks of treatment, Marcus has recovered significantly, and his treating physician deems that he now has capacity to make informed decisions about his care.

Involuntary Medications: Guidelines and Considerations

A feature of many psychiatric illnesses is a lack of insight into the need for treatment. You may need to secure a court order for involuntary treatment if a patient refuses medication and their symptoms put them or others at risk or hinder their ability to meet basic needs.

Criteria for Involuntary Psychiatric Medications

You'll need to present evidence supporting these four criteria:

- *Patient's incapacity to consent:* The patient is unable to understand the need for treatment due to their psychiatric condition.
- *Anticipated benefits of the medication:* There's a clear likelihood of benefit from the medication that outweighs any harm.
- *Lack of less intrusive effective alternatives:* Other less restrictive options (eg, psychotherapy) are unlikely to suffice or be effective.
- *Risk to self or others/inability to meet basic needs:* The patient's symptoms place themselves or others at significant risk, or severely hinder their ability to care for themselves.

Court Order Considerations

- Remember, patients have a right to refuse treatment, no matter how delusional they may be. The standard of evidence for court-ordered medication is higher than for involuntary commitment. A court might uphold the involuntary commitment but deny the request for involuntary treatment, unless you're able to convincingly demonstrate all four criteria mentioned above.
- The court will review the efforts you made to inform the patient about the treatment, so make sure you've provided written materials about risks, benefits, side effects, and/or alternatives.

Informed Consent Process

- Give patients easy-to-understand written material. Keep it simple and provide translated versions if needed to accommodate patients' diverse backgrounds.
- Offer reasonable alternatives. A patient's refusal of olanzapine over concerns of weight gain doesn't warrant involuntary treatment, as you can offer an alternative medication without that side effect. But if a patient refuses an antipsychotic due to delusions, like believing there's a chip in their head that needs to be removed with a knife, this justifies involuntary treatment for their safety.

Administering Involuntary Treatment

- Always try the polite approach first: "Would you like your medication?" If the patient refuses and you've got the green light for involuntary treatment, you can order a backup IM medication, eg, "Administer olanzapine 5 mg IM for each refusal of oral olanzapine."
- If there's no IM option for the prescribed med, you'll need to have a backup plan with an equivalent that comes in IM form. For example, if you prescribe risperidone and it is refused, you can administer an IM formulation of olanzapine or haloperidol as an alternative.

Patients' Rights

Throughout this process, keep the patient's rights front and center.

- In many states, patients have the option to appeal the court's decision through a second hearing. Assist with the necessary paperwork for this appeal if requested by the patient.
- Review the patient's situation regularly to see if involuntary medications are still justified.

How to Evaluate Capacity to Make Decisions

Conducting a capacity evaluation is a critical aspect of health care, particularly when you're faced with patients who may not be able to make informed decisions about their treatment. Any physician can evaluate a patient's capacity, but psychiatric clinicians are often consulted to assist with cases where mental illness or cognitive impairment might be influencing the patient's decision-making abilities.

Criteria for Capacity Documentation

Communicate a consistent choice

- Can the patient communicate? In some cases, such as catatonia or delirium, the patient may not be able to meaningfully communicate anything at all, in which case no further evaluation can occur and you will advise that the patient (at least temporarily) lacks decision-making capacity.
- Can the patient express a consistent yes/no decision? If they constantly change their mind, that's a red flag.
- Ask: "Have you made a decision?" "What have you decided?"

Understand the relevant information

- The patient should be able to convey an understanding of:
  - *Diagnosis:* "In your own words, what do you believe is wrong with your health?"
  - *Symptoms:* "Can you describe some symptoms of your condition?"
  - *Recommended test/treatment:* "What is our suggested next step? How might it help you?"
  - *Potential risks:* "What are some risks of the test/treatment?"
  - *Available choices:* "Can you list all the treatment options available to you?"

Appreciate the situation and its consequences

- This involves understanding the options, risks, benefits, outcomes, and alternatives.
- Ask: "What are the pros and cons of each option?" "What could happen if you do or don't follow the recommended plan?"

Use reason in decision making

- The patient's decision should be a product of logical reasoning and align with their values and beliefs.
- Ask: "How did you come to this decision?" "Why do you favor one option over another?"

Additional Points

- Don't generalize a patient's capacity assessment for one decision to all other medical decisions. The threshold for capacity varies based on the benefits and risks of a treatment (eg, a patient may have capacity to consent to a chest x-ray, but not to brain surgery).
- Capacity is not static. Periodically reassess a patient's capacity, as it can evolve with the patient's condition and understanding.

Steps to Take if a Patient Lacks Decision-Making Capacity

Review a health care proxy or power of attorney document

Hopefully, there will be such a document in the medical record, which specifies an agent empowered to make health care decisions if the patient lacks capacity (see the "Health Care Proxy and Power of Attorney" fact sheet in this section).

Reach out to family or surrogates

Get in touch with the patient's next of kin or surrogate decision maker. A medical social worker can help if locating family or surrogates gets tricky.

Emergency situations

If you're in a crunch with no surrogate in sight, or if there's just no time to find one due to the urgent nature of the treatment, you as the primary physician can go ahead with what you believe is best for the patient. This falls under the "emergency exception" rule. Document your decisions and actions in the medical record as soon as you can.

When family isn't available or willing

If you can't locate next of kin, or the ones found aren't able or willing to be involved, reach out to bioethics or risk management. They can help set up a committee for unrepresented patients.

Confidentiality and Release of Patient Information

Patient confidentiality is a fundamental principle in psychiatric care. You need to be very careful about how and when you share details of patients' protected health information (PHI). Typically, you should only disclose PHI with the patient's consent or in specific situations where the law allows or requires it. However, misunderstandings about the law, in particular about the Health Insurance Portability and Accountability Act (HIPAA), sometimes prevent essential communication for patient care.

HIPAA

HIPAA sets national standards for protecting patient information. It governs how PHI is used and disclosed by health care providers, health plans, and other covered entities.

Permitted disclosures without authorization

- You can share PHI for treatment purposes, such as coordinating care with other providers.
- It's also okay to disclose PHI for payment activities, like billing, and for health care operations, such as quality assessments and improvement activities.
- Always try to limit the information shared to the minimum necessary.

Patient rights under HIPAA

- Patients have the right to access their medical records and request corrections if needed.
- Patients also have the right to request a record of certain disclosures of their PHI.
- Patients can request restrictions on how their information is used or shared. However, you're not always required to agree to these requests, especially in situations where not sharing the information could likely result in serious harm to the patient or others.

Common HIPAA Myths

- *Myth:* You need patient consent before contacting their outpatient providers.
  - *Fact:* HIPAA allows you to share PHI with other health care providers for treatment purposes without needing the patient's explicit consent, although it's good practice to get consent when you can.
- *Myth:* You can't talk to social service agencies (eg, substance abuse treatment programs, community mental health centers) about discharge planning without the patient's consent.
  - *Fact:* You can share PHI with social service agencies if it's directly related to the patient's treatment or care coordination.
- *Myth:* You can't talk to a patient's family members without their consent.
  - *Fact:* HIPAA allows you to share information with family members if the patient is incapacitated or in an emergency where they pose a serious and imminent threat to health or safety, as is often the case for patients admitted on psychiatric holds. However, if the patient is capable of making informed decisions and objects to sharing information, you must respect their wishes unless there's a specific legal or safety reason to override them.

You can find HIPAA privacy rules and protections for the PHI of patients being treated for mental health conditions at this website: www.tinyurl.com/33ekrd2p

Using Release of Information (ROI) Forms

- In inpatient psychiatric settings, you'll typically use ROI forms to document patient consent for sharing their PHI.
- To comply with HIPAA, these forms must clearly specify what information will be disclosed, who will receive it, and the purpose of the disclosure; they must also include an expiration date and the patient's signature.

Power of Attorney (POA) and Access to Health Information

- *General POA:* A general POA usually covers financial or legal decisions. The POA must specifically authorize access to a patient's medical records or PHI. Without this, the designated person can't review or obtain medical records.
- *Medical POA (health care proxy):* A medical POA lets the designated person make health care decisions, including accessing PHI, but only if the patient can't make their own decisions. If the patient is capable, you'll need their explicit consent to share any information.

Patient Competency and Consent

- *Competent patients:* You need to respect a competent patient's preferences about sharing their medical information, even if someone else holds a POA. The patient must explicitly consent to share their health information.
- *Incompetent patients:* If a patient can't make informed decisions, a medical POA or legal guardian/conservator can authorize the release of the patient's PHI. Make sure to verify the validity and scope of the POA or guardianship by obtaining a copy of the documentation, either faxed or delivered to the hospital.

Situations Permitting Disclosure Without Consent

- *Emergencies:* You can disclose information without the patient's consent if it's necessary to prevent serious harm to the patient or others, like in imminent threats or medical emergencies.
- *Court orders:* If a valid court order requires the release of patient information, you must comply. Always consult with the hospital's legal department or risk management team to clarify the scope of what needs to be disclosed and to ensure only necessary information is shared.
- *Public health reporting:* Some situations, such as reportable diseases like tuberculosis or cases of abuse or neglect, require disclosure to public health authorities without the patient's consent.

Documentation and Legal Compliance

- Always document any disclosure of patient information in the patient's medical record. Include the date, what was disclosed, and why.
- Even though HIPAA allows you to share information for treatment, always document your rationale, especially if you're sharing the information without the patient's explicit consent. Note the patient's capacity, the urgency of the situation, and the potential impact on their care and safety.

Health Care Administration and Compliance

Medicare and Medicaid: Overview and Billing

Many psychiatric inpatients are covered by Medicare or Medicaid, and some ("dual eligible" patients) are covered by both. These are essential sources of coverage for many psychiatric inpatients, especially in facilities serving low-income populations. In geriatric psych facilities, nearly 100% of patients are covered by these insurances. As a clinician, you don't need to know the intricacies of insurance policies, but since these two public programs have an outsize influence in hospitals, you should learn the basics of whom they cover and how they work.

Medicare

Who is eligible for Medicare?

- Anyone 65 or older.
- Anyone who is disabled (as defined by the Social Security Administration) and who has been receiving Social Security Disability Insurance checks for 24 months.

What are the different types of Medicare?

- *Part A* (Mnemonic: Remember **A** for **A**dmission to a hospital): Covers hospitalization, skilled nursing facilities (rehab), home health care, and hospice. Does not cover nursing home stays—those are covered by Medicaid. Everyone gets Part A at 65 as long as they have worked and paid taxes into the system. Part A is free for most people.
- *Part B* (Mnemonic: Remember **B** for **B**and-Aid): Covers physician services, diagnostic tests, ambulances, and outpatient surgery. It is optional, and if a person wants it they must pay a premium, although it's not very expensive. The premium covers only about one-third of the actual insurance cost; the government picks up the rest of the tab. In addition to the premium, there's a 20% copay on most services covered by Part B. If a person forgoes obtaining Medicare Part B, their individual insurance may not cover the costs for services that Part B would typically cover.
- *Part C* (Mnemonic: Remember **C** for **C**ommercial Medicare) *or Medicare Advantage:* Private insurance offered by various commercial companies; wraps Part A, B, and D benefits into a single product. There are hundreds of Medicare Advantage plans available, although each one covers a limited region, so any given person will typically be choosing from less than 40 plans. Each plan charges its own premium, copay, etc, and the coverage will also vary.
- *Part D* (Mnemonic: Remember **D** for **D**rug): Provides payments for prescription drugs. There are many plans to choose from, and the average premium in 2024 was about $56 per month. Different plans have different deductibles and copays. The infamous Part D "donut hole" (or coverage gap) works like this: A patient's plan will pay for the first $5,030/year of medications. Once the patient reaches this limit, they enter the coverage gap and will have to pay 25% of the cost of their medications until they reach the catastrophic coverage threshold, which is $8,000 in 2024. After that, Part D kicks in again and will cover most of the remaining costs.

Medicare: Psychiatric hospital implications

- *Coverage/payment:* Medicare covers psychiatric hospitalization through Part A. The basic benefit is up to 90 days per benefit period and up to 190 days of lifetime coverage. Medicare pays the hospital a per-diem rate according to the Inpatient Psychiatric Facility Prospective Payment System. In 2024, the per-diem rate was $895.63/day. This is a bundled payment covering all the services provided during an inpatient stay, including psychiatric services.
- *Utilization review:* Medicare has no "concurrent review," meaning that unlike many insurance plans, neither you nor your social worker (or utilization review staff) will have to keep asking an insurance reviewer for more days of coverage. You can concentrate on treating your patient, and if a longer admission is necessary, so be it. However, you're not completely off the hook, because the government may still conduct postadmission audits to ensure a patient's hospital stay was medically necessary. If the documentation of the patient's need for inpatient care is weak, the Centers for Medicare & Medicaid Services (CMS) can demand to be reimbursed the amount of money they paid the hospital.
- *Certification of need:* You might be familiar with the annoying requirement that you sign a certification form periodically for your Medicare patients. Many hospitals still require an inked signature, and the forms must be signed by a physician—psychiatric nurse practitioners are not allowed to sign them. However, if you don't recall ever signing these forms, your hospital might use an automated system that handles certifications as part of the admission and billing workflow. So what are these forms about? Medicare requires that you certify the need for an inpatient stay at the time of admission and no later than the 12th day of admission. It's partly an antifraud measure—you are being held accountable for the decision to admit a patient and to extract a large amount of money from the government for ongoing psychiatric care. More relevant to patient care, this also means that throughout the admission, you must demonstrate in your daily notes that inpatient treatment is needed and can be "reasonably expected to improve the patient's condition or for diagnostic study."
- *Quality metrics:* At most hospitals, you are required to document that you fulfilled various elements of quality care. This is part of Medicare's quality reporting program, in which hospitals can get paid a little bit more if they prove that these practices were done. Each year, Medicare might add new quality measures that hospitals must track and report on. On the plus side, sometimes Medicare removes a reporting requirement when there is no justification for it. For example, in 2024, CMS removed the requirement that we report on patients discharged on multiple

antipsychotics—because new evidence showed that many patients do better with combination antipsychotic treatment. Examples of the quality requirements that you may still have to report in your notes include:
  - Screening for substance abuse, including alcohol and tobacco use, and providing appropriate treatment.
  - Screening for metabolic disorders with measures like weight, blood pressure, and blood lipid levels.
- *Discharge planning:* Medicare covers both rehab facilities and home health care, which makes discharge planning easier for certain patients, especially those in geriatric psych hospitals. However, as mentioned earlier, it doesn't cover nursing home care.

Medicaid

Who is eligible for Medicaid?

- Low-income individuals and families.
- Pregnant women.
- Children.
- Individuals receiving Supplemental Security Income.
- People with disabilities.
- Elderly individuals requiring long-term care.

In addition to these federally mandated groups, states can choose to expand coverage under the Affordable Care Act. These expansions can include adults without dependent children and those with incomes up to 138% of the federal poverty level. States can also raise income thresholds for children and pregnant women and provide extra coverage for individuals with specific medical needs, like chronic illnesses or mental health disorders. However, not all states have adopted these expansions, so eligibility will vary significantly depending on where you live.

What are the different types of Medicaid?

- *Traditional Medicaid:* Covers the basics, including inpatient and outpatient hospital services, physician services, laboratory and x-ray services, and home health services. Some states offer additional optional benefits, like dental care, vision services, physical therapy, and prescription medications.
- *Medicaid managed care:* Many states have transitioned to this model, where Medicaid contracts with private insurance companies to provide coverage. There are numerous Medicaid managed care plans available, each typically covering a limited region. Depending on where you live, patients might have five to 10 plans to choose from, but this number can vary significantly. In larger states like California, New York, and Texas, there can be many more options. Each plan has its own premiums, copays, and coverage details.

Medicaid: Psychiatric hospital implications

- *Coverage/payment:* Medicaid covers psychiatric hospitalization, with typical amounts ranging from $700 to $900 per day; this reimbursement varies not only across states but also regionally within states. Medicaid often pays hospitals through a per-diem rate that covers all services provided during the inpatient stay, including psychiatric care.
- *Administrative days:* Many states differentiate between "acute days" and "administrative days." You can place patients on "administrative status" when they no longer require acute psychiatric care but remain hospitalized due to a lack of appropriate discharge placement or while waiting for community-based services. Reimbursement rates for administrative days are lower since the level of care required is less intensive.
- *Utilization review:* Unlike Medicare, Medicaid often requires preauthorization for psychiatric admissions and ongoing concurrent review. You probably hear about this requirement regularly from your hospital's utilization review team, reminding you to provide solid documentation to justify your patients' ongoing need for hospitalization. Be prepared for periodic postadmission audits involving random chart reviews to verify the medical necessity of hospital stays. If your documentation does not adequately support the medical necessity of a stay, your state's Medicaid agency can require your hospital to reimburse the payments received.
- *Certification of need:* Like Medicare, Medicaid requires certification of the medical necessity for inpatient psychiatric care. This involves periodic documentation by the treating psychiatrist to justify the ongoing need for hospitalization. While some states require specific certification forms, others allow detailed documentation in the patient's medical records to fulfill this requirement.
- *Quality metrics:* Like Medicare, Medicaid programs may also have quality reporting requirements. These can include measures such as screening for substance abuse and mental health conditions, monitoring and managing metabolic disorders, and ensuring timely follow-up care post-discharge.
- *Discharge planning:* Medicaid covers a range of post-discharge services, including home health care, outpatient services, and sometimes community-based mental health services. However, coverage for long-term residential care can be limited, and availability of services varies widely by state.

State-specific names for Medicaid

While Medicaid is a federal program, many states have branded their Medicaid programs with unique names. Some examples include:

- *California:* Medi-Cal
- *Colorado:* Health First Colorado
- *Maine:* MaineCare
- *Massachusetts:* MassHealth
- *Missouri:* MO HealthNet
- *New Jersey:* NJ FamilyCare
- *Oklahoma:* SoonerCare
- *Oregon:* Oregon Health Plan
- *Pennsylvania:* Medical Assistance
- *South Carolina:* Healthy Connections
- *Tennessee:* TennCare
- *Washington:* Apple Health

Utilization Review (UR) and Compliance

UR is a fairly painful aspect of health care bureaucracy, but unfortunately you need to understand how it works and to engage with it on a daily basis. As a psychiatrist, understanding and effectively engaging in the UR process helps to ensure that your patients receive the appropriate level of care and that the hospital is reimbursed for the services provided.

A Brief Glossary

- *Hospital utilization reviewer (HUR):* This staff member, usually a social worker or a nurse, ensures that the medical record supports the medical necessity criteria laid out by insurance companies. They typically attend morning reports and team meetings.
- *Insurance utilization reviewer (IUR):* The insurance company counterpart to the HUR, the IUR's job is to determine whether to authorize more days for your patients. Usually, all contact is between the HUR and IUR.
- *Peer reviewer:* In cases of disagreement about authorization, the insurance company may ask a peer reviewer (usually a psychiatrist) to review a case. This may involve you discussing the case with the reviewer.

Understanding Medical Necessity Criteria

At the core of the UR process are the medical necessity criteria that must be met for a patient to be admitted and remain in an inpatient psychiatric setting. These criteria typically include:

1. The presence of a DSM-5 psychiatric diagnosis that can be expected to benefit from inpatient treatment.
2. Clear evidence that the patient is a danger to themselves or others, unable to care for themselves, or experiencing significant complications from their condition or treatment.
3. The patient will benefit from inpatient treatment—ie, you have a realistic plan for improvement.
4. The patient must be on a locked unit—ie, they can't be safely assessed or treated at a lower level of care, such as in a partial hospitalization or outpatient program.

The UR Process

When a patient is admitted to your unit, your hospital's administrative staff will get an initial authorization, typically lasting three to seven days, depending on the insurance. Throughout the hospitalization, your HUR will communicate with the treatment team to gather information about the patient's progress, treatment plan, and discharge readiness. To justify continued authorization for additional days, the HUR clinician will present the case to the IUR. If the IUR denies more days, then you may be asked to have a meeting with the peer reviewer to plead your case.

Since the HUR rarely meets with patients, the source of information will be either the medical record or verbal reports during team meetings.

Documentation

Mental status exam

- Use direct quotes when possible. Insurance reviewers like to hear direct quotes from patients because they tend to clearly illustrate how bad the pathology is. Saying "Patient expresses suicidal ideation daily" is much less compelling than writing "Patient said 'I'm going to cut my throat with those scissors,' referring to scissors he saw in the OT cart."
- Give specifics on certain crucial aspects of the mental status exam. Rather than simply checking off "auditory hallucinations" on a list of symptoms, add a specific one-liner such as "Patient hears two voices yelling at her saying that she is a prostitute."

Assessment

- Clearly describe the DSM diagnoses, including specifiers like "severe," "recurrent," etc.
- Describe whether the patient is improving.
- To describe the need for a continued stay, use words and phrases such as:
  - "Patient still has suicidal ideation."
  - "Judgment is impaired."
  - "Poor insight into illness."
  - "Needs continued inpatient monitoring."
  - "Has ongoing symptoms of psychosis, including hallucinations and disorganized speech."
  - "Meds are in the process of being adjusted."

Plan

Rather than simply reporting plans for medication adjustment (which can be done outpatient), add other plans to justify an inpatient stay, such as "Monitor level of suicidal ideation" or "Family meeting planned for tomorrow to review discharge and suicide risk management plan."

Coordination
Insurance reviewers will be looking at the entire medical record, not just at your notes. If you document incoherent thought process and agitation, but nursing or occupational therapy notes paint a picture of an irritable person who can carry on normal conversations, this inconsistency will raise red flags. When treating a patient whose authorizations are being contested, make sure to read other disciplines' notes and discuss any inconsistencies in the team meeting.

Peer-to-Peer Calls
A peer-to-peer call will occur if the insurance reviewer has presented the case to a psychiatrist who is skeptical that the patient still needs to be hospitalized. You will be talking to another psychiatrist, typically someone who has their own busy practice and has lots of clinical experience. Doing reviews for insurance companies can be a lucrative side gig, but it can also add variety to a clinician's schedule. While some reviewers may come across as gatekeepers trying to deny coverage, most are ethical and willing to compromise depending on your case and presentation.

How to Shine During Peer-to-Peer Calls
- Realize that a clinical review is a negotiation. You are using your knowledge and power of persuasion to convince the reviewer to authorize more days of treatment.
- Prepare answers to these questions:
  - *Why does the patient need to be hospitalized now?* Argue for the imminent possibility of danger to self or others, or complications needing treatment.
  - *What are you trying to accomplish with the hospitalization?* Avoid being vague. If a patient comes in for suicidality because of losing a job, don't say that the plan is to "treat her depression." Say: "I am going to further evaluate why she is suicidal and will be using a multipronged approach"; "I'll treat specific depressive symptoms with the goal of improving her sense of self-worth"; "I'll work on diminishing suicidal thoughts by having a family meeting and working out a plan for her to be able to save money as she looks for another job"; etc.
  - *How will you treat the patient?* Discuss specific doses so the reviewer sees that your plan is realistic: "I am going to start the patient on 100 mg of Seroquel and gradually increase the dose to 400–500 mg until there is a response or there are side effects." If you are using something nonstandard, you need to justify it. Pregabalin (Lyrica) is a nonstandard choice for anxiety, but for a person with an addiction to benzos, it may be a good choice.
  - *What are your plans for discharge?* Talk about discharge plans during the review. Be specific. Rather than saying "Plan to send the patient to outpatient treatment," specify the program or clinic to show that you know whom to call and that you are confident the clinic will accept the referral.
- Prepare a well-organized, succinct, compelling presentation. The reviewer will evaluate whether your presentation is organized, whether you understand the patient's history and symptoms, and whether your plan meets clinical guidelines.

Tips for Negotiating with Reviewers
- Before the review, request a copy of the list of criteria for medical necessity.
- Have a backup plan for lesser services that you're willing to accept.
- Have reasonable arguments to back up your request.
- Ask for a reasonable number of days. Don't be timid. Typically, ask for five days and justify why you need them.
- Don't get angry or unpleasant. It likely won't achieve anything and could harm future dealings with the reviewer.
- If the reviewer denies your request, ask if you can be approved for half that number of days, and explain that you will treat the patient as efficiently as possible.
- If you disagree with the denial, request an appeal, preferably right away while the patient is in the hospital.

Vignette: When You and the Reviewer Disagree—the Power of Vivid Details
A provider is requesting extra days for a psychotic and aggressive patient. The conversation goes as follows:
- *Provider:* "We're trying to stabilize his medication and help him develop some insight into how sick he has been."
- *Reviewer:* "Why can't you do that in a partial hospitalization program?"
- *Provider:* "He's still too dangerous. If you could see him, you'd know what I mean."
- *Reviewer:* "From what you've told me, this patient does not meet the medical necessity criteria for continued hospitalization. Can you describe him further?"
- *Provider:* "He's so scary that the patients and staff are afraid to be alone in a room with him. I've been in practice for 15 years, and he is the scariest patient I've ever seen. His eyes dart around; he does not maintain eye contact. He's threatening. He's thrown furniture around the ward. He looks like he's going to explode at any minute."
- The reviewer agrees and approves three more days.

Coding and Billing Protocols

Coding inpatient psychiatric visits is a way of briefly describing how much work you did and therefore how much money the insurance company should pay for the visit. The coding rules were developed by the American Medical Association (AMA) and the Centers for Medicare & Medicaid Services (CMS) and are published as the Current Procedural Terminology (CPT®) codes. While electronic health records are increasingly automating the process of coding your visits, it is still ultimately up to you to decide on the code. The more accurate you are, the more effective your hospital's billing staff will be and the more financially healthy your hospital will remain. This fact sheet will help you navigate the coding process, focusing on the time-based approach for inpatient psychiatry notes.

Understanding Coding Methodologies

There are two ways in which you can code your inpatient visits with patients:

Key components

The key components approach involves documenting specific elements of the patient encounter. These include history, examination, and medical decision making. Each component must meet certain criteria to justify the billing code. This method can be the more complex and rigid of the two, often requiring painstaking documentation of multiple facets of the patient interaction.

Here is an example for a high-complexity initial evaluation (CPT code 99223):

- *History:* Document a comprehensive psychiatric and medical history, including a review of systems.
- *Examination:* Conduct a detailed mental status examination and any relevant physical examinations.
- *Medical decision making:* Describe the complexity of data reviewed, the diagnoses considered, and the treatment plan.

Time-based (preferred)

While hospitals vary, the time-based approach is usually preferred for inpatient psychiatry notes because it aligns more closely with the nature of psychiatric care, where counseling and care coordination are often the primary activities. Use this approach when more than 50% of your time is spent on these activities.

Documentation Requirements

For time-based coding, it's essential to document:

- The total time spent on the unit/floor, which will include time spent interacting with your patient and time spent talking to nursing, other unit staff, and the patient's collaterals.
- A detailed description of counseling and care coordination activities (see below for details of what this means).

You will generally have a boilerplate series of phrases that you can use in your documentation templates. For example, for a 70-minute initial visit, the required description of the visit in order to support time-based coding might be: "I spent 70 minutes today on the unit/floor, including a face-to-face visit with the patient, of which over 50% of the time was spent counseling and/or coordinating care. Activities included discussing diagnostic results, providing brief psychotherapy, and recommending coping skills."

Time that Counts Toward Counseling/Care Coordination

Counseling and care coordination can include a variety of activities:

Counseling activities

- Describing diagnostic results and impressions.
- Providing brief psychotherapy (eg, cognitive behavioral therapy, supportive therapy).
- Discussing treatment options, compliance, and avoidance of risky behaviors.
- Recommending coping or other life skills.

Care coordination activities

- Communicating with other clinicians or agencies regarding the patient's condition and needs (eg, phone calls with outpatient providers, reviewing medical records).

Time that DOES NOT Count Toward Counseling/Care Coordination

Some clinicians are confused about the requirement that "at least 50%" of time spent with patients must be counseling or care coordination—since essentially all our time with patients involves talking, asking questions, and doing some counseling. However, the more "medical" aspects of your patient interviews are not considered counseling. These are:

- Taking a psychiatric/social history—eg, your standard series of focused questions about psychiatric symptom history, medication trials, impact of job, family, significant others, etc.
- Conducting the mental status exams and any aspect of the physical exam that you also document.

Initial and Subsequent Visit Codes

Initial visit (eg, initial evaluation visits, or psychiatric history and physical)

- *99221:* 30 minutes.
- *99222:* 50 minutes.
- *99223:* 70 minutes.

Subsequent visits (eg, progress note visits)

- *99231:* 15 minutes.
- *99232:* 25 minutes.
- *99233:* 35 minutes.

Prolonged Time

For complicated patients, you may well spend more than the maximum billable allotment of 35 minutes for a subsequent visit. If you spend at least an extra 30 minutes (a total of at least 65 minutes), you can and should bill for this, using the "prolonged time" code and providing appropriate documentation:

- *99356:* 35–74 minutes extra time.
  - *Example:* "In addition to time spent providing direct care to the patient, I spent an extra 30 minutes in prolonged service discussing the patient's care with her outpatient psychiatrist."

Discharge Notes

Billing for discharge visits can also be based on time:

- *99238:* Less than 30 minutes.
- *99239:* More than 30 minutes.
  - *Example:* "More than 30 minutes was spent by the attending psychiatrist coordinating the patient's discharge from the unit. This included discussing follow-up care with the outpatient psychiatrist, arranging community resources, and ensuring medication continuity."

The Joint Commission and Psychiatric Hospitals

You may have received that dreaded text first thing in the morning: "The Joint Commission has just arrived for a site visit. Please consult your supervisor for further information." Suddenly, everyone's on edge. What should you do? And why is this such a big deal?

What Is The Joint Commission?

The Joint Commission, a nonprofit founded in the 1950s, evaluates hospital quality. Originally, it was a joint effort among various health care organizations like the American Medical Association and the American Hospital Association, hence the name. They used to be called JCAHO, pronounced "jayco," until they rebranded as The Joint Commission in 2007.

Do Hospitals Have to Be Certified by The Joint Commission?

No, but about 80% of hospitals seek accreditation from them. Why? One major reason is that The Joint Commission has "deemed status" from the Centers for Medicare & Medicaid Services. This means hospitals accredited by The Joint Commission meet Medicare and Medicaid certification requirements, crucial for receiving federal reimbursements.

What Is the Process of Joint Commission Accreditation?

- *Application and self-study:* Hospitals apply by submitting a detailed self-study and paying an initial fee.
- *Site survey:* The Joint Commission conducts an unannounced site survey. If issues are found, a corrective action plan is required. Follow-up surveys may occur, but generally, full surveys are every three years.

Common Issues Found During Joint Commission Surveys

1. *Documentation*
    - *Incomplete/inaccurate records:* Missing or incomplete patient records, from initial assessments to ongoing notes.
    - *Inconsistent care plans:* Care plans not regularly updated or lacking specific goals.
    - *Poor medication documentation:* Missed doses, medication changes not documented properly.
2. *Environment of care*
    - *Ligature risks:* Unaddressed ligature points.
    - *Safety hazards:* Unsecured furniture, faulty equipment.
    - *Cleanliness and maintenance:* Facility cleanliness and maintenance issues.
3. *Patient rights and safety*
    - *Inadequate suicide risk assessments:* Insufficient regular suicide risk assessments.
    - *Improper use of restraints and seclusion:* Mismanagement and poor documentation.
    - *Patient rights violations:* Failing to obtain consent or address complaints.
4. *Staff competence and training*
    - *Lack of proper credentialing:* Not ensuring staff credentials are current.
    - *Insufficient training:* Lack of ongoing education on new protocols and procedures.
    - *Competency evaluations:* Lack of regular evaluations to ensure staff competence.
5. *Medication management*
    - *Lack of medication reconciliation:* Improper reconciliation at admission, transfer, and discharge.
    - *Poor storage and handling:* Improper labeling and storage of medications.
    - *Insufficient monitoring for side effects:* Inadequate monitoring and documentation of side effects.
6. *Performance improvement*
    - *Lack of data use:* Not using data to drive improvements.
    - *Inadequate improvement plans:* Ineffective performance improvement plans.
7. *Patient care and treatment*
    - *Lack of assessment and reassessment:* Irregular or incomplete assessments.
    - *Poor treatment planning:* Lack of individualized, regularly updated treatment plans.
    - *Poor coordination of care:* Ineffective multidisciplinary team communication and care planning.

Tips for Frontline Psychiatrists

- *Stay prepared:* Keep your documentation thorough and up to date.
- *Engage in training:* Participate in ongoing education and competency evaluations.
- *Focus on patient safety:* Regularly assess suicide risk and use restraints properly.
- *Collaborate effectively:* Work closely with your multidisciplinary team for coordinated care.

Quality Measures in Psychiatric Care

If you work in a psychiatric hospital, you've likely gotten emails about deficiencies in your medical records, which might come from the hospital compliance department or your medical director. While these emails can be annoying, they're just responses to laws and regulations that every psychiatric hospital must follow to stay open and receive insurance reimbursements. Here's a primer on quality and reporting requirements in psychiatric hospitals—including what, if anything, you need to do to help your hospital comply.

Specific Quality Programs: Who Makes the Rules?

There are two national quality programs that apply to most psychiatric hospitals: the Inpatient Psychiatric Facility Quality Reporting (IPFQR) program and the Hospital-Based Inpatient Psychiatric Services (HBIPS) program.

IPFQR

- *Created and enforced by:* The Centers for Medicare & Medicaid Services (CMS).
- *Importance:* Hospitals meeting these requirements get fully reimbursed for their services from Medicare. Noncompliant hospitals get penalized by 2%, which can add up to millions in lost revenue.

HBIPS

- *Created and enforced by:* The Joint Commission.
- *Importance:* HBIPS measures overlap with IPFQR measures but serve different purposes. IPFQR is a CMS initiative linked to federal reimbursement, while HBIPS is part of The Joint Commission's accreditation process. Hospitals that don't comply with HBIPS may lose their Joint Commission accreditation.

Quality Measures: What You Need to Know and Do

While hospitals vary in terms of which quality measures are emphasized, here is a list of key measures your hospital may collect, along with actions you should take. As you'll see, many of the measures fall more under the responsibility of nursing or other staff, but psychiatrists play a crucial role in ensuring these measures are properly documented.

HBIPS-1

Screening for violence risk, substance use, psychological trauma history, and patient strengths.

- *Your role:* During your initial evaluation, document history of substance use and history of trauma. While you will also ask about history of violence, formal screening for violence potential is often handled by nurses, who use validated measures like the Brøset Violence Checklist to assign a risk level for patients based on their words and behaviors. Listing patient strengths is also often a nursing or social worker task.

HBIPS-2, 3

Hours of physical restraint and seclusion use.

- *Your role:* Make sure to enter restraint and seclusion orders properly and write a brief note documenting the reason for restraints. Nursing has their own pile of paperwork, which will specify the number of hours patients have been in restraints or seclusion.

HBIPS-5

Justification for patients discharged on multiple antipsychotic medications.

- *Your role:* As part of the discharge workflow, most electronic health records (EHRs) have been prompting you to choose a reason why you are discharging a patient on more than one antipsychotic (when relevant). However, as of 2024, CMS has removed this measure, since recent studies have shown that combination antipsychotic treatment improves symptoms in many patients (www.tinyurl.com/bdhkeh9t). If the HBIPS-5 measure still appears in your hospital's discharge measures, it could be due to a lag between CMS' discontinuation of the measure and your hospital's implementation of this change, delays in your hospital's updating of EHR systems, or the hospital's internal decision to continue monitoring certain measures.

HBIPS-6

Post-discharge continuing care plan creation.

- *Your role:* Document the discharge care plan in your discharge summary, including prescriptions given and follow-up appointments. Social workers and other staff will usually take the lead in documenting a comprehensive discharge plan, and hospitals will vary in what they require you to document.

HBIPS-7

Transmitting post-discharge care plans to the provider at the next level of care.

- *Your role:* Administrative staff or case managers usually handle the transmission of discharge plans to the appropriate outpatient providers. But you need to complete your discharge summary in a timely fashion so your staff has something to transmit.

SMD

Screening for metabolic disorders in patients on antipsychotics.

- *Your role:* For your patients taking any antipsychotic medications (even those with few metabolic side effects), you must monitor weight, glucose levels, and lipid profiles. Blood pressure might be included in this list as well. Nursing staff will oversee weight and vitals, but you will have to order the labs.

Tobacco use treatment

- *Your role:* Document whether your patient uses tobacco; if so, have a discussion with them about whether they want help quitting. Depending on their wishes, recommend one of a range of tobacco cessation options, such as counseling, support groups, nicotine replacement therapy, or medications like varenicline or bupropion.

Alcohol use disorder treatment

- *Your role:* Screen for alcohol use disorders and document any treatment provided. This includes counseling, referral to specialized services, or pharmacotherapy.

Immunizations

- *Your role:* Some states mandate documentation that patients were offered certain immunizations, like influenza and pneumococcal vaccines. Encourage patients to accept these vaccines and order them if necessary. Note that in some states, registered nurses can administer these vaccines without a doctor's order.

Hospital Safety Protocols

How to Use Precaution Orders

Precaution orders help ensure the safety and well-being of patients and staff. Here's an overview of common precaution orders as well as examples of what they entail in terms of additional monitoring and intervention.

Assault Precautions

- *Purpose:* To protect staff and other patients from individuals who may exhibit aggressive or violent behavior.
- *Details:*
  - Close observation of patients.
  - Restriction of access to potential weapons such as pens and plastic utensils.
  - For patients who are particularly unpredictable or violent, having staff work in pairs for added safety.

Elopement Precautions

- *Purpose:* To prevent patients from leaving the facility without authorization.
- *Details:*
  - Increased monitoring during times when doors might be open.
  - Ensuring all exits are secured and constantly monitored to prevent unauthorized departure.

Fall Precautions

- *Purpose:* To prevent falls in patients at risk due to factors like medication side effects, mobility issues, or cognitive impairment.
- *Details:*
  - Daily fall risk assessments by nursing staff.
  - Assistance with walking, transfers, and toileting.
  - Assessment for and provision of mobility aids such as wheelchairs or walkers as needed.

Hypersexual Precautions

- *Purpose:* To manage and mitigate inappropriate sexual behaviors.
- *Details:*
  - Close monitoring to prevent inappropriate behaviors like sexual advances or touching.
  - When possible, assigning caregivers of the same gender to patients to reduce triggers and inappropriate conduct.

Isolation Precautions (Standard, Contact, Droplet, Airborne)

- *Purpose:* To prevent the spread of diseases by isolating infectious patients.
- *Details:*
  - Hand hygiene before and after patient contact.
  - Use of personal protective equipment such as gloves, gowns, and masks.
  - Placement of infectious patients in private rooms or cohorting with similar patients when necessary.
  - Immediate cleaning and disinfecting in cases of blood or body fluid exposure.
  - Prompt reporting of exposure incidents to the infection control team.

Medication Compliance Precautions

- *Purpose:* To ensure patients take their medications as prescribed and prevent them from hoarding or hiding pills, which can lead to overdose or other safety issues.
- *Details:*
  - Monitoring patients during medication administration, ensuring each dose is swallowed and not "cheeked" (hidden in the cheek to spit out later).
  - When appropriate, using liquid formulations or dissolvable tablets to minimize the risk of cheeking.

Seizure Precautions

- *Purpose:* To protect patients who are at risk of seizures.
- *Details:*
  - Ensuring patient beds have padded and raised bed rails.
  - Observing patients for signs of impending seizures, such as auras or unusual behaviors, to allow for prompt intervention.

Suicide Precautions

- *Purpose:* To protect patients who are at risk of self-harm or suicide.
- *Details:*
  - Conducting checks every 15 minutes or maintaining constant observation.
  - Removing potentially harmful objects from patient rooms.
  - Frequent interaction with patients to assess their mental state and provide emotional support.

Managing Sexual Activity Incidents on the Inpatient Unit

Sexual attraction—and even sexual activity—sometimes occurs among individuals staying together in a psychiatric inpatient unit. Nevertheless, many psychiatric hospitals lack policies on patient-to-patient physical contact. This sheet describes the steps to take when sexual contact occurs on the inpatient unit, whether consensual or nonconsensual.

How to Respond to Sexual Contact

- First, determine what type of sexual activity occurred. In most cases on inpatient units, sexual activity occurs between fully clothed individuals and involves kissing, hugging, and fondling. Actual sexual intercourse is rare. You will generally have a good idea of what happened from the reports of the unit staff who discovered the activity, but interview the patients yourself to get their sides of the story.
- Separate the patients and place them under 1:1 supervision while you evaluate each privately.
- The patients should not change clothing or take showers during this time, as physical evidence may be needed.
- Inform the hospital's risk management office of the incident.
- Determine the patients' capacity to consent.
  - All individuals—including those with severe mental illness or intellectual disability—have sexual consent capacity once they reach the age of consent as established by their state.
  - Patients on psychiatric holds also retain sexual consent capacity; the exception is if a court previously determined that a patient lacks capacity, such as in probate conservatorship.
  - The following principles have typically been used to determine sexual consent capacity:
    - *Knowledge:* Does the patient demonstrate basic knowledge and understanding of the sexual act in question?
    - *Rationality:* Does the patient demonstrate reasoning ability, including weighing the risks and benefits of sexual activity and appreciating its potential consequences (eg, STI transmission, pregnancy)?
    - *Voluntariness:* Is the patient able to decide to engage in sexual activity without coercion or undue influence? Do they understand they have the right to say no (withdraw consent) any time during sexual activity?
  - Capacity to consent is on a continuum: An individual may have the capacity to consent to activities with a low level of risk, like cuddling and kissing, but not intercourse, which carries a higher level of risk.
  - If the patients report that the sexual activity was consensual and both have the capacity to consent, there is no need for further intervention, other than to inform them of the risks of unprotected sex and review hospital policies regarding sexual activity on the unit.
  - Offer screening and prophylactic interventions in cases of sexual intercourse.
    - Pregnancy test; if negative, repeat in two weeks.
    - For emergency contraception, consult with OB-GYN.
    - Tests for STDs: HIV, hepatitis panel, syphilis, gonorrhea/chlamydia, trichomoniasis. If initial tests are negative but infection cannot be ruled out, repeat syphilis test at six weeks and three months; repeat HIV test at six weeks, three months, and six months.
    - Postexposure prophylaxis: HIV (consult with medicine team), hepatitis B vaccination.
    - Empiric antibiotic treatment:
      - Chlamydia/gonorrhea: Single dose ceftriaxone 500 mg IM plus doxycycline 100 mg PO 2x/day for seven days.
      - Trichomoniasis: Metronidazole 500 mg PO 2x/day for seven days.

How to Manage Nonconsensual Sexual Incidents

- If the patients claim the sexual activity was consensual but one or both lack the capacity to consent, immediately contact the surrogate decision makers for the patients lacking capacity to determine the steps they wish to take.
- If a patient reports the activity was not consensual, this constitutes sexual assault.
  - Ensure the patient is safe and is kept separated from the alleged perpetrator.
  - If the patient wants to press charges, contact the police and arrange for a private meeting.
  - Depending on the nature of the contact, a rape kit should be offered via the hospital's sexual assault response team. If your hospital lacks this service, the patient may be transferred briefly to another hospital.
  - Offer the patient counseling, given the psychological impacts such activity may have. Counseling can also help even in cases where the sexual activity was consensual.
  - Patients have the right to refuse the recommended examinations and interventions unless they lack the capacity to make informed decisions. In those cases, identify a surrogate decision maker.
  - Document all details of the incident, clinical evaluations, and interventions in the medical record. Include information on the location, timing, individuals involved, witnesses, clinical evaluations (including for capacity), interventions offered and completed, follow-ups, and referrals.
  - Debrief with the team to review staff's management of the incident, with the goals of minimizing future incidents and maintaining patient safety.

Workplace Violence Prevention and Safety

It's likely you'll encounter aggressive or violent situations in psychiatric EDs and inpatient units. They're part and parcel of the job, but that doesn't mean you're left without tools to handle them. Several training programs, like AVADE® and offerings from the Crisis Prevention Institute, are designed to teach employees how to stay safe in high-risk environments. Surprisingly, the Occupational Safety and Health Administration doesn't mandate these trainings, but several states do. Regardless of mandates, sign up for trainings if your hospital offers them and make an effort to engage in regular refresher sessions. You can learn very effective self-defense techniques in the role-playing scenarios that these programs offer. Here are some key points.

Awareness
- Be aware of patients' histories, including triggers and previous aggressive incidents.
- Pay attention to patients' body language. Agitation, pacing, clenched fists, or a tense posture can be precursors to aggression.
- Listen for changes in tone or volume that might indicate rising stress or aggression.

Avoidance
- Employ de-escalation strategies to defuse potential conflicts (see the "How to Verbally De-Escalate an Aggressive Patient" fact sheet in the Agitation Management section).
- Ensure there is enough space in consultation areas to prevent patients from feeling trapped.
- Minimize exposure to stimuli like loud noises or bright lights for agitated patients.

Defense
- Learn techniques to protect yourself without harming the aggressor.
- Techniques include:
  - *Blocking:* Learn how to block an incoming hit without engaging in a counterattack.
  - *Release techniques:* If grabbed, know how to break free using minimal force.
  - *Positioning:* Keep yourself in a stance that allows for mobility and balance, ready to move away quickly if needed.
  - *Containment:* Learn techniques to contain a patient if they pose an immediate risk.

Escape
- Familiarize yourself with the layout of the unit, including exits and safe zones.
- During consultations, position yourself nearer to exits than patients.
- Avoid places where you could be trapped.
- Understand protocols for discreetly signaling emergencies, like panic buttons, alarms, or coded messages. Wearable emergency alert buttons provide a fast way to signal for help.

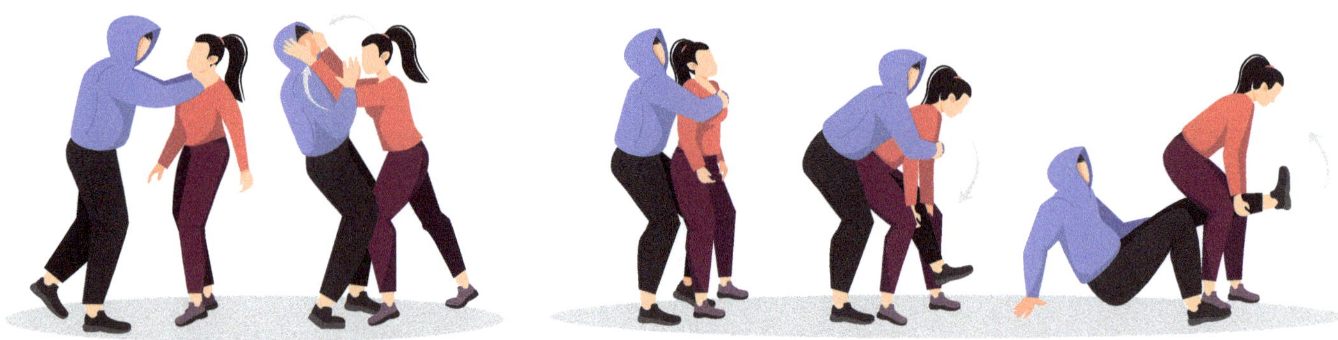

Minimizing PTSD from Workplace Trauma

Working on inpatient psychiatric units comes with a significant risk of developing PTSD. The incidence of PTSD among staff is about 9%, which is two to three times the national average of 3%–5%. This rate is even higher if you work with forensic patients or if you're a nurse. Nearly all psychiatric nurses have encountered direct or indirect exposure to critical events, and over half have faced physical assaults by patients.

How to Determine if You Have Workplace-Induced PTSD

While diagnosing PTSD in your patients is often straightforward, it's not so easy to know if you have it yourself. Most of us have experienced scary situations with patients—whether verbal aggression, physical threats, or actual assaults. We are likely to feel rattled and jittery afterward due to the release of adrenaline and cortisol. But usually, we calm down and are then able to go about our days. Here are some signs that you may be developing PTSD symptoms:

- *Anxiety:* You feel highly anxious at the thought of returning to work.
- *Work withdrawal:* You find excuses to spend as little time on the unit—or around the predatory patient—as possible.
- *Absenteeism:* You start taking extra days off to recover.
- *Reliving the trauma:* You find yourself thinking about and picturing the incident when you are away from the hospital.
- *Isolation:* You find yourself avoiding social situations because you are too preoccupied to relax around others.
- *Depression/anxiety:* Over half of those who meet PTSD criteria also exhibit symptoms of depression or anxiety.

Following a Traumatic Event

- To reduce your risk of developing PTSD, participate in a debriefing session, ideally within a few hours of the event.
- Keep in mind that a single debriefing session can cause retraumatization if not paired with individual counseling, which is often available through workplace employee assistance programs.
- If the traumatic event qualifies as a work-related injury, you may be eligible for additional support and benefits through workers' compensation, which can cover medical and psychological treatments needed for recovery.

Additional Strategies to Lower PTSD Risk

- *Maintain routine work activities:* This acts as a form of exposure therapy.
- *Engage in social interaction:* Spend time with others and talk about your experiences.
- *Practice mindfulness:* Techniques like muscle relaxation, meditation, and regular stress level assessments can help.
- *Make daily decisions:* Even small decisions can help foster a sense of control.
- *Normalize experiences:* Understand that recurring thoughts, dreams, or flashbacks are normal and typically diminish over time.

Supporting a Colleague Who Has Experienced Trauma

- *Offer help and support:* Be proactive in offering a listening ear and practical assistance.
- *Respect their privacy:* Don't pressure the colleague to discuss the incident if they are unwilling.
- *Validate their experience:* Avoid downplaying the experience and express a genuine willingness to understand and empathize with the colleague.

Routine Meetings and Team Support

Monthly staff meetings can reduce PTSD risks by fostering team cohesion and providing a platform for voicing concerns and receiving support.

Reportable Events: Documentation and Compliance

Reportable events, also known as safety events, adverse events, near misses, safety intelligence reports, or serious incidents, refer to any occurrence that diverges from standard care or poses a potential threat to the safety of patients, staff, visitors, or the hospital. These events range from incidents resulting in harm (adverse events) to near misses that could have caused harm but did not. While most of these events are reported by nursing or other staff, hospitals are encouraging providers to get more involved in safety reporting. These reporting systems involve software that you will typically be required to learn as part of standard employee training. This fact sheet will guide you through the essentials of safety event reporting.

Types of Reportable Events

- *Medication errors:* Wrong dosages, incorrect medications, adverse drug reactions.
- *Patient safety events:* Falls, suicide attempts, aggression toward others, elopement attempts.
- *Staff safety events:* Assaults by patients, injuries while restraining patients, needlestick injuries.
- *Environmental hazards:* Broken equipment, unsafe building conditions, fire safety issues.
- *Privacy breaches:* Unauthorized access to patient records, breaches of confidentiality.
- *Compliance issues:* Deviations from treatment protocols, unprofessional conduct.

Why Report?

- To improve patient care and prevent recurrences by identifying factors leading to safety events.
- To adhere to various local and federal mandates regarding patient safety and event reporting, including regulations from the Centers for Medicare & Medicaid Services, regulations under the Health Insurance Portability and Accountability Act, and standards set by The Joint Commission.

How to Report

1. *Address immediate dangers:* Take immediate action to secure the scene and ensure the safety of all involved. For example, if you see that a sharp object was left in a patient care area, remove it and collaborate with nursing to come up with an immediate plan to prevent a recurrence.
2. *Complete an event report form:* Access the reporting portal via the hospital's intranet and fill out the event report form with all relevant details:
   - *What, when, where, who:* Document the specifics of the event as soon as possible.
   - *Event description:* Focus on factual details; avoid subjective interpretations or assigning blame. The goal is to enhance safety, not to place fault.
   - *Categorize the incident:* Determine the nature of the event (eg, medication error, fall, privacy breach). This helps direct the report to the appropriate department.
   - *Assign a harm score:* This can range from "no harm" to "unsafe condition," "near miss," "temporary harm," "severe permanent harm," and "death."
   - *Describe the interventions that were performed:* These include medical, procedural, or safety measures, like administering a medication, implementing a new safety protocol, or repairing faulty equipment.
   - *Maintain confidentiality:* Do not disclose personal information of patients or staff members unnecessarily.
3. *Submit the report:* Follow hospital protocols to submit the report to the designated department or individual, which may include department heads, safety officers, or quality control teams.

Agitation Management

How to Verbally De-Escalate an Aggressive Patient

When patients become agitated and threatening, we often think first about chemical or physical restraints, particularly if staff safety is at risk. But coercive interventions can be degrading and might escalate the agitation and violence. Verbal de-escalation techniques can be very effective in calming a patient and potentially eliminating the need for forceful interventions. In this guide, we review the key principles of verbal de-escalation.

First, Create the Right Attitude

- Before you say much, try to adopt an attitude of friendliness and support. The patient is angry because they feel everybody is against them; you want to show that you are for them.
- Be aware of your countertransference. Most patients who require de-escalation can behave unpleasantly. They have likely already been verbally abusive or insulting, often with foul language and racist or sexist themes. Don't take the insults personally. Remember that this behavior is part of their illness.

Make Empathic and Caring Statements

- Identify their feelings and tell them you understand and want to help.
  - "You seem angry; is there something that you want but you're not getting? Maybe I can get it for you."
  - "You're pretty steamed. Let me know what's going on; I really do want to help you feel better."
- Take their side. "From what you've told me, it's clear you've been struggling and other people have been treating you terribly."
- Be the "good cop" if they've identified a "bad cop." "I can see you feel like you were mistreated by the staff in the emergency department—if that's true, we're going to make sure it doesn't happen to you up here on the inpatient unit."
- Listen.
  - "Have a seat and talk; I'll listen."
  - "Let me see if I understand you correctly."
  - "What do you want to have happen?"
  - "I want to help you get that."
- Try to find an area of agreement. "I agree that it's uncomfortable to be in the emergency department; I would feel the same way."
- Show concern. "How have you been sleeping? How's your appetite been?"

Make the Physical Situation Safer

- Respect the patient's personal space. Stay at a distance of two leg lengths—this keeps you far enough away that the patient will not feel hemmed in and you will be safe from punches or kicks. You and the patient should have room to quickly exit the encounter if either of you feels uncomfortable.
- If the patient is pacing, posturing, or standing, encourage them to sit down. Try to move the encounter away from public spaces. Having tense conversations in front of others might increase their sense of humiliation, which can escalate their anger.
  - "Do you mind if we find a place to sit down and talk? It's hard to have a good talk standing up in the hallway in front of everyone."
- Make sure you feel safe. Don't let a dangerous patient talk you into sitting with them alone. You may be tempted to agree to this as it may feel like a sign of trust, but you'll regret it if they start to escalate in a small room.
  - Clarify your need for staff in a way that is respectful and not insulting. "I want to talk to you, but I want to make sure I'm safe, so let's start by having one of our aides join the conversation."
  - Create space between you—at least an arm's length.
  - If you are sitting in a room, keep the door open and sit at the threshold. Feel free to explain why with humor. "Just in case you get annoyed with me and want to chase me away, this makes it easier."

Offer Food, Drink, or Other Comfort

- "Do you want a cup of water or juice? I'm thirsty and I'd be happy to get you something too."
- "Would you like a blanket?"

Provide Choices Whenever Possible

- "Do you want the medication in a pill form or in a shot?"
- "Would you like to talk about this now, or would you prefer to wait until you feel more comfortable?"

Express Optimism and Let the Patient Know Things Will Get Better

- "I realize you don't think this medication will help you, but I've seen a lot of people who've come in for similar reasons as you, and they've gotten better with it."

- If the patient states they want to get out of the hospital, give them clear goals—eg, appropriate impulse control and adherence to treatment—and assure them that, if they reach those goals, they will be discharged.

Allow Them to Feel Like They've Done Something Positive, Even After a Restraint Episode

- "You're doing a great job advocating for yourself."
- "You're really setting some limits and making it clear to us what's okay and what's not okay with you. I respect that."

How to Respond to Inappropriate Demands to Leave Immediately

- "You can't leave now, but let's sit down and talk about a discharge plan that's safe for you and everyone else."
- "It's legally impossible for me to discharge you right now. The law requires that you have a mental health evaluation before discharge."
- "We have a legal obligation to observe people for up to three days before discharge."

Be Concise and Repetitive When You Need Immediate Compliance, and Lay Down the Law When Appropriate

- "I need to keep you safe."
- "Please take a seat now."
- "Stop hitting the window."
- "Hitting others or damaging property here is unacceptable."
- "Racist language is not allowed here."

What to Say When Seclusion or Restraints Are Imminent

- "Would you like to take a time-out in the quiet room, or would you like a medication?"
- "Would you like to take a pill to calm down or receive an injection?"

Things to Avoid

- Don't keep an agitated patient waiting.
- Don't tell the patient to calm down or lower their voice. Instead, find out why they need to shout (eg, why they are angry). "You seem angry; is there anything I can do to help?"
- Don't order; ask. "Can I ask you to stop pounding on the wall?"

How to Medicate an Agitated Patient

While empathetic listening, validating emotions, and scheduled medications effectively calm many agitated patients, they don't always succeed. This fact sheet offers a guide on medication strategies for acute agitation in ED and psychiatric inpatient settings, specifically targeting agitation from primary psychiatric conditions such as schizophrenia, schizoaffective disorder, or bipolar disorder manic episodes. The overarching goal is to calm patients without over-sedating them.

How to Discuss Medications as the Patient Is Beginning to Escalate

As a patient begins to escalate, you have an opportunity to prevent the need for IM medications or restraints by doing all possible to first verbally de-escalate (see "How to Verbally De-Escalate an Aggressive Patient" fact sheet in this section). If verbal de-escalation doesn't sufficiently calm the patient, consider offering voluntary meds. You can engage the patient in a dialogue about meds at this early stage, and here are some suggested questions.

- "Is there any medication that helps you at times like this?" Most patients have experience with anti-agitation meds and may well have specific preferences.
- "I think you'd benefit from medication right now—how about some Ativan [or other med]?" Say this to a patient who is somewhat reluctant to take meds. This phrasing conveys a strong recommendation but still allows the patient to choose.
- "Would you prefer pills or an injection? The injection will kick in and you'll feel better twice as fast." Most patients prefer oral meds at this stage, but others prefer injectables—perhaps because they know how quickly they work.

IM Medications

These are usually used for severely agitated and potentially violent patients who need rapid tranquilization. The time to effect is around 15 minutes. It's important to prioritize medications that calm rather than sedate whenever possible.

- Ziprasidone (Geodon) 20 mg. Calming and widely used in emergency settings for agitation. Emergency physicians favor it for its effectiveness without excessive sedation. Probably underused by psychiatrists.
- Olanzapine (Zyprexa) 5–10 mg. Effective, but you must be cautious when combining it with IM lorazepam due to the risk of excessive sedation and respiratory depression.
- Haloperidol (Haldol) 5–10 mg, with lorazepam (Ativan) 2 mg and/or diphenhydramine (Benadryl) 50 mg. While historically popular, we generally recommend haloperidol as a later option due to its potential side effects, such as oversedation and dystonia.
- Chlorpromazine (Thorazine) 50–200 mg. Some clinicians swear by high-dose IM chlorpromazine for the most difficult and violent patients.

Oral Medications

- Appropriate for mild to moderate agitation.
- Oral meds take 20–30 minutes to kick in.
- Orally disintegrating tablets (ODTs) may have a faster time of onset than standard oral pills.

Benzodiazepines

You can often start with a benzodiazepine—usually lorazepam, but ask the patient if they have any preferences among benzos. Some patients ask for clonazepam (Klonopin), diazepam (Valium), or alprazolam (Xanax).

Typical agitation doses:

- Alprazolam: 2 mg.
- Clonazepam: 2 mg.
- Diazepam: 10 mg.
- Lorazepam: 2 mg.

Antihistamines

Both hydroxyzine (Vistaril or Atarax) and diphenhydramine can be sedatives, though they are often not thought to be "strong" enough for de-escalation. Nonetheless, some patients benefit.

- Hydroxyzine: 50 mg.
- Diphenhydramine: 50 mg.

Antipsychotics

There are many antipsychotics, and many patients will express a preference. The options seem to rotate in and out of favor, depending on the year, the institution, or the practitioner. Here are some commonly used oral options.

- Olanzapine ODT (Zyprexa Zydis) 5–10 mg. Often the preferred option, the Zydis formulation dissolves on the tongue within seconds and is very hard to "cheek"; may work a bit faster than swallow-only pills since some is absorbed through the oral mucosa.
  - Other ODTs to consider include aripiprazole ODT and risperidone ODT—though Zyprexa Zydis is generally more helpful for rapid control of agitation.
- Chlorpromazine (Thorazine) 50–100 mg. Similar to olanzapine in effect, and a little more sedating—but watch for side effects like QT prolongation and orthostatic dizziness.
- Haloperidol (Haldol) 5–10 mg. An old standby; very effective, but may cause dystonia, so it is often given with diphenhydramine and/or lorazepam to prevent that side effect.
- Quetiapine (Seroquel) 25–200 mg. While quetiapine works well, the dosing is much more variable, making it a bit more difficult to dose. Best used in patients who request it specifically.

How to Minimize Use of Restraints

The use of restraints ensures a quick end to any escalation of agitated or aggressive behavior, but restraint-free approaches can also defuse the situation while safeguarding patients' safety and dignity.

Understand Agitation and Aggression

Understanding agitation and aggression's root causes—delirium, dementia, substance abuse, severe mental disorders, environmental stressors, unmet needs—is key to effective management. Once you recognize these factors, they'll guide your steps to reduce the need for restraints, as detailed below.

Nonpharmacological Interventions: The Preferred First Line

Modify the environment to minimize stimuli

- *Reduce noise:* Provide earplugs, install sound-absorbing materials, encourage quiet conversations, and lower the volume of alarms and devices.
- *Control light:* Ensure adequate natural light during the day and reduce artificial light at night to help maintain a natural circadian rhythm.
- *Simplify surroundings:* Keep patients' rooms tidy and uncluttered, with clear paths for movement.
- *Maintain familiarity:* Personal items, like photos or a favorite blanket, can provide comfort and a sense of familiarity.
- *Control temperature and ventilation:* Keep the room comfortable.
- *Provide visual cues:* Clear signage for important areas such as bathrooms and exits can reduce confusion and stress. The use of calming colors and artwork creates a more relaxed atmosphere.
- *Offer private spaces:* Where possible, provide spaces where patients can have privacy or quiet time away from others.

Implement structured routines

- Establish predictable daily patterns such as mealtimes, sleep times, and activity times.
- Use visual aids like charts or calendars to help patients anticipate daily activities.
- Keep patients informed about any changes in their schedule to reduce anxiety.
- Integrate calming activities like reading or listening to music into the daily routine.

Initiate therapeutic activities that engage patients

- Cognitive activities (eg, puzzles, memory games, reading, drawing, interactive games on tablets).
- Physical activities (eg, dancing, tai chi, chair yoga).
- Music therapy (eg, karaoke, drumming).
- Pet therapy with certified therapy animals.
- Reminiscence therapy, encouraging patients to talk about their past through photographs, music, or life story books.
- Art therapy.
- Gardening or horticulture therapy.

Verbal de-escalation techniques

- Practice patience, empathy, and active listening (see the "How to Verbally De-Escalate an Aggressive Patient" fact sheet in this section).
- Create a therapeutic alliance to defuse potentially volatile situations.

Pharmacological Interventions: When Needed, Use Them Wisely

In instances when nonpharmacological measures fall short, pharmacological interventions may be necessary. Align your medication choice with the underlying condition and monitor for potential side effects. Options often include antipsychotics, benzodiazepines, and mood stabilizers.

Minimizing Restraints: A Team Effort

Reducing restraints requires a collaborative effort. Key steps include:

- Encouraging a culture shift within institutions.
- Addressing staff fears about safety.
- Providing continuous staff education.
- Regularly revisiting and reviewing restraint episodes.
- Encouraging open communication among staff.
- Developing individual care plans for patients known to become agitated or aggressive.
- Providing adequate staffing levels.
- Establishing clear policies regarding when and how to use restraints, based on the principle of using restraints as a last resort.

Physical Restraints and Seclusion: Guidelines and Safety

Occasionally, some of your patients will become so agitated or violent that they will need restraints for the safety of themselves and others. Often you will find out about these situations after the fact because nursing staff will have already initiated the restraint. In this fact sheet, we detail what your involvement should be in the process.

Types of Restraints

There are four types of restraints commonly used, many of which may occur simultaneously (eg, a patient may often receive mechanical and chemical restraints along with a brief period of seclusion). Generally, nursing staff will decide which restraint is necessary since they are the ones on the scene who have the most continuous contact with the patient.

Chemical restraint

This is when a patient is forced to take a medication against their will. A common misconception is that chemical restraints apply to forced injections only—but an oral medication can also be a chemical restraint if there is a coercion component. If a patient is getting agitated and you tell them they must take either a pill or a shot, and they agree to take a pill, this is considered a restraint even if the patient ended up taking the pill—because you essentially forced them to make that decision.

Physical restraint or physical hold

This means that a patient is held briefly, usually by both arms, in order to facilitate an IM injection or to escort them to locked-door seclusion. Many hospitals are encouraging use of these types of restraints as opposed to mechanical restraints because they are less traumatizing to the patient.

Mechanical restraint or hard restraint

This occurs when an agitated patient requires leather or cloth restraints applied to their wrists, ankles, or waist.

- Four-point restraints: This method secures all four extremities—both arms and legs—to a bed or chair. It is used in severe situations where there is a substantial risk from a patient's behavior.
- Two-point restraints: This method involves restraining two extremities, either both arms or both legs. It is used when a patient's behavior can be safely contained with less restriction.

Locked-door seclusion

This means that a patient is told that they must stay in the quiet room until they calm down. The element of choice is crucial—if a patient decides of their own accord to go into the quiet room, with the understanding that they can leave when they want, then this is *not* considered to be a restraint.

Training and Competency

Federal and state guidelines require all psychiatric hospital staff (including you) to undergo training in how to assess and manage violent patients. Make sure you understand and comply with your hospital's requirements.

During the Restraint

Order the restraint

If you enter the order into the electronic health record after the restraint has occurred, make sure to ascertain exactly what type of restraint was used so that your order accurately reflects what happened. Most medical record systems allow you to check off the various categories of restraints.

Order medications if needed

Decide on what medication to give as part of the restraint process. (For more details on meds for agitation, see the "How to Medicate an Agitated Patient" fact sheet in this section.) While each patient is different and may respond best to a particular medication, the most common chemical restraint meds are:

- Haloperidol (Haldol) 5 mg, often combined with lorazepam (Ativan) 1–2 mg. These are often given IM if the patient is refusing oral meds, but some patients will take them orally. To mitigate the risk of extrapyramidal symptoms (EPS), diphenhydramine (Benadryl) 50 mg or benztropine (Cogentin) 1–2 mg are also often included, though lorazepam typically suffices for EPS.
- Chlorpromazine (Thorazine) 50–200 mg is also effective and can be given either IM or PO.

Be present to support your staff and patient

While nursing and psych tech staff typically will oversee the hands-on aspects of the restraint, it's best practice for you to come onto the unit and be part of the restraint "code." What does this mean?

- Support staff by verbally agreeing with their assessment and actions: "Yes, I agree that he needs four-point restraints now, thank you."
- If your hands-on assistance is needed, be prepared to participate under the direction of the charge nurse or nurse manager, who will usually be running the code.

- Interact with the patient as needed during the restraint process, endorsing limits and explaining why the restraint is happening: "John, we're here to help you through this tough moment, and our priority is to keep everyone safe. This is temporary, and we'll work with you to find better ways to help you feel safe." The patient may yell and scream at you and staff, including obscenities or racial slurs. Try to model a firm and compassionate stance: "I know you are angry and you are saying things that reflect your anger. We're doing everything we can to make you feel calmer and better."

Do a face-to-face evaluation within one hour of the restraint

This federal and state regulatory requirement was instituted many years ago after rare incidents in which some patients died in restraints because they were not examined promptly. During your face-to-face evaluation, confirm that the patient was not injured, that vital signs are stable, and that the restraint is still required due to the behavior. There are also protocols at all hospitals requiring nursing to monitor patients, typically every 15 minutes.

Write a restraint note

Most hospitals require that you use a restraint note template to document the restraint, and each institution may have unique guidelines for what to include in the note and when the note must be written. Make sure you are educated about your hospital's policy.

Debrief with staff

While policies vary from hospital to hospital, staff are usually required to hold a debriefing session after applying restraints to discuss how the incident was handled and whether there was any room for improvement. As the provider, you may or may not be included in these debriefs.

After Restraints Have Been Removed

Debrief with your patient

Meet with your patient to discuss why the restraint occurred and come up with strategies for how to prevent future restraints (eg, medication adjustments, coping skills).

Create a behavior plan in collaboration with staff

Creating a written plan for behavioral expectations will help prevent restraints. See the "Sample Behavioral Management Plan" fact sheet in the Psychotherapy on the Inpatient Unit section for more details.

Nonviolent Physical Restraints

You'll occasionally use these. Monitoring requirements are less stringent than for violent restraints, and orders can be valid for up to 24 hours.

- Nonviolent ambulatory restraints (for patients who are at risk of elopement and must be transported to a different area of the hospital or to an external location, like a courthouse).
- Soft restraints (made from cloth, vinyl, or foam and mainly used on wrists or ankles to prevent self-harm or harm to others; they're mostly used for patients with delirium or dementia who might try to remove IV lines, catheters, or feeding tubes).
- Other types (eg, body vests, often used for patients at risk of falling or attempting to leave the facility unsupervised, and mittens, used to prevent patients from picking at wounds or pulling out medical devices).

Suicide and Self-Injurious Behaviors

How to Identify and Respond to Self-Injurious Behaviors

Self-injurious behaviors (SIB) are among the most pressing concerns you will face on an inpatient psychiatric unit. They require a balance of swift medical intervention, empathy, and stringent safety measures. Here we review practical tips for preventing and managing SIB.

Assess Risk for SIB

- Common diagnoses associated with SIB include borderline personality disorder, developmental disorders, and major depression with psychosis or suicidality.
- Patients with a prior history of SIB are at high risk of engaging in these behaviors on the unit.

First, Ensure the Patient Is Safe

- Remove any objects that a patient might use for self-harm. This includes sharp objects, belts, and shoelaces.
- Review the level of observation in patients with a history or risk of SIB. Depending on the severity, this can range from 15-minute checks to continuous 1:1 supervision.
- For patients who have injured themselves, see the "Medical Management of Self-Injurious Behaviors" fact sheet in this section for specific evaluation and management recommendations regarding common self-injuries.

Therapeutic Interventions

Work with your unit's social worker, psychologist, and occupational therapist to provide these interventions:

- Cognitive behavioral therapy to address negative thought patterns and develop healthier coping mechanisms.
- Dialectical behavior therapy, especially for patients with borderline personality disorder, to improve emotional regulation and reduce self-harming behaviors.
- Mindfulness exercises and stress reduction techniques to help manage impulses.
- Skill-building sessions focusing on communication, interpersonal skills, and emotional self-awareness.
- Working with the patient to create a safety plan. Identify triggers and develop coping strategies, like listening to music, practicing deep breathing, or talking with a trusted nurse.

Medication Management

- Consider prescribing antidepressants, such as selective serotonin reuptake inhibitors, for patients with underlying depression contributing to SIB.
- In cases of severe mood swings or bipolar disorder, mood stabilizers or second-generation antipsychotics may be appropriate.
- If you prescribe sedative-hypnotics for acute anxiety or agitation, monitor their use to avoid dependency.

Additional Tips

- Listen actively and validate the patient's feelings. By making the patient feel understood, you reduce the sense of isolation that often accompanies SIB.
- Encourage distraction techniques, such as art therapy, journaling, exercise, or group therapy.
- Involve the patient's family or support system in their care plan, where appropriate and with the patient's consent. This creates an extended support network for the patient during and after hospitalization.

Medical Management of Self-Injurious Behaviors

While we do our best to prevent inpatients from injuring themselves on the unit, it is impossible to prevent very determined self-destructive patients from engaging in certain common self-injurious behaviors. When they occur, you will likely get a medicine consult to help with management, but you should also understand the basic evaluation and medical management of these common self-injuries. (Also see the "How to Identify and Respond to Self-Injurious Behaviors" fact sheet in this section for psychiatric management of self-injurious behaviors.)

Self-Cutting

Typical scenarios

Most often, self-cutting on inpatient units involves patients with borderline personality disorder who repurpose items found in common areas for self-injury. Examples include plastic utensils and staples from magazines. Patients may also simply use their fingernails to scratch deeply.

Medical treatment

- Start with cleaning the wound using an antiseptic solution and assess the severity. Deep or bleeding cuts might require stitches or staples.
- If the patient used a dirty or rusty item, consider a tetanus shot, particularly if you're uncertain about their last immunization.
- Prescribe antibiotics, like cephalexin (Keflex) or trimethoprim/sulfamethoxazole (Bactrim), to prevent infections; instruct the patient on wound care and signs of potential infection.

Self-Strangulation

Typical scenarios

Self-strangulation attempts usually arise from extreme emotional distress or psychotic episodes. Patients might use items like bed sheets, clothing, or cords.

Medical treatment

- Ensure the patient's airway is open and monitor for breathing difficulties.
- Examine the neck for injuries and provide immediate care for symptoms like bruising or swelling.
- Monitor patients closely following the attempt for delayed complications like airway swelling.
- Conduct a thorough psychiatric assessment due to the high risk associated with strangulation.

Self-Hitting

Typical scenarios

Self-hitting usually involves patients striking their own body with their hands or objects. It may be directed at the head, limbs, or torso.

Medical treatment

- Inspect the hit areas for damage such as swelling, open wounds, or bruises. Imaging may be required for suspected fractures.
- Provide pain relief, ranging from over-the-counter painkillers to prescription meds.
- Use cold packs or compression to reduce swelling or bruising.

Ingesting Harmful Substances

Typical scenarios

This behavior often occurs impulsively, with patients ingesting available substances like cleaning agents or medications.

Medical treatment

- If you suspect a patient has ingested a toxic substance, seek emergency medical assistance immediately. Do not induce vomiting unless specifically instructed by medical professionals or poison control.
- Contact a poison control center for specific advice (eg, the National Capital Poison Center online at www.poison.org or by telephone at 800-222-1222).

Interference with Healing Wounds

Typical scenarios

Patients may interfere with healing wounds due to compulsive behavior, a desire to prolong care, or psychiatric symptoms like hallucinations.

Medical treatment

- Clean and dress the wound. If the patient persistently interferes with a wound, use protective measures like bandages, dressings, or casts.
- Monitor the wound for signs of infection or delayed healing and adjust treatment as necessary.

Assessing Suicide Risk

Assessing suicide risk is one of the most critical tasks you'll face on an inpatient psychiatric unit. Many units, often in response to Joint Commission requirements, mandate the inclusion of suicide risk and protective factors in progress notes or treatment plans. Here we review how to assess and manage suicide risk and recommend the appropriate level of nursing observation.

Identify Key Risk Factors

- *Common risk factors:* Look for chronic mental health conditions, previous suicide attempts, substance use, and acute stressors (eg, recent loss, major life changes).
- *Pay attention to dynamic factors:* Agitation, hopelessness, severe anxiety, or a sudden change in mood can all signal an elevated risk of suicide.

Use Standardized Assessment Tools

- *Columbia Suicide Severity Rating Scale (C-SSRS):* This tool helps you assess the severity and immediacy of suicide risk. Regularly use it to evaluate ideation, intent, and planning. www.tinyurl.com/mu2964kp
- *SAFE-T (Suicide Assessment Five-step Evaluation and Triage):* A comprehensive approach that covers risk and protective factors and guides your intervention strategy. https://store.samhsa.gov/sites/default/files/sma09-4432.pdf

Conduct the Clinical Interview

- *Establish rapport:* Build trust by showing empathy and asking open-ended questions. This encourages the patient to share their thoughts and feelings honestly.
- *Ask direct questions:* Don't shy away from asking about suicidal thoughts, plans, or intent. For instance, "Have you thought about how you would hurt yourself?"
- *Assess lethality:* Evaluate how specific and lethal the patient's plan is, and how accessible the means are.

Stratify Risk

- *Low risk:* Suicidal thoughts without a specific plan or intent. Strong protective factors are present.
- *Moderate risk:* Vague plan with some feasibility. Protective factors exist but may be weakened.
- *High risk:* Specific, feasible plan with intent to act soon. Protective factors are minimal or absent.

Document Everything

- *Record all findings:* Document the patient's statements, observed behaviors, and your assessment of their risk level. Include scores from any standardized tools used.
- *Keep it detailed:* Clear documentation is crucial for continuity of care and legal protection.

Communicate and Intervene

- *Coordinate with the treatment team:* Share your findings and collaborate on a care plan. Ensure that everyone involved understands the patient's risk level and the interventions planned.
- *Create a safety plan:* Work with the patient to develop a plan that addresses their triggers and outlines coping strategies, such as who to call when in crisis or what to do to stay safe.
- *Involve family if appropriate:* With patient consent, include their family or support system in safety planning for an additional layer of protection.

Table 1: **Suicide Risk and Protective Factors**

Risk Factors For Suicide	Protective Factors
Age: adolescents and young adults; elderly individuals	Core values/religion
Agitation or severe anxiety	Engagement in treatment/safety planning
Chronic pain or other serious condition	Engagement in work or school
Command hallucinations to hurt self	Immediate social supports
Current intoxication	Marital status
Family history of suicide	Planning for the future
Gender: males>females	Restricted access to highly lethal means
Gun present in the home	Self-protective behaviors/attempts to secure resources for self
Highly impulsive behavior	
History of extreme/lethal behaviors	
History of past suicide attempt	
History of past self-injurious behavior	
History of recent psychiatric hospitalizations	
Hopelessness	
Major depressive episode	
Mixed affective episode	
Noncompliance with treatment	
Psychosis	
Race: White individuals; Indigenous populations	
Recent alcohol/drug use	
Recent loss or other significant negative event	
Recent preparatory behavior for suicide	
Refusal to engage in safety planning	

Suicide Risk Levels and Nursing Interventions

Low risk

- Observation at 30-minute intervals.
- Permitted off-unit activities, supervised by a nurse.
- Full access to recreational activities, including those requiring items like scissors and pens.

Medium risk

- Observation at 15-minute intervals.
- Confined to the unit.
- Supervised access to recreational activities, with certain limitations.

High risk

- Continuous visual observation.
- Institute 1:1 observation if you deem this to be necessary.
- Strictly no access to recreational activities involving sharp or potentially harmful objects.

Creating a Patient Safety Plan

Once a patient who experienced suicidal thoughts is feeling better and is ready for discharge, help them create a safety plan so they can be prepared in case their emotional state deteriorates at some later point. For kids, share this plan with the child's parents and make sure it's easy to find (eg, by having it stored on the child's phone). Here's a sample blank safety plan.

My Safety Plan

Triggers/warning signs that tell me when to use my plan (like feeling tense or having thoughts of dying):

____

____

Reasons for living (things to look forward to, like being with family, friends, pets; life goals):

____

____

Things I can do to safely feel better (like practicing relaxation skills or listening to calming music):

____

____

People/places/activities that provide distraction:

____

____

Ways to make my environment safe:

____

____

People who I can call for help and to feel safe:

1. Name: ______________________ Phone number: ______________________
2. Name: ______________________ Phone number: ______________________
3. Name: ______________________ Phone number: ______________________

Professionals/agencies that I can call for help and to feel safe:

1. Name: ______________________ Phone number: ______________________
2. Name: ______________________ Phone number: ______________________

Emergency room phone/address: ______________________

Suicide prevention lifeline: 988
Crisis text line: Text HOME to 741741

I have participated in the development of this safety plan with my mental health provider.

Recipient signature: ______________________ Date: ______________________

Guardian signature*: ______________________

Provider signature: ______________________ Date: ______________________

**for patients who are minors or have appointed guardians*

Protocols Following a Patient Suicide

Suicide in a psychiatric inpatient unit is rare, occurring in about one out of 1,000 inpatients. The most common cause is by hanging, and unfortunately the standard 15-minute checks can't prevent it, since it only takes about five minutes for constriction of the carotid artery to cause lethal hypoxia to the brain. Inpatient suicides not only deeply impact the staff and other patients but also evoke intense scrutiny from external agencies. Here's how you can navigate this difficult situation.

Immediate Response

- Ensure the safety of other patients and staff. Remove any immediate hazards from the area.
- Ensure that medicine is immediately consulted, even if it seems obvious that the patient has died.
- Typically nursing will have called a code blue (or your hospital's equivalent) before you even learn about the event.

Other Personnel to Alert

- Notify the unit supervisor or head of the department about the incident.
- Connect with hospital administration to ensure they're aware and can provide necessary support.
- Bring in law enforcement to initiate their investigation.

Breaking the News to the Family

- Make sure the patient's family or next of kin are informed in a sensitive and timely manner.
- A senior psychiatrist or hospital administrator, accompanied by a member of the therapy team or a social worker, might be the best choice for this difficult task.

Caring for Your Team

- Schedule a debriefing for your staff so they can share feelings and concerns.

Supporting Other Patients

- Host group discussions or therapeutic sessions to help patients process the incident.
- Be mindful of the risk of copycat suicides. Keep a close watch on patients, especially those emotionally linked to the deceased or those at heightened risk.

Investigation and Review

- Conduct an internal review to understand the circumstances leading up to the suicide. This will help identify if any gaps in care or procedure contributed to the event.
- Depending on jurisdiction and hospital policy, an external review might be necessary.

Documentation

- Make sure all relevant records, notes, and documentation concerning the patient's care are thorough and current.

Legal Considerations

- Consult with the hospital's legal team or legal counsel regarding potential liability and any required disclosures or reports.

Long-Term Responses

- Review suicide prevention protocols with staff to reinforce education and safety measures; update these as necessary.
- Consider organizing a memorial or tribute for the deceased patient, in alignment with the family's wishes. This can help provide closure for both staff and patients.

How to Manage Deliberate Foreign Body Ingestion

Patients who deliberately swallow objects are among the most challenging you'll work with. Deliberate foreign body ingestion (DFBI) is costly and resource intensive, in part because of these patients' extremely high rate of repeated swallowing attempts: Over 80% of DFBI presentations occur in patients with prior ingestions. Pens, toothbrushes, and batteries are among the most commonly ingested items.

Common Causes of DFBI

- *Malingering:* DFBI in institutionalized settings, like jails, is often for secondary gain. Incarcerated individuals who swallow foreign objects are more likely to select highly injurious items, like sharp metallic objects, which require transfers to hospitals and prolonged treatment.
- *Borderline personality disorder (BPD):* Swallowing foreign objects can reflect a variety of pathologies in BPD. It may resemble other forms of self-injury (eg, cutting, burning) in which patients gain temporary relief from emotional pain by redirecting focus onto physical sensations or ensuing medical interventions. BPD patients may also find that this behavior allows them to achieve interpersonal goals, forcing staff to show them care and attention that they desperately crave.
- *Psychosis:* About a quarter of DFBI patients have a history of psychosis, and delusions/command hallucinations can prompt swallowing behavior.
- *Pica:* Refers to the repeated consumption of nonnutritive substances (eg, dirt, paint) and is most often diagnosed in children, pregnant women, and those with iron deficiency. In adulthood, pica primarily occurs in cases of severe intellectual disability, autism spectrum disorder, and schizophrenia.

Management of DFBI

Imaging (first step)

- Noncontrast CT (better than x-rays; if the ingested object is radiolucent, x-rays are of no use).

Medical guidelines

- Sharp objects (knives, razor blades), batteries, packages of narcotics, or objects that could obstruct or perforate the esophagus: Emergent surgical removal (within six hours).
- Sharp objects that have already progressed to the stomach or duodenum, or objects greater than 6 cm in length and/or greater than 2.5 cm in diameter: Removal by endoscopy within 24 hours.
- Blunt objects with rounded edges (eg, coins, buttons), smaller than 2.5 cm in diameter, and/or smaller than 6 cm in length: Nonemergent removal.
- Small, blunt, nontoxic objects: Monitor for spontaneous passage. Once objects reach the stomach, most will pass in four to six days. Seek surgical consultation if the object fails to progress after 72 hours or the patient develops symptoms of perforation, obstruction, or peritonitis.

Preventing repeated DFBI incidents

- Minimize access to swallowable items (eg, utensils, pens, combs, toothbrushes).
- Specific management principles vary depending on the subtype:
  - *Malingering:* Minimize the secondary gain; keep transfers for hospital treatment as brief as possible.
  - *BPD:* Utilize dialectical and cognitive behavioral therapy; target impulsivity and self-injurious behavior with pharmacotherapy (eg, use mood stabilizers or naltrexone).
  - *Psychosis:* Treat with antipsychotic medications.
  - *Pica:* Selective serotonin reuptake inhibitors can be helpful.

Danger to Others

Assessing and Managing Homicide Risk

Responding to Threats of Homicide

When a patient threatens to kill someone, immediate action is necessary:

1. Evaluate the patient's intent, capability, and history of violence or aggression. Consider the specificity of the threat, including details about the potential victim and the plan.
2. Ensure the safety of the patient, staff, and others by implementing appropriate security measures within the unit.

Legal Considerations

- Familiarize yourself with your state's laws regarding the duty to warn and protect third parties. These laws often require health care professionals to take reasonable steps to warn identifiable victims of threats. (See the "Handling Tarasoff Obligations" fact sheet in this section for more details.)
- While patient confidentiality is important, exceptions are made when there is an immediate threat to the safety of others. If you're not sure what to do, consult with the hospital risk management team.

Assessment and Diagnostic Evaluation

- Ask about any history of violent behavior or previous threats.
- Assess for substance use, which can increase the risk of acting on homicidal ideations.
- Evaluate for symptoms that may contribute to homicidal thoughts, such as delusions, hallucinations, or severe impulsivity.
- Consider stressors or triggers that may increase the risk of violence.

Questions to Guide Assessment

- "Have you thought about harming others recently?"
- "Do you have a plan to harm someone? Can you tell me about it?"
- "What makes you feel like you want to hurt others?"
- "Have you ever acted on these thoughts before?"
- "What do you think might stop you from acting on these thoughts?"

Managing Homicide Risk

- Develop a detailed safety plan involving the patient, staff, and possibly the patient's family, focusing on de-escalation strategies and triggers for homicidal ideation.
- Medications can help to manage underlying psychiatric conditions or acute agitation—such as antipsychotics or mood stabilizers.
- Engage the patient in psychotherapy aimed at addressing violent ideation, improving impulse control, and developing coping strategies.
- If there is a credible threat, collaborating with law enforcement may be necessary, following legal guidelines and institutional policies.

Handling Tarasoff Obligations

The 1968 case of Tatiana Tarasoff and Prosenjit Poddar in Oakland, California, brought significant changes to mental health law. After Tarasoff and Poddar's relationship ended, a distressed Poddar told his therapist he planned to kill Tarasoff. Despite the therapist's warning to police, Tarasoff wasn't informed and was later murdered by Poddar. This led to the creation of "Tarasoff warnings," requiring mental health professionals in California and other states to warn individuals about or provide protection from their patients' threats.

Duty to Warn vs Duty to Protect

- *Duty to warn:* If you're faced with a patient expressing a clear intent to harm someone, you're legally bound to warn the intended victim.
- *Duty to protect:* In some states, the law requires that you take whatever steps are necessary to protect the intended victim. You can warn them, but you can also protect the intended victim by, for example, placing the patient on an involuntary psychiatric hold. This option has the advantage of not breaching patient confidentiality.

Do Tarasoff Obligations Apply to You?

Tarasoff laws are in place in 26 states and Puerto Rico, often with local variations. To get specifics, check out this webpage from the National Conference of State Legislatures: www.tinyurl.com/mves5y29

Evaluating Risk

Your patient might express violent fantasies but have no intention of following through with them. How do you decide whether a patient's threats are serious enough to warrant action?

- Look for red flags that increase the likelihood of a threat leading to actual violence: prior violence, substance use, and untreated mental illness.
- The more positive responses to these questions, the greater the urgency for you to act:
  - Is the threat clear and imminent?
  - Is the patient able to carry out the threat?
  - Has the patient engaged in preparatory actions, such as buying a weapon or rehearsing a planned attack?
  - Is the intended victim identifiable?

What Do You Do if You Have No Contact Information for the Intended Victim?

- If you know family members of the patient who might have the intended victim's contact information, consider reaching out to them.
- Conduct an online search.
- Let the police department know if you are unable to reach the intended victim.

Documentation

- Document all your efforts to warn or protect the intended victim.
- Describe the patient's threat using verbatim quotes.
- If you contact the police, take down the name and badge number of the officer you spoke with.

COMMON PSYCHIATRIC CONDITIONS

Anxiety Disorders

Screening for Common Anxiety Disorders

Many patients whom you will admit to the hospital have significant anxiety. Often this is anxiety related to depression or psychosis, but sometimes it is an actual anxiety disorder. In this fact sheet, we discuss an efficient and rapid method for screening and making a provisional diagnosis of an anxiety disorder.

Diagnostic Criteria in Brief for the Major Anxiety Disorders

- *Generalized anxiety disorder (GAD):* Six months of worry plus three of the following: insomnia, fatigue, irritability, restlessness, poor concentration, muscle tension.
- *Panic disorder:* Recurrent panic attacks plus one month of worrying about a recurrence or showing a change in behavior to avoid an attack.
- *Social anxiety disorder:* Persistent fear of social situations, avoidance due to anxiety.
- *Obsessive-compulsive disorder (OCD):* Presence of obsessions and/or compulsions that are time-consuming and cause significant distress or impairment.
- *PTSD:* Exposure to traumatic event, presence of intrusion symptoms, avoidance of trauma-related stimuli, negative alterations in cognition or mood, and marked alterations in arousal and reactivity.
- *Simple phobia:* Excessive fear or anxiety about a specific object or situation, which is avoided or endured with intense anxiety.

What to Ask to Establish Diagnoses

Begin with a high-yield screening question related to each potential diagnosis; follow up with more specific questions as needed.

GAD

- *Screening question:* "Are you a person who worries almost all the time about all kinds of things?"
- *Follow-up questions:* "What do you worry about?" "Have you felt tense, restless, or irritable for the past six months?" "Do you have trouble sleeping and feel fatigued during the day?" "Is your concentration affected?"

Panic disorder

- *Screening question:* "Have you ever had a panic or anxiety attack?"
- *Follow-up questions:* "What does it feel like when you have a panic attack?" "Do you worry about having another attack?" "Have you made any changes in your life to avoid these attacks?"

Social anxiety disorder

- *Screening question:* "Do you feel very anxious or uncomfortable in social situations?"
- *Follow-up questions:* "Describe the anxiety you feel." "Do you avoid these situations due to your anxiety?"

OCD

- *Screening question:* "Do you have obsessive thoughts, like worrying about germs, or repetitive behaviors, like washing your hands over and over?"
- *Follow-up questions:* "What are these thoughts or behaviors?" "How much time do you spend on these thoughts or behaviors in a day?" "Do they cause you distress or interfere with your life?"

PTSD

- *Screening question:* "Have you ever experienced or witnessed a very traumatic event?"
- *Follow-up questions:* "Do you often think about this event when you don't want to?" "Do you avoid anything that reminds you of the event?" "Have you noticed any changes in your mood or behavior since the event?"

Simple phobia

- *Screening question:* "Do you have a strong fear of a specific object or situation?"
- *Follow-up questions:* "What is the object or situation you fear?" "Do you avoid it?" "How does your fear affect your daily life?"

Obsessive-Compulsive Disorder (OCD)

OCD can be severely debilitating, with some individuals' lives becoming consumed by their compulsions. Their response to treatment can be frustratingly slow, but the advantage of inpatient units is the opportunity for intensive daily treatment, which can accelerate this improvement.

Diagnosis

- *Obsessions:* Distressing recurring thoughts, images, or urges.
- *Compulsions:* Repetitive, ritualistic behaviors that the person feels driven to perform in response to obsessions.

Common Obsessions

- *Contamination:* Worries about germs, dirt, or toxins. "If I touch that doorknob, I might get a deadly disease."
- *Fear of harm to oneself or others:* "I might have left the stove on and now the house might burn down."
- *Need for symmetry or exactness:* "All the pencils on my desk need to be perfectly parallel."
- *Religious or moral fears:* Often referred to as "scrupulosity." "What if I have bad thoughts during my prayers?"
- *Unwanted sexual or violent thoughts:* "What if I harm my child?" or "What if I act on a taboo sexual urge?"

Common Compulsions

- *Washing and cleaning* (eg, washing hands many times in a row, or excessive showering).
- *Checking:* Repeatedly making sure something is off, locked, safe, etc (eg, a stove or a door).
- *Repeating:* Doing something over and over a certain number of times or until it feels "just right" (eg, going in and out of a door several times).
- *Ordering/arranging* (eg, arranging books by size or color, or ensuring shoes are paired perfectly).
- *Mental rituals:* Counting, praying, or repeating certain words in one's mind to counteract or neutralize a distressing thought (eg, counting to 10 every time one has a bad thought).

Treatment

- *Cognitive behavioral therapy with exposure response prevention (CBT-ERP):* A therapeutic approach that involves gradually exposing individuals to their feared objects or obsessive thoughts, teaching them to refrain from their habitual compulsive responses.
- *Medications:* Close monitoring in an inpatient setting allows for faster dose increases, especially since doses for OCD often lean toward the higher side.
  - Selective serotonin reuptake inhibitors (SSRIs), such as fluoxetine (Prozac) 40–80 mg daily, fluvoxamine (Luvox) 200–300 mg daily, sertraline (Zoloft) 200–300 mg, or paroxetine (Paxil) 40–60 mg daily.
  - Clomipramine (Anafranil) 100–250 mg daily.
- A combination of CBT-ERP and medication offers the best outcomes.
- Track progress with the Yale-Brown Obsessive-Compulsive Scale (Y-BOCS).

Interventions for Treatment-Resistant OCD

- Switch to a different SSRI or switch to clomipramine or venlafaxine.
- Greatly increase the dose of the SSRI (eg, fluoxetine up to 120 mg daily or sertraline up to 400 mg).
- Augment with second-generation antipsychotics, such as aripiprazole (titrate to 15–30 mg daily), olanzapine (5–10 mg daily), or risperidone (2–6 mg daily).
- Augment an SSRI with clomipramine (be cautious of serotonin syndrome and drug interactions.)
- Augment an SSRI with one of a range of glutamate modulators, such as lamotrigine, pregabalin, topiramate, memantine, amantadine, or riluzole.

Interventions for Refractory OCD

- *Transcranial magnetic stimulation:* Depending on your facility's resources.
- *Surgical interventions:* Liaise with neurosurgical teams regarding potential suitability for deep brain stimulation, cingulotomy, or anterior capsulotomy.

Panic Disorder

Panic disorder is a common and treatable condition characterized by recurrent, unexpected panic attacks and ongoing fear of future attacks. These episodes of intense fear can come on suddenly and can include physical symptoms such as chest pain, palpitations, dizziness, or shortness of breath. Understanding how to effectively manage panic disorder is crucial for helping patients regain control over their lives.

Diagnosis

To diagnose panic disorder, a thorough evaluation is necessary to rule out other medical conditions and confirm that the patient's symptoms align with DSM-5 criteria:

- Recurrent, unexpected panic attacks that involve an abrupt surge of intense fear or discomfort.
- At least one of the attacks has been followed by one month or more of persistent concern or worry about additional panic attacks or their consequences, or a significant maladaptive change in behavior related to the attacks.
- The disturbance is not attributable to the physiological effects of a substance or another medical condition and is not better explained by another mental disorder.

Initial Assessment

When assessing a patient for panic disorder, make sure to:

- Obtain a detailed medical history to rule out other conditions that can mimic panic symptoms, such as hyperthyroidism, cardiac arrhythmias, or drug withdrawal.
- Assess for comorbid psychiatric conditions like depression, other anxiety disorders, or substance use disorders, which are common in patients with panic disorder.
- Evaluate the impact of panic disorder on the patient's daily life, including any avoidance behaviors or functional impairments.

Treatment

Effective management of panic disorder typically involves a combination of pharmacotherapy and psychotherapy, tailored to the patient's needs and preferences.

Pharmacotherapy

- *Selective serotonin reuptake inhibitors (SSRIs):* SSRIs are considered the first-line treatment for panic disorder due to their efficacy and favorable side effect profile. Common choices include fluoxetine, sertraline, and escitalopram. Start with a low dose and gradually increase to minimize the risk of initial increased anxiety.
- *Serotonin-norepinephrine reuptake inhibitors (SNRIs):* SNRIs, such as venlafaxine, are also effective in treating panic disorder. Like SSRIs, they should be started at a low dose and titrated up as needed.
- *Benzodiazepines:* Benzodiazepines, such as clonazepam or lorazepam, can be used for short-term management, particularly during the early phase of treatment or for acute relief. However, due to the risk of dependence, they should be used cautiously and are not recommended as a long-term solution.
- *Tricyclic antidepressants (TCAs):* TCAs like imipramine can be effective but are generally considered second-line due to their side effect profile. They can be an option if SSRIs or SNRIs are not effective or tolerated.
- *Other medications:* In some cases, adjunctive treatments like beta-blockers (eg, propranolol) can help manage the physical symptoms of panic attacks, such as palpitations or tremors.

Psychotherapy

- *Cognitive behavioral therapy (CBT):* CBT is the most evidence-based psychotherapeutic approach for panic disorder. It involves helping patients understand the relationship between their thoughts, feelings, and behaviors, and teaching them skills to manage and reduce their anxiety.
  - *Psychoeducation:* Patients are educated about the nature of panic attacks and the fight-or-flight response, which helps demystify the experience and reduce fear.
  - *Exposure therapy:* Gradual exposure to panic-inducing situations, combined with relaxation techniques, helps reduce avoidance behaviors and desensitize patients to triggers.
  - *Cognitive restructuring:* Patients learn to identify and challenge the catastrophic thoughts that contribute to panic, replacing them with more balanced and realistic perspectives.
- *Mindfulness and relaxation techniques:* Mindfulness meditation, deep breathing exercises, and progressive muscle relaxation can be helpful adjuncts to CBT, reducing overall anxiety levels and helping patients remain calm during panic attacks.

Trauma-Related Disorders

Many of your patients will most likely have been exposed to significant trauma, such as adverse childhood experiences, domestic or sexual violence, and the hardships associated with homelessness or substance use. In this fact sheet, we describe a practical approach to diagnosing trauma-related conditions and assessing the extent to which your patient's daily functioning is significantly affected by past trauma.

DSM-5 Criteria for PTSD

- Symptoms last for more than one month.
- Mnemonic: **R**emembers **A**trocious **N**uclear **A**ttacks (Must meet all of the following criteria to qualify; suggested probing questions follow criteria).
  1. Exposure to traumatic event: Directly experiencing, witnessing, or learning about a traumatic event involving a close family member or friend: "Have you experienced any traumatic events that have stuck with you, like being attacked or surviving a disaster?"
  2. **R**emembers: **R**emembers or **r**eexperiences intrusive distressing memories, dreams, or flashbacks of the event: "Does the experience come back to haunt you? In what ways?"
  3. **A**trocious: **A**voidance of stimuli associated with the traumatic event, such as avoiding certain activities or thoughts, or having amnesia for the event: "Do you find yourself avoiding things that you associate with the memory?"
  4. **N**uclear: **N**egative changes in cognition and mood, such as exaggerated negative beliefs about oneself or the world, inability to have positive emotions, diminished interest in various activities, or a sense of foreshortened future.
  5. **A**ttacks: **A**rousal and reactivity, such as irritable behavior and angry outbursts, hypervigilance, exaggerated startle response, concentration problems, or sleep disturbance: "Since the trauma, have you noticed major mood changes, like not caring about anything or not seeing a future for yourself? Have you been more on edge, more irritable, or had insomnia?" (These questions apply to items 4 and 5.)

DSM-5 Criteria for Acute Stress Disorder

- Symptoms last for three days to one month after exposure.
- Symptoms are similar to PTSD criteria, except shorter duration.

Criteria for Complex PTSD

- Symptoms can last for years.
- Not an official DSM-5 diagnosis.
- Refers to long-lasting effects of prolonged and repeated trauma, occurring over many months or years.
- Typical symptoms include persistent depressed mood, feeling permanently damaged or worthless, persistent distrust, interpersonal difficulties, chronic suicidal thoughts, and physical symptoms without a clear organic cause.

Diagnostic Interviewing Tips

- *Establish trust:* Begin by building rapport and establishing a safe and supportive environment for the patient.
- *Provide trauma-informed care:* Be sensitive and mindful of the patient's trauma history. Avoid retraumatization by carefully navigating discussions about the traumatic event.
- *Specific inquiry:* Use open-ended questions to allow the patient to describe their experiences, then follow up with more specific questions based on the DSM-5 criteria.
- *Collateral information:* Consider obtaining information from significant others or previous medical records, with the patient's consent, to gather a comprehensive history.

Treatment

First-line medications

- Selective serotonin reuptake inhibitors (SSRIs): The primary choice for treating PTSD, effective in reducing symptoms like reexperiencing, avoidance, and hyperarousal.
  - *Sertraline (Zoloft):* 50–200 mg daily.
  - *Paroxetine (Paxil):* 20–60 mg daily.

Second-line medications

- Serotonin/norepinephrine reuptake inhibitors (SNRIs): For patients who do not respond to or tolerate SSRIs.
  - *Venlafaxine (Effexor XR):* 37.5–225 mg daily.
- Alpha-1 adrenergic blockers:
  - *Prazosin:* Especially beneficial for nightmares and sleep disturbances, but also can diminish daytime hyperarousal. Start at 1 mg at bedtime; can be titrated up gradually to usual maintenance dose of 2–6 mg. To treat daytime symptoms, can use 1–2 mg up to four times a day. Side effects include hypotension and sedation.

- Alpha-2 agonists for hyperarousal and anxiety:
  - *Clonidine:* Start with 0.1 mg BID; can increase to 0.2 mg BID or TID, either standing or PRN. Side effects include hypotension and sedation.
  - *Guanfacine:* Start 1 mg HS; can increase to 4 mg HS.

Adjunctive and alternative medications

- *Second-generation antipsychotics:* For severe symptoms or psychotic features.
  - Add quetiapine (starting at 25 mg, titrating up as needed) to an SSRI or SNRI.
  - Add any of the following: Risperidone (Risperdal), olanzapine (Zyprexa), ziprasidone (Geodon).
- *Mood stabilizers:* Lithium or valproate for mood swings or bipolar symptoms.
- *Anticonvulsants:* Lamotrigine or gabapentin for mood instability, anxiety, or insomnia.
- *Benzodiazepines:* With caution, for acute anxiety or insomnia.
- *Tricyclic antidepressants:* Amitriptyline or imipramine for panic attacks, nightmares, or chronic pain.
- *Monoamine oxidase inhibitors:* Phenelzine for patients who don't respond to other treatments, but be sure to educate about dietary restrictions.
- *Other antidepressants:* Mirtazapine for sleep and appetite issues; trazodone for sleep disturbances.
- *Novel therapeutics:* Ketamine in specialized settings for rapid symptom relief.
- *Over-the-counter options and supplements:* Melatonin for sleep regulation; omega-3 fatty acids for mood and anxiety.

Considerations for special populations

- *Substance use disorders:* Avoid potentially habit-forming medications like benzodiazepines.
- *Elderly patients:* Use lower starting doses and titrate slowly.
- *Comorbid conditions:* Tailor medication choices to address comorbid psychiatric conditions effectively (eg, use a second-generation antipsychotic for a patient with PTSD who also exhibits symptoms of schizophrenia).

How to Manage Anxiety with Nonaddictive Medications

Many patients with substance use disorders suffer from anxiety and agitation. A common challenge on inpatient units is to steer such patients away from benzodiazepines and toward alternatives. In fact, some patients themselves express concern about dependence and specifically ask for non-habit-forming medications. This fact sheet provides guidance on managing anxiety with nonaddictive medications, offering effective options for those at risk of substance misuse.

How to Discuss Your Unwillingness to Prescribe Benzodiazepines

The best strategy here is to be very direct, eg:

- "You need treatment for anxiety, but you have a substance use issue, so we are going to use nonaddictive antianxiety medications."
- "I understand that Klonopin has worked for you before, but considering your long-term anxiety and the risk of dependence, we should explore nonaddictive options instead."

Common Nonaddictive Medications for Anxiety

Selective serotonin reuptake inhibitors (SSRIs)

First-line treatment for generalized anxiety disorder (GAD), panic disorder, and obsessive-compulsive disorder (OCD). Suggested SSRIs include fluoxetine (20–60 mg/day), sertraline (50–200 mg/day), and escitalopram (10–20 mg/day). Regular monitoring for common side effects like sexual dysfunction, nausea, and sleep disturbance is recommended.

Serotonin/norepinephrine reuptake inhibitors (SNRIs)

Useful in GAD and panic disorder, SNRIs like venlafaxine (75–225 mg/day) and duloxetine (60–120 mg/day) are good alternatives to SSRIs. Monitor for side effects like dry mouth, constipation, and excessive sweating.

Pregabalin (150–600 mg/day)

It's an alternative to SSRIs and SNRIs for GAD. Watch out for dizziness, sleepiness, and potential for misuse in those with a history of substance abuse.

Buspirone (20–60 mg/day)

It can be effective in GAD, especially for patients who have had negative experiences with SSRIs or SNRIs. Some common side effects are dizziness and nausea.

Beta-blockers

Drugs like propranolol (20–40 mg taken before anxiety-inducing situations) can manage acute episodes of anxiety, particularly situational anxiety. Useful for treating the physical symptoms of anxiety, such as a racing heart or trembling.

Hydroxyzine (25–100 mg/day)

An antihistamine with anxiolytic properties. Suitable for short-term use or as an adjunct treatment. Be cautious about potential side effects like sedation and dry mouth.

Other antidepressants

Certain tricyclics like imipramine (50–200 mg/day) and monoamine oxidase inhibitors (MAOIs) like phenelzine (45–90 mg/day) are sometimes used. While effective, their side effects and dietary restrictions (especially for MAOIs) make them less preferred choices.

Second-generation antipsychotics

Quetiapine (50–300 mg/day) can be used when other treatments fail or in cases of comorbid bipolar disorder. Monitor for potential metabolic side effects.

Choosing and Managing Benzodiazepines

Benzodiazepines can be a tricky class of meds to manage, especially in an inpatient setting where patients might have complex needs or a history of substance use. Here's a guide to help navigate through this process.

Evaluating the Need for Benzos

- Start by evaluating why the patient needs a benzo. Common indications include severe anxiety, acute agitation, alcohol withdrawal, seizure management, or severe muscle spasms.
- Check the patient's history with benzos and other substances. Do they have a history of substance use disorder? If so, tread carefully.
- Have any of these nonbenzodiazepine options been tried and failed?
  - *Selective serotonin reuptake inhibitors (SSRIs), serotonin/norepinephrine reuptake inhibitors (SNRIs):* Worth considering first, given their safety and efficacy profile.
  - *Buspirone:* Another option, especially for patients who don't respond well to SSRIs or SNRIs or experience side effects from those meds.
  - *Hydroxyzine:* Useful and quick-acting for anxiety; also helps with insomnia.
  - *Propranolol:* Helps manage the physical symptoms of anxiety, like tremor and rapid heart rate.
  - *Antipsychotics (eg, quetiapine):* Can be effective for severe anxiety and agitation.
  - *Gabapentinoids:* Gabapentin and pregabalin are particularly useful for patients with comorbid pain syndromes.
- Weigh the immediate benefit of symptom relief against the risks of tolerance, dependence, and potential misuse.

Choosing the Right Benzo

Short-acting benzos (good for acute, short-term use)

- *Lorazepam (Ativan):* Quick onset, useful for acute agitation or severe anxiety. Also a go-to for alcohol withdrawal.
- *Oxazepam (Serax):* Slower onset, less abuse potential, good for elderly patients or those with liver impairment.

Long-acting benzos (good for tapering or maintenance)

- *Diazepam (Valium):* Fast onset, long half-life, useful for alcohol withdrawal and muscle spasms.
- *Clonazepam (Klonopin):* Longer duration, good for anxiety and panic disorders.

Dosing Tips

- Always start with the lowest effective dose and titrate up slowly. This helps minimize side effects and dependence risk.
- For acute symptoms, use PRN dosing. This limits overall exposure and reduces the risk of developing tolerance.
- For persistent anxiety or agitation, patients might need scheduled dosing. Reassess regularly to see if the dose can be tapered down.

Handling Requests for Higher Doses

- Evaluate why the patient is asking for more. Increased anxiety or agitation? Developing tolerance? Seeking euphoria?
- Use nonpharmacological strategies first. Deep breathing exercises, cognitive behavioral techniques, or even distracting activities (eg, reading, calling a friend, doing stretching exercises) can help.
- Be cautious about increasing doses and explain the risks of tolerance and dependence. Having a frank discussion about the goals of treatment and long-term plans can often help.
- Consider adding or switching to a different class of medication if the current regimen isn't cutting it. An adjunctive medication like gabapentin or a second-generation antipsychotic like quetiapine can also be beneficial.

Monitoring and Follow-Up

- Regularly reassess the patient's symptoms and the need for ongoing benzo use. Look for signs of improvement or worsening.
- Educate the patient about the risks associated with long-term benzo use, including tolerance, dependence, and potential cognitive effects.
- If you decide to taper off the benzo, do it slowly to avoid withdrawal symptoms, and take into account the duration of benzodiazepine use and the medication's half-life:
  - *Short-term use (weeks to a few months):* Patients may tolerate a faster taper, reducing by 25% every one to two weeks.
  - *Long-term use (several months to years):* Patients will require a slower taper, reducing by 10%–15% every one to two weeks, and potentially 5%–10% every two to four weeks if withdrawal symptoms occur.
  - *Short-half-life benzodiazepines (eg, alprazolam):* Patients on these benzodiazepines may experience more frequent and severe withdrawal symptoms. To mitigate this, switch to a longer-acting benzodiazepine like diazepam or

clonazepam before beginning the taper. This approach provides a smoother and more gradual reduction of benzodiazepine levels in the body.
  - *Long-half-life benzodiazepines (eg, diazepam):* These benzodiazepines can sometimes be tapered more quickly due to their prolonged action, which provides a natural buffer against withdrawal symptoms. However, individual response varies, so adjust the tapering pace as needed.
- When tapering, the rate of reduction can typically be faster for the first 50% of the dose and then slower for the remaining 50% to minimize withdrawal symptoms.

Considerations for Specific Populations

- *Elderly:* Use lower doses due to increased sensitivity and risk of falls, cognitive impairment, and paradoxical agitation. Consider oxazepam or lorazepam due to shorter half-lives and safer metabolism.
- *Liver impairment:* Use oxazepam or lorazepam as they do not require hepatic oxidation for metabolism.
- *History of substance use:* Be extremely cautious. Consider nonbenzodiazepine alternatives and involve addiction specialists if needed.

Table 2: **Comparative Table of Benzodiazepines**

Benzodiazepine	Brand Name	Approximate Equivalent Dosages Compared to Lorazepam (mg)	Half-Life (hours)	Common Use	Typical Dose
Alprazolam	**Xanax**	0.5	6–20	Anxiety, panic disorders	0.25–0.5 mg PO every 6–8 hours PRN
Chlordiazepoxide	**Librium**	10–25	5–30 (longer due to active metabolites)	Anxiety, alcohol withdrawal	10–25 mg PO every 6–8 hours PRN
Clonazepam	**Klonopin**	0.5–1	18–50	Anxiety, panic disorders	0.25–1 mg PO every 12 hours PRN
Diazepam	**Valium**	5–10	20–100 (longer due to active metabolites)	Anxiety, muscle spasms, alcohol withdrawal	2–10 mg PO/IM/IV every 6–8 hours PRN
Estazolam	**ProSom**	1–2	10–24	Insomnia	1–2 mg PO at bedtime
Flurazepam	**Dalmane**	15–30	40–250 (longer due to active metabolites)	Insomnia	15–30 mg PO at bedtime
Lorazepam	**Ativan**	1	10–20	Acute agitation, severe anxiety, alcohol withdrawal	0.5–2 mg PO/IM/IV every 4–6 hours PRN
Midazolam	**Versed**	1–2	1.5–4	Procedural sedation, acute agitation	1–5 mg IV/IM
Oxazepam	**Serax**	15–30	4–15	Mild to moderate anxiety, elderly patients, those with liver impairment	10–30 mg PO every 6–8 hours PRN
Temazepam	**Restoril**	15–30	5–15	Insomnia	15–30 mg PO at bedtime
Triazolam	**Halcion**	0.25	1.5–5.5	Insomnia	0.125–0.25 mg PO at bedtime

Source: Ashton CH. *Benzodiazepines: How They Work and How to Withdraw* [aka The Ashton Manual]. Newcastle-upon-Tyne, England: Newcastle University, 2002. https://www.benzo.org.uk/manual/

COMMON PSYCHIATRIC CONDITIONS

Bipolar Disorder

Bipolar Disorder Diagnostic Interview

The most challenging aspect of diagnosing bipolar disorder is establishing a history of a manic or hypomanic episode. Patients with bipolar disorder spend much more time in depressed episodes and may not clearly recall having had a manic episode. Furthermore, the symptoms of mania overlap with other syndromes, such as borderline personality disorder, psychosis, anxiety, and ADHD.

DSM Criteria

There are two common types of bipolar disorder:

- *Type 1:* A history of episodes of depression and mania.
- *Type 2:* A history of episodes of depression and hypomania.

Mania

One week of elevated mood plus three out of seven **DIGFAST** symptoms (four if irritable mood):

- **D**istractibility.
- **I**ndiscretion (high-risk behaviors).
- **G**randiosity.
- **F**light of ideas.
- **A**ctivity excess.
- **S**leep not needed.
- **T**alkativeness.

Hypomania

Same as mania criteria, except the distinct mood only needs to last for four days and the episode does not cause marked impairment in functioning.

Depression

Two weeks of depressed mood plus four out of eight **SIGECAPS** symptoms for two weeks. (See the "How to Diagnose Major Depressive Disorder" fact sheet in the Common Psychiatric Conditions section, Depressive Disorders subsection, for more details.)

Diagnostic Interviewing Tips

Quick screening questions for a history of mania

"Has there been a time of several days when your mood felt great and you slept only two or three hours a night, or even less, but still had a lot of energy?"

Sometimes people will say that they have "mood swings" and believe this means they have bipolar disorder. This may mean that they go from feeling depressed to feeling normal (which does not qualify as bipolar disorder). To clarify this issue, ask something like: "When you felt better, did people say, 'You look like you're feeling pretty well' or did they say, 'Wow, you're acting sort of different or strange'?"

Follow-up questions when the screen is positive

If you believe that your patient's answers to your screening questions indicate a probable manic (or hypomanic) episode in the past, your next step is to ask about each of the DIGFAST symptoms, referring repeatedly to the most severe manic period they can recall: "Now I want to ask you some questions about things you were doing during that week last year when you felt manic."

- *Distractibility:* "During that period, was it hard for you to concentrate on one thing at a time?"
- *Indiscretion (high-risk behaviors):* "As you look back over that period, do you recall doing anything that could have caused trouble for you or your family? Did you find yourself involved in doing things that you wouldn't ordinarily do? Things that you look back on now as showing poor judgment or being risky?"
- *Grandiosity:* "During that period, did you have a sense that you were smarter or more attractive than others, or did you have the sense that you could accomplish a lot more, or had special powers or skills that others don't have? That you were much more capable and more confident, above what is normal for you at your baseline?"
- *Flight of ideas:*
  - "During that period, did you find that you had lots of ideas going through your mind? Were they good ideas? Did you feel that your mind was accelerated, like it was in fifth gear and you couldn't slow it down?"
  - You may need to distinguish this from anxious thinking by asking, "You said you had a sense that your mind was going quickly—was it that you were worrying or ruminating over and over again?"
- *Activity excess:*
  - "Did you have the sense that you wanted to keep moving or that you were physically uncomfortable if you were just sitting still? Did you sense that you were very fidgety?"
  - "Did you find yourself much more active than usual? If I had been with you, would I have found you to be much more active than is normal for you?"
- *Sleep not needed:* "Did you find that you didn't need as much sleep as usual? Were you able to get by on only a couple of hours of sleep a night?"
- *Talkativeness:* "Did you have the sense that it was hard to stop talking once you started? Or did you find yourself interrupting people?"

How to Medicate Manic Episodes

This sheet guides you in how to use medications to rapidly treat patients with severe mania. Many of these patients have bipolar disorder; others may have schizoaffective disorder, bipolar type; still others may have arrived on your unit with a murky psychiatric history but with agitation, racing thoughts, and other hallmarks of mania.

Identify Target Symptoms and Goals

Typical therapeutic goals include slowing down racing thoughts and flight of ideas; normalizing excessively euphoric or irritable mood; improving insight and reality testing if there are psychotic delusions; improving sleep; slowing down hyperactivity; and decreasing impulsivity and intrusiveness.

Medication Treatment

Medication choices

- Start with both a mood stabilizer (MS) and an antipsychotic (AP), since generally the combination is more effective than either one alone. You can also start a benzodiazepine or add one later to augment response if needed. If the first combination of meds doesn't work within several days, increase doses or switch to another MS/AP/benzo if needed.
- MS choices:
  - Start with either lithium or valproic acid.
    - Lithium: Start with 600–900 mg daily (either BID or HS) and increase to achieve a serum level of 0.8–1.2, which will often require about 1200–1500 mg daily.
    - Valproic acid (Depakote): Start with a loading dose of 20 mg/kg, then titrate based on clinical response and serum levels, aiming for 50–125 µg/mL. Can also start with 750 mg once a day, in divided doses if using immediate release, and increase dose every two to three days as tolerated up to 1500–3000 mg daily.
  - Carbamazepine (Tegretol) is second line. Start with 200 mg twice daily, then titrate based on clinical response.
- AP choices:
  - There are no definitive data showing that any particular AP is superior for mania.
  - Anecdotally, the "biggest guns" for rapid control of mania are olanzapine, quetiapine, or haloperidol—but each has a high side effect burden.
  - A reasonable philosophy is to start with a medication that will be most tolerable for long-term treatment.
  - Common APs:
    - Aripiprazole, 10–15 mg daily, increase up to 30 mg daily (divided doses).
    - Olanzapine, 10–15 mg HS, increase up to 25 mg daily (divided doses).
    - Quetiapine, 50–100 mg HS, increase up to 600–800 mg daily (divided doses).
- Benzodiazepine choices:
  - Lorazepam (start 1 mg TID, increase up to 3 mg TID) or clonazepam (start 1 mg BID, increase up to 3 mg BID).

Treatment-resistant mania options

- Clozapine, either alone or in combination with MS.
- Other meds with less evidence of efficacy in mania but sometimes tried: Allopurinol, tamoxifen, lamotrigine (Lamictal), gabapentin (Neurontin), topiramate (Topamax), zonisamide, tiagabine, oxcarbazepine (Trileptal), verapamil.
- Blue-blocking or orange-tinted glasses, worn from 6 pm to 8 am.
- Electroconvulsive therapy (though it is difficult to get consent in manic patients).

Tips on choosing meds for specific patients

- Renal disease? Avoid lithium.
- Liver disease? Avoid valproic acid or carbamazepine.
- Obesity? Avoid olanzapine, quetiapine, and clozapine.
- History of extrapyramidal symptoms? Avoid aripiprazole and risperidone.
- Women of childbearing age? Avoid valproic acid.
- Pregnant women? Avoid valproic acid, plus avoid lithium in the first trimester.
- Ask about how the patient's family members have responded to specific drugs.

Tips on convincing patients to take meds

Many manic patients have poor insight into symptoms and will challenge you to explain why they need to take medications. Avoid directly challenging their delusions or feelings; instead, try to acknowledge their perspectives while still gently guiding them toward treatment.

- "You have a lot on your mind and a lot to share, but you're talking so quickly that it's hard for us to understand you. This medication can calm your mind and make it easier to connect with people."

- "You're feeling on top of the world, but that can make it challenging to make safe choices. This medication can help balance things out and make you feel calmer and more grounded."
- "You have a lot of energy, which feels great but is also exhausting. This medication can help you channel that energy so that you'll feel better and will get more sleep."
- "I see that things feel intense for you right now. I want to help and ensure you're safe. This medication can help you feel calmer and less overwhelmed."
- "You have interesting ideas and lofty goals. These meds won't take away your beliefs, but they will help you focus in a way that's more beneficial to you and others."
- "These meds may allow us to prevent a depressive episode once your energy runs out."

How to Treat Bipolar Depression

Bipolar depression is the depressive phase of bipolar disorder, and it presents very similarly to regular major depression. The key is to recognize it and to be cautious about using antidepressants.

Diagnosis and Assessment

- Ask about a history of mania in all patients with depression (see the "Bipolar Disorder Diagnostic Interview" fact sheet in the Common Psychiatric Conditions section, Bipolar Disorder subsection).
- Depressive symptoms in bipolar depression tend to be more severe and are more likely to include poor energy, increased sleep, inertia, and psychomotor slowing.
- Rapid cycling (at least four distinct mood episodes per year) is common. Note that all these episodes can be depression and still qualify.

Treatment

- Mood stabilizers:
  - *Lamotrigine (Lamictal):* Helpful but works slowly (typically six to eight weeks) due to slow titration schedule to prevent Stevens-Johnson syndrome. Start at 25 mg daily for two weeks, then 50 mg daily for two weeks, then 100 mg for one to two weeks, then 200 mg. Reduce dosing by 50% for patients who are also on valproic acid (Depakote).
  - *Lithium:* Proven efficacy in both the manic and depressive phases. Monitoring serum lithium levels is essential; aim for a therapeutic range of 0.6–0.8 mEq/L (lower than the target dose in mania).
- Antipsychotics: The following are FDA approved for bipolar depression.
  - These two may be the most effective but have a higher side effect burden:
    - *Quetiapine (Seroquel):* Both immediate-release and extended-release formulations have evidence of efficacy in bipolar depression. Start at 50 mg daily and titrate up to 300 mg daily over one week.
    - *Olanzapine/fluoxetine combination (Symbyax):* An FDA-approved option, but watch for potential side effects like weight gain. Start with one capsule daily in the evening.
  - These three are also effective and are better tolerated:
    - *Lurasidone (Latuda):* Start with 20 mg once daily; can increase based on response, tolerability up to 120 mg daily.
    - *Cariprazine (Vraylar):* Start at 1.5 mg daily; can be titrated up to 6 mg daily.
    - *Lumateperone (Caplyta):* Typically 42 mg once daily.
- Antidepressants:
  - Any antidepressant, plus a mood stabilizer (eg, lithium, lamotrigine) or antipsychotic to avoid mood destabilization.
  - Risk of antidepressant-induced mania, from low to high, is: bupropion < SSRIs < SNRIs < tricyclics. Start bupropion low (75 mg); raise slowly (by 75 mg/week).
- Electroconvulsive therapy.
- Other possibilities (less evidence but can be tried):
  - *Pramipexole (Mirapex):* Start at 0.25 mg at night; raise by 0.25 mg every week to 1–2 mg at night. Most common side effect: Nausea.
  - *Armodafinil (Nuvigil) or modafinil (Provigil):* 50–250 mg in the morning.
  - *Valproic acid:* Start at 250 mg twice daily, titrating to achieve serum concentrations of 50–125 µg/mL.
  - Natural remedies:
    - *L-methylfolate:* 7.5–15 mg daily.
    - *Omega-3:* 1–3 g EPA+DHA daily; choose formulations with an EPA:DHA ratio of greater than 1.5:1.
    - *Inositol:* 12–18 g daily.
    - *N-acetylcysteine:* 600–1200 mg twice daily.
  - *Light therapy:* Start 15 minutes/day and increase to target time of 1 hour/day.

Psychoeducation

- Tell your patient that you think they have bipolar disorder. Define it simply, saying something like, "Bipolar disorder refers to people who have periods of depression with occasional times of feeling very high, even too high."
- Encourage medication compliance:
  - *Not curative:* "Bipolar disorder is lifelong. We don't cure it, but we have medications that can help treat it, and our goal is to extend your period of wellness as long as we can."
  - *Analogy of diabetes:* "Bipolar disorder, like diabetes, is lifelong. If you have diabetes, you have to stay on medication, but it's not enough to just take meds—you have to eat right, get exercise, and check your blood glucose. In both illnesses, you have to be an active participant in your care by adhering to a routine and structure."
  - *General positive response to mood stabilizers:* "Most patients who take and stay on their mood stabilizer have stable moods for the first time in their lives. Imagine what you could do if you had a stable mood!"

COMMON PSYCHIATRIC CONDITIONS

Depressive Disorders

Differential Diagnosis of Depressive Disorders

Major Depression

- Depressed mood + **SIGECAPS** symptoms (four of eight).
- **SIGECAPS: S**leep, **I**nterest, **G**uilt, **E**nergy, **C**oncentration, **A**ppetite, **P**sychomotor, **S**uicide.

Bipolar Depression

- Depression plus history of mania or hypomania.
- Use mood stabilizers/antipsychotics.

Depression with Mixed Manic Features

- Depression plus three of:
  - Elevated mood.
  - Grandiosity.
  - More talkative.
  - Flight of ideas.
  - Increased energy.
  - Excessively active in an impulsive way.
  - Decreased need for sleep.
- Use antidepressant plus mood stabilizer/antipsychotic.

Melancholic Depression

- One of the following:
  - Anhedonia.
  - Lack of mood reactivity.
- And at least three of the following:
  - Early-morning awakening.
  - Worse mood in the morning.
  - Excessive guilt.
  - Depression that is subjectively different from grief or loss.
  - Severe weight loss or loss of appetite.
  - Psychomotor agitation or retardation.
- Consider tricyclic antidepressants.

Atypical Depression

- Mood reactivity (mood brightens in response to positive events).
- Two or more of the following:
  - Increased appetite or weight gain.
  - Hypersomnia.
  - Leaden paralysis. Ask, "Do you get so depressed that you feel too tired to even move?"
  - Rejection sensitivity. Ask, "When you get disappointed or rejected, does that really affect you or are you able to shrug it off?"
- Consider monoamine oxidase inhibitors.

Psychotic Depression

- Delusions, often of a paranoid or nihilistic nature, with themes typically about personal inadequacy, guilt, disease, death, or deserved punishment.
- Hallucinations of voices putting the patient down, saying disparaging or critical things.
- Consider antipsychotics/electroconvulsive therapy.

Ruminative Depression

- Persistent, intrusive thoughts, typically about personal inadequacies, regrets, and worries about the future.
- Consider selective serotonin reuptake inhibitors/cognitive behavioral therapy.

How to Diagnose Major Depressive Disorder

Diagnostic Criteria

For you to diagnose the presence of a major depressive episode, DSM-5 requires you to establish that your patient has had depressive mood or anhedonia **plus** four out of eight **SIGECAPS** symptoms for at least two weeks:

- **S**leep decrease.
- **I**nterest decrease.
- **G**uilt.
- **E**nergy decrease.
- **C**oncentration decrease.
- **A**ppetite decrease.
- **P**sychomotor retardation or agitation.
- **S**uicidality.

Tips for Exploring Each Symptom

Mood

- "How has your mood been over the last two weeks?"
- "Have you felt so depressed that you felt like your entire life has been affected by your mood?"
- Note that people will experience a "depressed mood" in different ways. Some typical terms that will resonate with many depressed patients include feeling sad, empty, irritable, discouraged, never happy, or desperate. Some patients will feel a constant sense of dread, nervousness, or anxiety, but with probing they may be found to be suffering from major depression as opposed to an anxiety disorder.

Sleep

- "Have you slept well or poorly over the last two weeks?"
- "Do you sleep too much or too little when you are depressed?"
- Depressed patients may have insomnia or hypersomnia, though insomnia is more common. Insomnia may be described as sleepless nights, and it may include early-morning awakening. Pay close attention to sleep habits because our meds are very good at improving them quickly. Insomnia is usually the first symptom to improve during an inpatient stay, typically on the first night.

Interest (loss of interest or pleasure)

- "Have you been able to enjoy doing anything over the last few weeks?"

Guilt, worthlessness, hopelessness

- "How has your self-esteem been?"
- "Do you feel that you are a good person?"
- "Do you still have hope?"
- "Have you felt guilty about things you've done or haven't done?"

Energy

- "How has your energy level been over the last couple of weeks?"

Concentration

- "Have you been able to focus on things well?"
- "How has your concentration level been?"

Appetite

- "Have you felt like eating? Have you lost weight lately?"
- "Have you been eating too much, just to feel good?"
- Consider adding Ensure to the meals of patients who have lost a lot of weight.

Psychomotor retardation or agitation

- This is usually diagnosed more by observation than by asking questions, but you can try questions like: "Have you felt like everything has become slowed down? Or have you felt unusually restless or agitated?"

Suicidality

- "Have you had thoughts of wishing you were dead?"
- "Have you been thinking about ways to kill yourself?"

Depression with Psychotic Features

Diagnosis

- DSM-5 criteria:
  - At least two weeks of unipolar major depression (eg, five out of nine **SIGECAPS** symptoms), plus hallucinations or delusions.
  - Suicide attempts are common (30%).
- Prevalence: Much more common than you might think—28% of people with depression have psychotic symptoms; 42% of patients hospitalized for depression have psychotic features.
- Interviewing tips:
  - Can be subtle and easy to miss.
  - Ask: "Many people with severe depression find that their mind starts to play tricks on them. Have you had any strange experiences, like hearing voices, or have you been worrying irrationally about things?"
  - Delusions may initially sound reasonable (eg, patient states, "The neighborhood kids have been noisy") but with probing questions they may reveal themselves (eg, patient believes that the kids are chanting that she is a prostitute). Delusions are often related to guilt about imagined sins or crimes.

Differential Diagnosis

- In schizophrenia and schizoaffective disorder, psychosis occurs in the absence of mood episodes.
- In bipolar disorder, the patient has a history of a manic or hypomanic episode.

Labs

- Tox screen, complete blood count, comprehensive metabolic panel, creatine kinase.
- Consider brain imaging.

Treatment

Antidepressant plus antipsychotic

- Choice of combinations:
  - Sertraline plus olanzapine is the most well-studied combination, but any combination should work. Others that are well studied include fluoxetine plus olanzapine; venlafaxine plus quetiapine; and amitriptyline plus haloperidol.
  - Sertraline or escitalopram plus aripiprazole or lurasidone are less-studied combinations, but they will generally work well and cause fewer side effects.
- Dosing is higher than for unipolar depression:
  - Start sertraline 50 mg plus olanzapine 5 mg daily; gradually increase to a target dose of sertraline 150 mg and olanzapine 15 mg daily.
  - Similar protocol for other antidepressants (eg, increase to three or four times the initial starting dose).
- Try lithium augmentation for treatment-resistant patients (those who have not responded after four to eight weeks).

Electroconvulsive therapy (ECT)

- Can be first line for severe cases, such as patients who are persistently suicidal, completely nonfunctional, or experiencing significant weight loss or other medical complications due to their depression.
- ECT typically elicits a faster response compared to medication, with noticeable effects often observed within two to three weeks vs four to six weeks with meds.

How to Choose Medications for Major Depressive Disorder

Patients Who Have Never Tried Antidepressants

Best first-line antidepressants for most patients

- Sertraline (best combination of efficacy and tolerability).
- Escitalopram (similar in tolerability to sertraline; citalopram can also be used).
- Bupropion (best side effect profile, but less helpful for anxiety).

Choice based on symptom profile/comorbidities

- Comorbid anxiety disorder, bulimia, premenstrual dysphoric disorder: Selective serotonin reuptake inhibitors (SSRIs).
- Comorbid ADHD or tobacco use disorder, or prominent lethargy and poor concentration: Bupropion.
- Comorbid pain conditions such as fibromyalgia, chronic musculoskeletal pain, and diabetic neuropathy: Duloxetine or amitriptyline.
- Prominent insomnia and poor appetite: Mirtazapine.

Choice based on possible side effects

- For patients concerned about sexual side effects: Use bupropion, mirtazapine, or vilazodone.
- To avoid weight gain: Avoid paroxetine and mirtazapine and consider bupropion.
- To avoid drug interactions: Avoid paroxetine, fluvoxamine, and fluoxetine.
- To minimize seizure risk (eg, in patients with alcohol use disorder): Avoid bupropion.

Patients Who Have Tried Antidepressants

History of medication response

- If the patient clearly responded to an antidepressant in the past, try it again.
- If a patient reports that a close family member responded well to a particular antidepressant, it's reasonable to try that one.

History of nonresponse to an SSRI

- If the patient has tried and failed one SSRI, you can try a different SSRI.
- Optimize dose—increase to up to four times standard SSRI starting dose (eg, Zoloft 200 mg, Prozac 80 mg).
- Switch to another class (eg, from an SSRI to bupropion or duloxetine).

Patients Who Have Tried and Failed Numerous Antidepressants

- Trial a less popular antidepressant (eg, a monoamine oxidase inhibitor or a tricyclic).
- Trial a newer antidepressant (eg, vortioxetine), but make sure patients can financially access it after discharge.
- Augment with another medication—this is often convenient and can yield a fairly rapid response.
  - Second-generation antipsychotics:
    - Aripiprazole: 5–10 mg daily.
    - Lurasidone: 20–120 mg daily.
    - Quetiapine: 50–300 mg daily.
  - Lithium: Usually 300–600 mg at bedtime.
  - Benzodiazepines: Though potentially addictive, they help speed up antidepressant response in patients with anxiety and insomnia.
    - Clonazepam: 0.5–1 mg BID.
    - Lorazepam: 1–2 mg BID.
  - Bupropion: Add to SSRIs, especially in patients with lethargy.
  - Stimulants: Methylphenidate can quickly mobilize patients with poor energy and concentration; start at 5 mg and titrate upwards.
  - Mirtazapine: Helpful for patients with insomnia and poor appetite; use 15–30 mg at bedtime.
  - Thyroid: Start T3 (triiodothyronine, or Cytomel) at 12.5–25 mcg/day and increase gradually toward a dose of 50 mcg/day.

Prolonged Grief Disorder

Prolonged grief disorder (PGD), previously known as complicated grief, occurs when the normal process of grieving becomes extended and disabling. The risk is particularly high when the death of the loved one occurs unexpectedly or under traumatic circumstances. In severe cases, individuals may require hospitalization due to an inability to function or suicidal thoughts.

Evaluation

DSM-5-TR criteria for diagnosis

- *Duration:* Symptoms persist for at least 12 months after the death of a close relative or friend (for children and adolescents, at least six months).
- *Symptoms:*
  - Persistent longing for the deceased and/or constant preoccupation with thoughts of the deceased.
  - Plus at least three of the following:
    - Feeling like a part of oneself has died.
    - Difficulty accepting the reality of the death.
    - Avoiding places or activities that trigger memories of the deceased.
    - Intense emotional pain related to the death.
    - Struggling to reengage in relationships and activities after the death.
    - Feeling emotionally numb.
    - Believing that life is meaningless because of the loss.
    - Experiencing profound loneliness because of the death.

Assessment tools

Consider using a tool like the Prolonged Grief Disorder (PG-13) Scale (www.tinyurl.com/yhnvnryf) to assess the severity and symptoms of prolonged grief and to help guide treatment.

Management Strategies

Psychotherapy

- *Grief counseling:* Involves active listening, empathetic responses, and facilitating the expression of feelings. Encourage patients to talk about the deceased and share memories.
- *PGD therapy:* Typically a 16-week outpatient therapy course, but you can integrate key elements into inpatient care, focusing on helping the patient understand and accept their grief, manage their emotions, set and pursue future goals, strengthen relationships, and use imaginal revisiting to process the loss and live with reminders of the loved one.

Medication management

- *Antidepressants:* Consider selective serotonin reuptake inhibitors or serotonin/norepinephrine reuptake inhibitors for managing symptoms of depression.
- *Anxiolytics:* Short-term use can help patients with severe anxiety related to the grief.
- *Insomnia meds:* Sleep problems are common in patients experiencing prolonged grief.

Supportive interventions

- *Psychoeducation:* Educate on the grieving process and healthy coping strategies.
- *Social support:* Encourage participation in the unit's support groups. Refer patients to community grief support groups for ongoing help following discharge.
- *Mindfulness and relaxation techniques:* Teach mindfulness practices, deep breathing exercises, or progressive muscle relaxation to help manage stress and emotional pain.

Cultural considerations

- Tailor interventions to align with the patient's cultural background and preferences. These might include providing a quiet space for prayer or meditation, allowing the presence of cultural or religious items in the patient's room, or facilitating rituals that can be done in an inpatient setting, such as reading from sacred texts like the Bible, Quran, Bhagavad Gita, or Torah.
- Offer the option of visits from the hospital chaplain, who can provide spiritual and emotional support to all patients regardless of their beliefs.

Electroconvulsive Therapy (ECT)

ECT is one of the most effective treatments in psychiatry, and it's important to keep it in mind for a variety of inpatients—especially those with treatment-resistant depression and psychotic depression. In this fact sheet, we are assuming that you are not the one actually administering the ECT treatment, but rather that you will be referring your patient to an ECT program either in your hospital or elsewhere. Thus, our focus will be on discussing ECT with your patient, coordinating with the ECT consultant, and managing your patient in between ECT treatments.

FDA Indications

Treatment-resistant or **severe depression (either unipolar or bipolar); catatonia.**

Off-Label Uses

Psychotic depression; **severe schizophrenia;** suicidality; **neuroleptic malignant syndrome; acute mania.**

How to Decide Who Might Benefit

- *Depressed patients:* Patients with treatment-resistant depression are the main candidates. Do a careful history to ensure that they have already tried the major classes of antidepressants to no avail; collaborate with outpatient providers to obtain this information. Depression with psychotic features is especially sensitive to ECT, and patients with ruminative thought processes, especially if they are constantly thinking about suicide, are good candidates.
- *Elderly patients:* ECT is often particularly helpful for the elderly with severe depression because medications may cause unacceptable side effects in this population. Some evidence suggests elderly patients may respond slightly better than younger patients.
- *Catatonic patients:* While ECT is very effective for catatonia that doesn't respond to medications, it can be hard to obtain consent for the procedure in a catatonic patient. A health care proxy or court order may be necessary. However, if benzodiazepines are not working, ECT can be lifesaving, and response rates are very high.

How to Broach the Topic of ECT with Patients

- *Introduce the concept:* "I'd like to chat about another treatment option for patients like you who haven't responded to medications or therapy. It's called electroconvulsive therapy, or ECT. Have you heard of it?"
- *Address myths and misconceptions, if the patient refers to them:* "Some people have heard scary things about ECT from movies like *One Flew Over the Cuckoo's Nest,* but modern ECT is very different—more refined and more scientific. It's actually considered to be the most effective treatment in all of psychiatry."
- *Describe the procedure:* "During ECT, you'll be under anesthesia, so you won't feel or remember the procedure. We place electrodes on one side of your head (which is called unilateral) or on both sides (which is called bilateral) and deliver a brief electric current lasting just a few seconds. This causes a short, therapeutic seizure. The whole process, including waking up from anesthesia, takes about an hour, and then you'll be brought back up to the unit. We usually do the treatments three mornings a week for three or four weeks, depending on the response. If you do very well, a taper or maintenance treatment might be suggested for a period of time to try to solidify the response and prevent relapse."
- *Describe potential side effects:* "Most people have some mild side effects, like headache or jaw pain. The biggest concern patients have is about memory loss. It is common to be more forgetful during the course of ECT, but this effect usually clears up within a couple weeks after the end of treatment. Sometimes, a few weeks after ECT is done, your memory might actually be better than before the ECT if your depression has improved. However, some patients are left with some gaps in their memory. Usually, the events closest to the course of ECT are most at risk, but rarely older memories can be lost. Sometimes these come back with time or prompting. And you'll be in charge every step of the way—if you want to stop the treatments at any time, you can do so."
- *Encourage questions:* "I know this is a lot to take in—let me know if you have any questions. If you want to proceed, we'll have our ECT specialist come up and do an evaluation to make sure it's the right treatment for you."

Working with the ECT Consultant

- In most inpatient settings, you will request consultation for ECT, and an ECT specialist will come to do a formal evaluation, order any necessary medical workup (or ask you to do that), and have the patient sign an informed consent.
- Since ECT specialists are in short supply and very busy, you want to make sure that your referral is appropriate. In your referral note, document the evidence for treatment resistance, including a list of medication failures. Document the severity of the symptoms and indicate why you think this patient is a good candidate. If your patient has a personality disorder, acknowledge that. There is controversy in the ECT field regarding efficacy of the treatment for patients with borderline or narcissistic personality disorder. Highlight any significant medical concerns, as they may need to be better studied or evaluated before treatment.

Pre-ECT Workup

No specific labs are required for all patients, but depending on the patient, the consultant may ask for specific procedures. This will typically include a medical consultation, and possibly labs and an ECG.

Medication adjustments related to ECT

If the patient is taking benzodiazepines or anticonvulsants, collaborate with the consultant on how to manage these medications as they can elevate the seizure threshold, rendering the ECT procedure ineffective. Often the recommendation will be to hold these medications (or lower the dose) on the night before the ECT treatment.

Managing ECT Patients on the Inpatient Unit

- ECT is typically done early in the morning, three days per week. Orders may include some or all of the following:
  - Medication holds or reductions the night before and the morning of the procedure.
  - NPO (nothing by mouth) after midnight.
  - Transfer to ECT suite.
- When patients return from ECT treatments, they will often have side effects such as grogginess, head or jaw pain, and transient memory loss. Order PRN medications like Tylenol.
- Care between treatments:
  - Evaluate symptoms of depression daily, either with a formal symptom scale or by simply asking patients to rate their depression on a scale of 1 to 10. Response usually begins after three to six treatments (one to two weeks), and patients receive seven to 10 treatments on average.
  - Ask about side effects and attend closely to them, as some patients may prematurely drop out of treatment not knowing that side effects are transient and treatable.
  - All psychiatric medications may be continued during ECT. Lithium doses may need to be decreased to minimize cognitive side effects, and benzodiazepines and anticonvulsants may need to be withheld the night before treatment—work closely with the ECT consultant on these decisions.
- After discharge, ECT may be continued on a maintenance basis (typically, patients will have weekly ECT for two to four weeks, then taper down to monthly or as required based on symptoms). Maintenance ECT lasts six months or more, depending on response and side effects.

Transcranial Magnetic Stimulation (TMS)

TMS is a noninvasive neuromodulation technique primarily used to treat major depressive disorder. Although it's mostly available on an outpatient basis, you might see it increasingly being offered in hospital psychiatric units. Patients often prefer TMS over electroconvulsive therapy (ECT) because it's noninvasive, there's no need for anesthesia, and it generally has fewer side effects. However, for some, it may be less efficacious than ECT.

How TMS Works

TMS uses a device that generates magnetic pulses, which are delivered through a coil placed on the patient's scalp. These pulses induce electrical currents in the brain tissue, particularly the dorsolateral prefrontal cortex, which is implicated in mood regulation. Each session lasts 20–30 minutes, and TMS is typically conducted five days a week over several weeks.

Side Effects

TMS is well tolerated, but common side effects include headaches, scalp discomfort, and nausea.

Effectiveness

Rates of response and remission vary widely across studies, with response rates of approximately 25%–65% and remission rates of 14%–37%. Some patients experience significant improvements with TMS, and considering how well tolerated it is, it might be worth trying in cases of treatment-refractory depression.

Insurance

Insurance coverage for TMS varies. Many insurance plans require documentation that the patient has not responded to multiple antidepressants and has tried other forms of treatment augmentation. Without insurance coverage, TMS is expensive at $200–$500 per session (and remember, a course of treatment typically consists of 20–30 sessions).

When to Recommend It

Consider TMS for patients who haven't found sufficient relief from depressive symptoms with traditional treatments like medication and psychotherapy. It's also a viable option for those who experience intolerable side effects from medications. For patients with obsessive-compulsive disorder, TMS can be a next step when first-line treatments are ineffective. Some studies suggest that it is also helpful for conditions like generalized anxiety disorder and PTSD, but these uses are still under investigation.

How to Discuss TMS with Patients

Begin by explaining that TMS is a noninvasive procedure that uses magnetic pulses to stimulate areas of the brain involved in mood regulation. Reassure patients that TMS is generally well tolerated and that no anesthesia is required. Outline the typical course of treatment, which usually involves daily sessions over several weeks, and set realistic expectations about the variability in response and remission rates. Make sure to also inform patients about potential costs and insurance coverage.

How to Manage Patients Who Were Receiving TMS Outpatient

For hospitalized patients who were receiving TMS prior to admission, obtain records of their treatment history, including the number of sessions completed, the frequency of treatment, and the patient's response. This information will help you decide whether to continue TMS during the hospital stay or to adjust the patient's treatment plan.

If TMS cannot be administered on the inpatient unit, monitor the patient closely for changes in their condition, particularly any exacerbation of symptoms due to the interruption of TMS. Also, communicate with the patient's outpatient TMS provider to plan for the potential resumption of TMS after discharge if the patient's condition has not sufficiently improved with inpatient treatment.

COMMON PSYCHIATRIC CONDITIONS

Developmental and Intellectual Disabilities

Intellectual Disabilities: Management in Inpatient Psychiatry

Patients with intellectual disabilities (ID) may be admitted to adult inpatient units for a range of issues, often related to self-harm or impulsive violence toward caregivers. This fact sheet offers a concise review of ID and provides guidelines for patient management in an adult inpatient unit.

DSM-5 Criteria

ID was formerly known by the stigmatizing term "mental retardation" and is characterized by significant limitations in both intellectual functioning and adaptive behavior, which manifest during the developmental period. The diagnosis is based on:

- *Intellectual impairment:* Measured through standardized IQ testing, typically an IQ score of 70 or lower. An IQ of 70 is two standard deviations below the mean IQ of 100—meaning that these individuals are in the lowest 2.3% of the population. Mild ID is defined as an IQ of 55–70, moderate is 40–55, severe is 25–40, and profound is below 25. A related term is "borderline intellectual functioning," defined as an IQ of 71–84.
- *Adaptive functioning deficit:* To meet the criteria, the intellectual impairment must interfere with functioning, such as the ability to graduate high school, maintain a job, or have significant social skills.

Psychiatric/Behavioral Issues

The most common comorbidities that bring ID patients into the inpatient unit are depressive disorders, anxiety disorders, autism, impulse control disorders, conduct disorders, and schizophrenia. Behavioral issues that you may have to manage include:

- *Aggression:* May include hitting, biting, or throwing objects; yelling, threats, or use of offensive language.
- *Self-injury:* Such as hitting oneself, head-banging, or biting oneself.
- *Hyperactivity:* Difficulty sitting still, running around the unit, or continuously talking.
- *Inappropriate social interactions:* Such as invading personal space, inappropriate touching, or making socially inappropriate comments.
- *Isolation:* Difficulty in forming connections, leading to withdrawal from social interactions.
- *Emotional dysregulation:* Rapid and unpredictable changes between emotional states such as happiness, irritability, and sadness.
- *Overreaction to stimuli:* Extreme reactions to sounds, lights, or textures, which can cause distress or disruptive behavior.
- *Rigidity:* Difficulty adapting to new routines or changes in the environment, leading to stress or agitation.

Initial Assessment

Validate the diagnosis through a thorough review of prior medical records and discussions with caregivers or family members. In interview, ID patients may present with slow speech; simple vocabulary; inability to understand complex language or follow your train of thought if you are speaking fast; or inability to process complex thoughts.

Interviewing ID Patients

- *Keep language simple:* Use clear and straightforward language. Avoid medical jargon or complex phrases.
- *Repeat and rephrase:* It might be necessary to repeat questions or rephrase them if the patient appears confused or nonresponsive.
- *Employ visual aids:* Use pictures, or demonstrate with body language, to support verbal communication.
- *Allow time:* Some ID patients may require more time to process information and respond. Do not rush them.

Teaching Coping Skills

- *Deep breathing:* Teach the basics of deep breathing by counting breaths, using visual cues, or incorporating tactile objects like a soft ball that they can squeeze and release.
- *Grounding techniques:* Use the "5-4-3-2-1" method or similar techniques to help ground them in the present moment. Adapt the method by utilizing textures or objects that the patient finds comforting or engaging.
- *Positive self-talk:* Introduce simple affirmations or comforting phrases that the patient can repeat to themselves.

Medication

Medications can be crucial to target specific symptoms and behaviors.

- Agitation/self-harm/aggression:
  - Mood stabilizers, such as lithium and valproic acid (Depakote).
  - Antipsychotics such as risperidone and aripiprazole.
- Depression/anxiety:
  - Selective serotonin reuptake inhibitors (SSRIs).
  - Benzodiazepines.
- ADHD symptoms (especially hyperactive/impulsivity):
  - Psychostimulants.
  - Alpha-2 agonists (eg, clonidine).

ADHD in Adults

Adult ADHD can become a contentious issue on the inpatient unit, primarily because the treatment of choice, psychostimulants, is a substance of abuse for some people. Some units have a blanket policy of not prescribing stimulants; in other cases, specific doctors decide to withhold stimulants as part of their own practice. There are rationales for both continuing and discontinuing these medications.

The Case for Continuing Stimulants

- Discontinuing stimulants will often cause a mild withdrawal syndrome of fatigue and depression, both of which can exacerbate the presenting psychiatric disorder.
- Patients who have severe inattention symptoms will concentrate poorly when they are off stimulants, and this will diminish their ability to benefit from therapeutic programs.
- Discontinuing stimulants implicitly communicates a mistrust of the outpatient prescriber's judgment.

The Case for Discontinuing Stimulants

- Stimulants are likely to destabilize major psychiatric syndromes that led to admission, such as bipolar disorder, psychosis, or agitation.
- Since ADHD is easily malingered, patients may claim they have ADHD just to receive a stimulant prescription and get high while they are admitted.

Recommended Approach

- Attempt to establish the diagnosis.
  - Recall that the key points for an adult ADHD diagnosis are:
    - Initial onset of symptoms by age 12.
    - Symptoms include either or both of the following two categories:
      - Inattentiveness and disorganization (eg, easily distracted, can't finish projects, can't concentrate on tasks).
      - Impulsivity and hyperactivity (eg, can't keep still, talks impulsively, makes rash decisions).
  - You can ask about these symptoms in a reliable patient—but inpatients often have comorbid conditions, such as psychosis, bipolar disorder, or substance use disorder, that make it hard to establish a valid diagnosis based on interview. Contact collaterals, such as outpatient providers and family members or significant others, who have known the patient for years and can usually provide more reliable information.
- Keep an open mind on prescribing stimulants—but don't be a pushover either.
  - If the outpatient provider has consistently prescribed stimulants, you should generally continue the same medication at the same dose during the inpatient stay. Exceptions to this rule include the following:
    - The symptoms prompting admission may have been worsened by stimulants (eg, psychosis, agitation, anxiety, mania).
    - There are clear signs of substance use disorder, either by history or by results of urine drug screening.
  - If the patient is requesting stimulants but there is no track record of an outpatient ADHD diagnosis or consistent refills of stimulants, we don't generally recommend starting them. Instead, offer a nonaddictive alternative, such as atomoxetine or bupropion. Some patients will get angry or irritated, insisting that stimulants are the only things that really help them. Here are some ways to respond to this:
    - "Diagnosing ADHD is difficult, and the best way to do it is in the outpatient setting where your doctor can do a full evaluation that may take several appointments. We can't do that here on the inpatient unit."
    - "Stimulants can be helpful, but they are also highly addictive—for that reason, we don't prescribe them unless we can talk to an outpatient prescriber who can assure us that you have the diagnosis and that you have used these meds responsibly."

Autism Spectrum Disorder

Patients with autism spectrum disorder (ASD) may be admitted to inpatient units for a variety of reasons. Sometimes the admission is due primarily to the ASD syndrome and related irritability and behavioral issues. Other times, the main problem is a comorbid condition, such as depression, bipolar disorder, or psychotic disorder, with the ASD being a contributing factor. Either way, ASD patients can be challenging, and this fact sheet will remind you of the basic features of ASD as well as some helpful treatment measures to implement.

DSM-5 Criteria

ASD is a neurodevelopmental disorder that typically begins in childhood and is diagnosed on a spectrum from mild (formerly termed "Asperger's syndrome") to severe. To meet the diagnostic criteria for ASD, patients must exhibit both social communication deficits and repetitive behaviors or interests. Here are key features of these two criteria.

Social communication and interaction deficits

- Social unawareness, poor socialization skills, or inability to respond appropriately to emotional cues.
- Atypical eye contact, ranging from poor to too intense and unchanging.
- Challenges in understanding social cues, conversational norms like small talk, and jokes.
- Difficulty interpreting others' emotions or viewpoints.

Restrictive, repetitive behaviors, interests, and activities

- Manifestations (rocking, flapping, twirling) when excited/anxious.
- Low tolerance to change or disruption in routine.
- Perseverative thinking.
- Intense, narrow interests.

Initial Assessment

Confirm the diagnosis

With recent publicity around the increased prevalence of ASD, people tend to throw around vague terms and say things like, "He's on the spectrum," "She's a little Aspy," "He's neuroatypical," and so on. Confirm the ASD diagnosis via a combination of interviewing the patient and gathering collateral information, eg, from family members or staff at group homes. You might find it helpful to use a screening tool like the Autism Spectrum Quotient (www.tinyurl.com/4wk5r8e8).

On interview, you may note the following:

- Eye contact anomalies: Avoidance, intense gaze, or gazing at areas other than your eyes.
- Language abnormalities: Unusual volume, pace, or monotonal speech.
- Intense, specific interests, especially in mechanical or scientific topics.

Assess for comorbid disorders

Common comorbidities include depression, anxiety, ADHD, and insomnia.

Environmental Modifications

- Predictable, structured environments can be helpful. Try to establish a routine, including mealtimes, activity times, and bedtimes.
- Noise, crowding, and so on can exacerbate irritability. If possible, provide a quiet and less stimulating environment.

Behavioral/Therapeutic Interventions

- Use positive reinforcement techniques to encourage appropriate behavior.
- Form a crisis intervention plan including de-escalation techniques and, if needed, safe physical restraint methods.
- For some adults with ASD, irritability can be reduced through brief cognitive behavioral therapy techniques targeting emotional regulation and stress management.

Medication

There are no medications for the core deficits of autism, but various medications can help with specific symptoms and comorbidities.

- Risperidone and aripiprazole are FDA approved for irritability in ASD (specifically for children), though other antipsychotics likely work too. Mood stabilizers (eg, gabapentin, oxcarbazepine, valproate, topiramate) are also options.
- SSRIs (or benzodiazepines) are helpful for anxiety, depression, obsessive-compulsive disorder, and repetitive behaviors.
- Methylphenidate or amphetamine salt stimulants work for ADHD symptoms in autism. Also try guanfacine or clonidine.
- Valerian, omega-3 fatty acids, melatonin, and lavender have been used, with varying success, for ASD-related symptoms.

Aftercare Planning

Before discharge, collaborate with the group home staff and family to prepare an aftercare plan that includes outpatient follow-up and any necessary adjustments to the living environment.

COMMON PSYCHIATRIC CONDITIONS

Eating Disorders

Anorexia Nervosa

Patients with anorexia nervosa often present with severe physical and mental health challenges that require coordinated care from an interdisciplinary team. Your role will involve diagnosing comorbid conditions, managing psychiatric symptoms, and collaborating with other health care professionals to support the patient's weight restoration and overall recovery.

Diagnostic Criteria

- Restriction of caloric intake relative to requirements, leading to a significantly low body weight for age and sex. While there is no specific weight cutoff, a BMI of <18.5 kg/m^2 is often used.
- Intense fear of gaining weight or becoming fat.
- Disturbance in the way one's body weight or shape is experienced.
- Specify one of the following subtypes:
  - *Restricting type:* During the last three months, the individual has not engaged in recurrent episodes of binge eating or purging behavior.
  - *Binge eating/purging type:* During the last three months, the individual has engaged in recurrent episodes of binge eating or purging (seen in up to 50% of anorexia patients).

Initial Assessment

- *Psychiatric:* In addition to confirming the diagnosis of anorexia, ask about common comorbidities such as major depression, anxiety disorders (especially obsessive-compulsive disorder), substance use disorder, and borderline personality disorder.
- *Medical:* Request a medical consult for a comprehensive history and physical. Typical symptoms related to extreme weight loss and its complications include fatigue, postural lightheadedness, palpitations, amenorrhea (in female patients), cold intolerance, hair loss, and bone fractures. Vital signs may show hypotension, bradycardia, and hypothermia, and fluid restriction can cause orthostasis. Labs should include electrolytes, fasting glucose, liver function, and complete blood count. Hypokalemia and hypomagnesemia are common in patients who purge and can lead to arrhythmia. Get an ECG if electrolytes are abnormal.

Interdisciplinary Treatment Protocol

Inpatient treatment of anorexia aims to restore your patient's body weight to a BMI range that is closer to normal.

- *Nutrition and weight restoration:* Request a nutrition or dietetics consult. A hospital nutritionist will recommend a diet plan for gradual weight restoration. In severe cases, you may have to initiate forced refeeding (see the "Forced Refeeding in Anorexia Nervosa" fact sheet in this subsection).
- *Meal supervision:* All meals and snacks are supervised by staff to ensure adherence to the meal plan. Patients may progress to more independence during the hospitalization.
- *Post-meal supervision:* Since many patients with anorexia purge following meals of any size, the usual protocol is to require supervision for one hour following meals so that they do not purge in private areas, such as their rooms or bathrooms.
- *Medical monitoring:* This will generally be overseen by the hospitalist and may include ECG, labs, vitals, and weights to monitor for refeeding syndrome and other medical stabilization. Inspect patients' pockets for objects they might have concealed to give the impression of a heavier weight.
- *Individual psychotherapy:* Cognitive behavioral therapy is often used, especially in short-term treatment settings. Its primary objectives are to identify disordered thoughts and behaviors related to food and weight, and to recognize and sidestep triggers that lead to restrictive eating, binging, or purging.
- *Family therapy:* Family-based treatment of anorexia is an evidence-based approach to weight restoration. Rather than focusing on addressing underlying family dynamics, this technique encourages parents to take a primary role in ensuring that their children eat adequate portions—eg, the parents actively supervise meals to ensure the child doesn't skip them or purge afterward.
- *Group therapy:* This can include support groups, psychoeducation groups, and mindfulness groups.
- *Aftercare planning:* Patients should have a transition plan for continued treatment after discharge, including outpatient counseling, nutrition plans, psychiatrist follow-up, and so on.
- *Pharmacotherapy:* Psychiatric medications are sometimes helpful for weight restoration and may improve comorbid psychiatric symptoms.
  - *Antipsychotics:* Olanzapine (typically dosed 2.5–10 mg daily) produces a modest amount of weight gain (around five pounds more than placebo over the course of a several-week inpatient admission) as well as reducing agitation and obsessional thinking (Han R et al, *Brain Behav* 2022;12(2):e2498). There's less evidence for other antipsychotics.
  - *Antidepressants:* Fluoxetine and other selective serotonin reuptake inhibitors help reduce depression and anxiety symptoms associated with anorexia—but they don't significantly impact weight gain. Mirtazapine (Remeron,

15–45 mg at bedtime) has the benefit of also stimulating appetite and improving sleep. Avoid bupropion and tricyclic antidepressants due to risks of seizures and arrhythmias, respectively.

- *Other options:* Several medications and supplements have limited and mixed data but are worth trying as second- or third-line agents.
  - Cyproheptadine is an antihistamine that has a similar pharmacological profile as mirtazapine and may improve weight gain and depressive symptoms in anorexia (target dose 8 mg QID, starting at 2 mg TID and titrated over three weeks).
  - Dronabinol is a synthetic cannabinoid that is FDA approved for weight loss in HIV/AIDS. Preliminary evidence suggests potential benefit for anorexia (2.5 mg twice a day).
  - Zinc levels are often low in anorexic patients. Supplementation with zinc gluconate 100 mg daily has been found to increase BMI.

Forced Refeeding in Anorexia Nervosa

Severe anorexia can lead to life-threatening complications. If you are not able to convince your patient to eat voluntarily, you may have to initiate forced refeeding.

Criteria for Forced Refeeding

- Presence of life-threatening electrolyte imbalances.
- Continuous weight loss despite therapeutic interventions, usually with a BMI <15 kg/m^2.

Legal Considerations Before Forced Refeeding

- *Capacity assessment:* You must confirm the patient's incapacity to make health decisions. Often anorexic patients will seemingly have the capacity to think logically but may be in denial that their condition is life-threatening (see the "How to Evaluate Capacity to Make Decisions" fact sheet in the Legal and Ethical Considerations section).
- *Health care proxy (HCP):* An HCP is a legal method granting someone else the ability to make medical decisions for the patient. Activating an HCP requires that you document your reasons for believing the patient lacks decision-making capacity (see the "Health Care Proxy and Power of Attorney" fact sheet in the Legal and Ethical Considerations section).
- *Guardianship:* If no HCP is present, guardianship might be initiated. Rapid emergency guardianship is available in urgent scenarios.
- *Ethics or medical review committee:* In the absence of an HCP or a guardian, hospitals can convene an ethics committee meeting to authorize emergency medical decision making.

Forced Refeeding Methods and Criteria

There are two options for forced refeeding: parenteral (via an IV line) and enteral (tube feeding directly into the GI tract). Enteral is the method of choice because there are fewer complications, but some patients will allow only parenteral feeding. Feeding method may be continuous or boluses, based on clinical goals and preferences.

- *Parenteral nutrition (or total parenteral nutrition [TPN]):* Nutrition is directly infused into the bloodstream, bypassing digestion. Risks include potential refeeding syndrome with swift weight gain and infections due to catheter.
- *Tube feeding:* A method that introduces food directly into the digestive system using tubes.
  - *Nasogastric tube (NG tube):* This is the most common refeeding procedure. A flexible tube is inserted through the nostril, down the esophagus, and into the stomach. It's used for short-term feeding, typically less than six weeks. The placement is generally straightforward and can be done at the bedside, but there's a risk of accidental placement in the lungs, which can cause complications.
  - *Gastrostomy tube (G or PEG tube):* A tube is inserted directly into the stomach through the abdominal wall. It's used for longer-term feeding (more than six weeks). Placement requires a surgical or endoscopic procedure but offers a more stable and long-term solution.
  - *Jejunostomy tube (J tube):* A tube is inserted into the small intestine. This method is suitable for those intolerant to stomach feedings.

Potential Complications of Nutritional Rehabilitation

- *Refeeding syndrome:* A rare but serious metabolic disturbance that is caused by electrolyte shifts, particularly in phosphate, and can lead to complications like cardiac failure, especially in those with a BMI <16 kg/m^2. It arises from aggressive nutritional replenishment, causing an abrupt switch from fat to carbohydrate metabolism, which leads to a rapid decline in electrolytes. Management/prevention: Begin refeeding gradually, monitor electrolytes regularly, and ensure thiamine supplementation. Restrict initial fluid intake. Monitor for symptoms like heart arrhythmias.
- *Refeeding edema:* Swelling observed during the refeeding process. Triggers include insulin's influence on sodium retention and possible hypoalbuminemia. Management strategies involve bed rest, leg elevation, and low-sodium diets. In extreme scenarios, diuretics such as furosemide are administered with caution.
- *Constipation:* A common side effect owing to decreased gastric motility as weight is regained. It typically resolves as oral intake continues.

Bulimia Nervosa

Patients with bulimia nervosa often present with complex challenges, including the cycle of binge eating and purging, as well as associated medical complications. The goal in the inpatient setting involves not only breaking the binge-purge cycle but also addressing the underlying psychological issues and preparing the patient for sustained recovery. This fact sheet outlines the essential steps in assessing and treating bulimia nervosa in an inpatient setting.

DSM-5 Diagnostic Criteria

- Recurrent episodes of binge eating.
- Recurrent inappropriate compensatory behaviors to prevent weight gain, such as vomiting, excessive exercise, fasting, or misuse of laxatives.
- Both of the above behaviors occur, on average, at least once a week for three months.
- Self-evaluation is unduly influenced by body shape and weight.
- The disturbance does not exclusively occur during episodes of anorexia nervosa.

Initial Assessment

- *Psychiatric:* Along with confirming the diagnosis of bulimia, inquire about comorbidities like depression, anxiety disorders, substance use disorders, and borderline personality disorder.
- *Medical:* Symptoms related to regular purging include electrolyte imbalances, dental erosion, and GI issues. Labs should evaluate electrolytes, kidney function, and liver enzymes. Hypokalemia is common, especially in patients who induce vomiting, leading to cardiac issues. An ECG is recommended if electrolyte abnormalities are detected.

Interdisciplinary Treatment Protocol

Inpatient treatment of bulimia aims to stop the binge-purge cycle and address the patient's underlying psychological issues.

- *Nutritional counseling:* Counseling is an essential aspect of treatment. The goal is not to restore weight, but to establish regular eating patterns without binging and purging.
- *Meal and post-meal supervision:* Supervised meals prevent binge episodes, and post-meal monitoring (typically for one to two hours) helps ensure no purging behaviors.
- *Medical monitoring:* This can include monitoring vitals, electrolytes, and any other medical concerns, typically overseen by a medical professional.
- *Individual psychotherapy:* Cognitive behavioral therapy is the primary evidence-based treatment for bulimia. Goals include recognizing and altering distorted thought patterns and behaviors related to eating.
- *Group therapy:* This can offer support, psychoeducation, and skills training.
- *Aftercare planning:* Having a plan for care following discharge is essential for maintaining recovery. This includes outpatient therapy, dietary guidance, and medical monitoring.
- *Pharmacotherapy:* Unlike anorexia, medications play a central role in treating bulimia.
  - First line: Selective serotonin reuptake inhibitor (SSRI) antidepressants have been approved for bulimia treatment. They can help reduce the frequency of binge-purge episodes and improve mood. Fluoxetine (Prozac) is the first-line agent, starting at 20 mg daily, with a target dose of 60 mg daily. Other SSRIs are also effective, and the target dose is higher than the usual antidepressant dose (eg, sertraline 150 mg daily, escitalopram 30 mg daily). Avoid paroxetine due to the risk of weight gain. Avoid citalopram due to the risk of QT prolongation.
  - Second line: Tricyclics (especially desipramine), topiramate, trazodone, monoamine oxidase inhibitors.
  - Avoid bupropion in bulimia due to an increased risk of seizure.

COMMON PSYCHIATRIC CONDITIONS

Insomnia

Sleep Disturbances in Inpatient Psychiatry

For patients in hospital psychiatric units, sleep disturbances are not uncommon. They may arise due to underlying psychiatric conditions or from external factors within the hospital setting. Proper diagnosis and management are critical to enhance the well-being and recovery of these patients.

Differential Diagnosis

- *Psychiatric:* Acute mania, psychosis, anxiety, depression, PTSD.
- *Medical:* Obstructive sleep apnea, restless legs syndrome, menopausal hot flashes/night sweats.
- *Additional considerations:*
  - Medication side effects (eg, from stimulants, antidepressants, or diuretics); antipsychotic-induced extrapyramidal symptoms like akathisia.
  - Environmental factors (eg, adjusting to a new environment, uncomfortable hospital beds, disturbances from other patients, being awakened by 15-minute checks).
  - Frequent daytime napping.

General Approach to Managing Insomnia

- Manage the underlying cause if you identify one. This can significantly improve sleep quality.
- Employ medication adjustments, behavioral interventions, environmental adjustments, or medical team referrals.
- For patients who nap a lot during the day, encourage them to remain active and participate in unit activities.

Sleep hygiene enhancements

- Create a consistent sleep schedule with calming bedtime rituals.
- Avoid caffeine in the afternoon or evening.
- Avoid large meals two to three hours before bedtime.
- Engage in physical activity during the day—just not immediately before bedtime.
- Minimize blue light exposure from devices one to two hours before bedtime.
- Work with unit staff to create a sleeping environment that is as comfortable and quiet as possible.

Cognitive behavioral therapy for insomnia (CBT-I)

CBT-I is an effective strategy even within the context of a psychiatric hospital. If a trained CBT-I practitioner is available, consider a referral. Otherwise, introduce the following basic techniques:

- Restrict bedtime to match the patient's actual sleep duration.
- Challenge and redirect negative sleep beliefs (eg, "This is terrible! If I can't sleep, I'll be completely nonfunctional tomorrow and my day will be totally wasted!").
- Encourage using the bed only for sleep; discourage activities like reading or watching TV in bed.
- Introduce relaxation techniques, such as deep breathing and progressive muscle relaxation.

Medications

- Consider when CBT-I is ineffective or inaccessible.
- Use on a short-term basis due to risks of daytime drowsiness and dependency, especially considering the already-complex medication regimens of many psychiatric patients.
- Watch for risk of drug interactions or exacerbation of psychiatric symptoms (eg, depression or confusion induced by sedative-hypnotics).
- Refer to the "Insomnia: Medication Management" fact sheet in this subsection for detailed guidance.

Insomnia: Medication Management

We have many insomnia medications to choose from—some FDA approved for this indication, others not. In inpatient psychiatry, theoretically we would solve insomnia issues by simply treating the underlying psychiatric disorder, but in the real world that doesn't always work. In this fact sheet, we lay out a long list of meds we typically consider, along with tips on how to choose among them.

Medication for Insomnia

Everything listed here is taken at bedtime except when otherwise noted.

- Benzodiazepine receptor agonists (BZRAs):
  - Eszopiclone (Lunesta): 1–3 mg.
  - Zaleplon (Sonata): 5–20 mg, can also be taken for middle-of-the-night awakenings.
  - Zolpidem (Ambien): 5–10 mg for men, 5 mg for women.
  - Zolpidem CR (Ambien CR): 6.25–12.5 mg.
  - Zolpidem SL (Intermezzo): 1.75–3.5 mg, taken for middle-of-the-night awakenings.
- Melatonin receptor agonists:
  - Ramelteon (Rozerem): 8 mg.
- Antidepressants:
  - Doxepin (Silenor): 3–6 mg.
  - Mirtazapine (Remeron): 7.5–15 mg.
  - Trazodone (Desyrel): 25–100 mg (off-label use).
- Antihistamines:
  - Diphenhydramine (Benadryl): 25–50 mg.
  - Doxylamine (Unisom): 12.5–25 mg.
- Antipsychotics:
  - Quetiapine: 25–100 mg (off-label use).
- Dual orexin receptor antagonists (DORAs):
  - Daridorexant (Quviviq): 25–50 mg.
  - Lemborexant (Dayvigo): 5–10 mg.
  - Suvorexant (Belsomra): 5–20 mg.
- Benzodiazepines:
  - Clonazepam (Klonopin): 0.5–1 mg.
  - Lorazepam (Ativan): 0.5–1 mg.
  - Temazepam (Restoril): 7.5–15 mg.
- Alpha-agonists:
  - Clonidine: 0.1–0.3 mg.
  - Prazosin: 1–5 mg.
- Over-the-counter options:
  - Melatonin: 1–5 mg.

Choosing a Medication for Insomnia

- *Sleep-onset insomnia:* Doxepin, ramelteon, trazodone, antihistamines, melatonin, BZRAs, DORAs.
- *Middle-of-the-night awakenings:* Zolpidem SL, zaleplon, doxepin.
- *Elderly patients:* Ramelteon, melatonin, trazodone, DORAs. Avoid antihistamines due to anticholinergic effects.
- *Patients with substance use disorders:* Avoid BZRAs and benzodiazepines.
- *Comorbid depression:* Trazodone, ramelteon, antihistamines. Be cautious with doxepin, BZRAs, and benzodiazepines due to overdose risk. Avoid DORAs due to links with new-onset suicidal thoughts.
- *Comorbid schizophrenia spectrum or mood disorders:* Quetiapine is often used, although other options (trazodone, antihistamines, ramelteon, melatonin) carry less risk for effects such as weight gain and metabolic syndrome.
- *Comorbid anxiety disorders:* Benzodiazepines, antidepressants.
- *Respiratory issues (eg, chronic obstructive pulmonary disease):* Ramelteon, trazodone, doxepin, melatonin.
- *Pregnant patients:* Diphenhydramine appears safe.
- *Budget constraints:* DORAs tend to be more expensive.

COMMON PSYCHIATRIC CONDITIONS

Neurocognitive Disorders

Major Neurocognitive Disorder: Evaluation

In this fact sheet, we outline the basic DSM-5 criteria for diagnosing major neurocognitive disorder (MND) and review the characteristics of the various subtypes of dementia. We also discuss our clinical approach for assessing and treating dementia.

DSM-5 Differential Diagnosis

DSM-5 criteria

Diagnosing MND requires establishing significant decline in at least one of the following neurocognitive domains:

- *Learning and memory:* Difficulty recalling events or information, especially acquiring and retrieving new information.
- *Complex attention:* Reduced ability to sustain focus, filter distractions, and manipulate information; reduced processing speed.
- *Social cognition:* Difficulty reading social cues and behaving appropriately; sometimes called "personality changes."
- *Perceptual-motor skills:* Difficulty interpreting visual information, impaired ability to coordinate movements, apraxia.
- *Language skills:* Deficits in speaking, comprehending spoken or written language, reading, or writing (eg, various forms of aphasia).
- *Executive functions:* Challenges with planning, organizing, initiating, and executing tasks; problems with reasoning and judgment.

Subtypes of MND: Recognizing the patterns

While it is useful to understand the subtypes of dementia, keep in mind that the majority of patients with MND have "mixed dementia," which is usually a combination of Alzheimer's and vascular dementia.

- Alzheimer's disease:
  - *Prevalence*: 70%–80% of dementias; affects about 10% of people over 65.
  - *DSM criteria*: Gradual and steady decline, with the key symptoms being memory impairment.
  - *Diagnostic tips:* Generalized cerebral atrophy on MRI; amyloid-beta deposits on PET scans.
  - *Treatment tips*: Start with cholinesterase inhibitors.
- Vascular neurocognitive disorder:
  - *Prevalence*: 10%–15% of dementias.
  - *DSM criteria*: Symptoms of dementia plus neurological signs/symptoms of cerebral vascular problems, such as strokes or blood vessel abnormalities.
  - *Diagnostic tips*: Symptoms correlate temporally with vascular events. An MRI typically reveals evidence of infarcts or white matter ischemic lesions. Suspect in dementia patients with hypertension, diabetes, or high cholesterol.
  - *Treatment tips*: In addition to standard dementia meds, encourage comprehensive treatment of hypertension and atherosclerosis.
- Frontotemporal dementia:
  - *Prevalence*: 5%–10% of dementias; more common in men.
  - *DSM criteria*: Gradual decline in social functioning and appropriate behavior in the absence of significant memory impairment.
  - *Diagnostic tips*: Patients exhibit major "personality changes" such as becoming abruptly angry, making inappropriate jokes, or other examples of behavioral disinhibition. MRI usually reveals atrophy in the frontal and temporal lobes.
  - *Treatment tips:* Consider selective serotonin reuptake inhibitors to curb impulsivity, as well as low-dose quetiapine.
- Dementia with Lewy bodies:
  - *Prevalence*: About 5% of dementias.
  - *DSM criteria*: At least two of the following: Fluctuating cognition, recurrent visual hallucinations, parkinsonian features (eg, bradykinesia, rigidity, resting tremor).
  - *Diagnostic tips:* REM sleep behavior disorder may occur; severe side effects on neuroleptics is a clue; cognitive impairment occurs before parkinsonism (as opposed to Parkinson's disease, in which motor symptoms occur before cognitive symptoms).
  - *Treatment tips*: Consider pimavanserin or low-dose quetiapine or clozapine for psychosis.

Clinical Evaluation of Dementia

Although DSM-5 lists a variety of cognitive functions that can be impaired in dementia, by far the most important aspect of the assessment is forgetfulness—specifically, rapid forgetting. In the forgetfulness of normal aging, we become slower at retrieving past information. However, in dementia, the hippocampus is so damaged that memories can no longer be stored, and this is the main target of your evaluation.

This evaluation is divided up into four phases: the patient interview, the informant interview, brief cognitive testing, and laboratory screening.

1. *Interview the patient*

   Many patients complain about memory loss and are worried about dementia, but only a small percentage of such patients actually have dementia. A diagnosis requires establishing that there is both memory loss and a significant life impact of the deficit.

   Start by asking about the time course of the memory loss. Has it occurred gradually over years (typical with dementia), or has it occurred rapidly over months (a red flag for organic causes)?

   Ask if the memory issues have been significant. Can they recall an instance where their memory issues have caused a problem in daily life? Have they missed appointments, forgotten important dates (eg, birthdays, anniversaries), gotten lost, or done anything that has put them in danger (eg, leaving the stove on or leaving the car door open when driving)?

2. *Interview family members or other informants*

   Interviewing informants is crucial; in fact, it is likely more sensitive in detecting dementia than interviewing the patients themselves. Use the IQCODE questionnaire to save time when interviewing informants (see "Short Form of the Informant Questionnaire on Cognitive Decline in the Elderly (Short IQCODE)" at: www.thecarlatreport.com/shortIQCODE.

   Ask informants how the patient is at the following, compared with 10 years ago:

   - Remembering things that have happened recently.
   - Remembering where things are usually kept.
   - Remembering things about family and friends, such as names, occupations, birthdays, or addresses.
   - Making decisions on everyday matters.
   - Handling financial matters.
   - Finding the right words when talking about things.
   - Knowing how to do everyday things around the house, such as cooking and cleaning.

3. *Perform formal cognitive testing*

   Use the Montreal Cognitive Assessment (MoCA), which takes about 10 minutes to administer (see: www.thecarlatreport.com/AdministeringMoCA). The MoCA is more sensitive than the Mini-Mental State Examination (MMSE). Look for rapid forgetting in Alzheimer's patients, especially in the list recall sections of the MoCA.

4. *Do lab work and neuroimaging*

   Ensure that certain lab tests have been done recently; if they aren't readily available, order them yourself. Below is a list of relevant tests and the pathologies each one assesses for:

   - *MRI:* Atrophy patterns (hippocampal, frontal, temporal lobes) indicating Alzheimer's, vascular dementia, or frontotemporal dementia; rule out tumors, infarcts, or hydrocephalus.
   - *Complete blood count:* Anemia, infection.
   - *Electrolytes:* Fluid/electrolyte imbalances, renal dysfunction.
   - *Thyroid panel:* Hypothyroidism, hyperthyroidism.
   - *Vitamin B12:* Vitamin B12 deficiency.
   - *Vitamin D:* Vitamin D deficiency.
   - *Syphilis serology:* Neurosyphilis.
   - *Erythrocyte sedimentation rate/C-reactive protein:* Inflammation, infection.
   - *Liver function tests:* Hepatic encephalopathy.
   - *Glucose:* Uncontrolled diabetes.
   - *Calcium:* Hypocalcemia/hypercalcemia.

   A psychiatrist can comfortably diagnose dementia in approximately 70% of cases. Refer to a neurologist when encountering younger patients, unexpected MRI findings, or unusual dementia patterns.

Major Neurocognitive Disorder: Medication Treatment

There is no cure for major neurocognitive disorder (MND), but several medications mitigate the progression of cognitive and functional decline. Most medications are FDA approved for Alzheimer's dementia but are often used off-label for other memory disorders. Educate patients and caregivers about the importance of medication adherence: Missing doses, even briefly, can cause significant memory deterioration, which may not be reversible even after resuming the medication. Side effects for all these meds mainly include GI issues, headaches, and abnormal dreams.

For Mild to Moderate Dementia: Cholinesterase Inhibitors

- *Donepezil (Aricept):*
  - Most data and experience are with this agent.
  - Start with 5 mg daily for a month; increase to 10 mg if well tolerated.
  - If the cognitive decline continues, increase to 15 or 20 mg daily.
- *Galantamine (Razadyne, Razadyne ER):*
  - Extended release: Start with 8 mg; increase to 16 mg after a month (equivalent to 10 mg of donepezil). If required, increase to 24 mg.
  - Immediate release (if patient experiences vivid dreams): Start with 4 mg; increase to 8 mg if tolerated.
  - Oral solution of 4 mg/mL is good for patients who have trouble swallowing pills.
- *Rivastigmine and rivastigmine patch (Exelon, Exelon Patch):*
  - Patch form is suitable for patients who have trouble swallowing medications.
  - More expensive than other agents and requires assistance to apply or remove.
  - FDA approved for dementia associated with Parkinson's disease.
  - Oral form: 1.5 mg twice daily with meals; increase after every four weeks up to 6 mg twice daily with meals.
  - Patch: Start with 4.6 mg/24 hours; potentially increase to 9.5 mg. The 13.3 mg dose is rarely used due to GI side effects.

For Moderate to Severe Dementia

- *Memantine IR, memantine XR (Namenda, Namenda XR):*
  - Immediate release: 5–10 mg daily or twice daily.
  - Extended release (if patient doesn't tolerate the immediate-release version): 7–28 mg daily. More expensive.
- *High-dose donepezil:*
  - Combine two 10 mg tablets or use the 23 mg version.

Alternative Approach Regardless of Dementia Severity

Use the same protocol regardless of the severity of dementia:

- Prescribe a combination of donepezil and memantine at the doses mentioned above.
- Or consider Namzaric, a combination pill of donepezil and memantine. Patients on memantine 10 mg twice daily and donepezil 10 mg daily would take 28/10 mg Namzaric QPM.

Reminder

Review your patients' medications for their potential cognitive impact. Agents that may worsen cognition include benzodiazepines, nonbenzo Z-drugs, and anticholinergic agents.

How to Identify and Manage Confusion and Delirium

The terms confusion, delirium, encephalopathy, and altered mental status (AMS) are often used interchangeably when describing a patient who has undergone a rapid cognitive change and is unable to think and concentrate normally. Psychiatrists are often asked to evaluate and treat acute confusion in patients who are medically ill. This fact sheet outlines a quick and systematic approach to assessment.

Clinical Assessment

History

Review the medical record and discuss with caregivers and family members. Did the symptoms emerge recently, or do they represent a long-standing condition like dementia? Were there any recent triggers, like health complications, initiation of new medications, or other medical conditions? When you read the nursing notes, is there evidence of fluctuating confusion (eg, worsening in the evening)?

Medical assessment

Review the chart for the medical workup, which will usually clearly delineate acute medical illnesses that may be causing delirium, such as infections, cardiac issues, respiratory failure, acute renal injury, and alcohol withdrawal.

Psychiatric assessment

- Spend a minute simply observing the patient before asking questions. Delirious patients may be rambling incoherently, struggling against restraints, attempting to pull out IV lines, and picking at the air as if hallucinating. Other times, the patient may be quietly delirious, providing few clues on simple observation.
- Interview:
  - *Attentional impairment*. Introduce yourself and engage in normal conversation. A delirious patient will quickly demonstrate distractibility (eg, their gaze may drift away, and they will not be able to concentrate long enough to provide a complete answer to questions).
  - *Cognitive impairment*. Do some kind of formal assessment, using either the Mini-Mental State Examination (MMSE) or the Montreal Cognitive Assessment (MoCA). However, delirious patients may lack the attention required to complete this testing. Common deficits are orientation, three-word recall, and tests of concentration such as spelling "world" backwards or reciting the months backwards.
  - *Hallucinations and delusions*. Both visual and auditory hallucinations (or simply misperceptions) are common; a tip-off is when your patient is looking all around the room. Delusions may be vague and somewhat paranoid, like the patient believing they are being harmed.

Standardized tool

The Confusion Assessment Method (CAM; www.tinyurl.com/j7ez5nc3) is a highly sensitive rating tool for diagnosing delirium. Although it was created for clinicians without psychiatric training, it is helpful for psychiatrists as well, especially those earlier in their career.

Treatment

Medical interventions

- For infections, start with antibiotics.
- If medications are the issue, adjust doses or consider alternatives.
- For metabolic issues, focus on hydration and correcting electrolytes.
- For vitamin or hormone levels, administer appropriate supplements or hormones to correct the deficiencies.
- Give these recommendations to the hospitalist team:
  - Keep the patient's environment well lit during the day and dark at night to help regulate sleep-wake cycles.
  - Watch for unmanaged pain as this can contribute to delirium.
  - Use calendars and clocks to assist with orientation and provide cognitively stimulating activities, like word search puzzles and art therapy. Facilitate visits from friends and family to support social interaction.
  - Encourage the patient to move and ensure walking aids are within reach.
  - If the patient needs hearing aids, glasses, or dentures, make sure they are available.

Psychiatric management

- If psychiatric conditions are at the root, focus on managing the underlying disorder, be it bipolar mania, major depressive disorder with psychotic features, or severe anxiety.
- Use antipsychotics or benzodiazepines cautiously as they can sometimes worsen delirium.
- Enhance sleep with nighttime medications such as melatonin (1–5 mg), ramelteon (8 mg), and trazodone (25–50 mg).

Behavioral and Psychological Symptoms of Dementia

Dementia patients often exhibit symptoms like agitation, aggression, wandering, psychosis, depression, and anxiety—collectively referred to as behavioral and psychological symptoms of dementia, or BPDS. While therapeutic approaches like art and music therapy can be highly effective, you'll sometimes need to prescribe medications to ensure safety. Here we'll delve into your pharmaceutical options. Start low, increase doses as needed or tolerated, and monitor closely for side effects.

Cholinesterase Inhibitors

These not only slow cognitive decline but also address behavioral issues. They're particularly beneficial for dementia resulting from Parkinson's or Lewy body disease.

- *Donepezil:* 5–20 mg daily.
- Galantamine:
  - *Sustained release:* 8–24 mg daily.
  - *Immediate release:* 4–8 mg daily.
- *Rivastigmine patch:* Start with 4.6 mg/24 hours; can increase to 9.5 mg.

Antidepressants

Suitable for mild to moderate agitation, restlessness, and anxiety.

- Selective serotonin reuptake inhibitors:
  - *Escitalopram:* 5–20 mg daily.
  - *Sertraline:* 12.5–75 mg daily.
- *Mirtazapine:* 7.5–15 mg at bedtime; also helps with insomnia.

Benzodiazepines

Use judiciously, given potential side effects like cognitive impairments and balance disturbances.

- *Lorazepam:* 0.25–0.5 mg as needed every four to six hours.
- *Clonazepam:* 0.25–0.5 mg once daily or at bedtime; also helps with REM sleep anomalies.

Antipsychotics

While there's an FDA warning about antipsychotics presenting increased mortality and stroke risk in the elderly, the absolute risk remains modest. These medications can be indispensable for patients exhibiting psychosis or aggression.

- *Risperidone:* 0.125–2 mg at bedtime.
- *Quetiapine:* 25–50 mg at bedtime; the better option for Parkinson's patients and patients with insomnia.

Mood Stabilizers and Anticonvulsants

- *Depakote:* 250 mg two to three times daily; good for impulsivity. Monitor for hyperammonemia.
- *Lithium:* 600–900 mg at bedtime; aim for blood levels of 0.4–0.8 mEq/L.
- *Gabapentin:* 100–300 mg three to four times daily; good for agitation.

Other Agents

- *Acetaminophen:* 500 mg BID or TID; surprisingly helpful, probably because it eases pain, which is often the underlying cause of agitation.
- *Opioids:* Use Roxanol liquid; start with 2.5 mg daily. Effective for pain-related agitation.
- *Trazodone:* 12.5–50 mg at midday or bedtime; for agitation and insomnia.
- *Prazosin:* Begin with 1 mg at bedtime and monitor for blood pressure changes. Good for treating agitation, particularly in patients experiencing nightmares or PTSD-related symptoms.
- *Clonidine patch:* Begin at 0.1 mg daily; good for anxiety and agitation, and the patch ensures compliance.
- *Dronabinol:* 2.5–5 mg once or twice daily; helps with agitation and promotes appetite.

Traumatic Brain Injury

Patients with a history of traumatic brain injury (TBI) often arrive at the psychiatric unit due to symptoms such as suicidality, aggression, or substance disorder issues. It's often difficult to know how the TBI—which may have occurred many years earlier—is related to the presenting psychiatric issues. These guidelines will help you more accurately evaluate these patients and come up with a treatment plan specific to their needs.

Vignette

John, a 45-year-old male, is admitted to the inpatient psychiatric unit for suicidal ideation. He sustained a severe TBI 10 years ago in a car accident. Since then, he has struggled with persistent mood swings, memory problems, and frequent headaches. His family reports that he has become increasingly irritable and withdrawn over the years.

Assessment

TBI can be a vague term and is sometimes used loosely, so it's helpful to understand the formal definitions, as well as the formal DSM criteria for neurocognitive disorder due to TBI. Patients and families may find it reassuring that there are formal diagnostic criteria, and knowing this can motivate patients to seek treatment.

Acute vs chronic TBI

- Timeline:
  - *Acute:* Occurs immediately after the traumatic event, typically within the first few hours to days.
  - *Chronic:* Symptoms persist or emerge after the initial injury phase, lasting for months to years.
- Symptoms:
  - *Acute:* Loss of consciousness, posttraumatic amnesia, disorientation, confusion, and acute neurological signs like seizures.
  - *Chronic:* Chronic cognitive impairment, persistent mood and anxiety disorders, PTSD, and long-term behavioral changes.

DSM-5 criteria: Major or mild neurocognitive disorder due to TBI

- *Evidence of a TBI:* History of head trauma with at least one of the following: loss of consciousness, posttraumatic amnesia, disorientation and confusion, or neurological signs (eg, neuroimaging showing injury, new-onset seizures, visual field cuts, anosmia, hemiparesis).
- *Neurocognitive impact:* Cognitive deficits in one or more domains (complex attention, executive function, learning and memory, language, perceptual-motor, or social cognition) that interfere with independence in everyday activities (major) or do not affect independence but require greater effort, compensatory strategies, or accommodation (mild).
- *Symptom time course:* The cognitive deficits present immediately after the TBI or after a recovery period and persist past the acute post-injury period.

Common psychiatric complications of chronic TBI

- *Depression:* Common in TBI patients, often exacerbated by physical limitations and cognitive impairments. Look for symptoms like persistent sadness, loss of interest, and changes in sleep or appetite.
- Anxiety disorders:
  - *Generalized anxiety disorder:* Persistent and excessive worry, often related to the TBI's impact on life.
  - *Panic disorder:* Recurrent panic attacks, sometimes triggered by reminders of the injury.
  - *PTSD:* Particularly common in cases where the injury involved trauma or violence. Look for reexperiencing symptoms, avoidance, hyperarousal, and negative alterations in mood and cognition.
- Cognitive impairments:
  - *Memory issues:* Difficulty with short-term and working memory.
  - *Attention deficits:* Problems with concentration and sustained attention.
  - *Executive dysfunction:* Impaired planning, decision-making, and problem-solving abilities.
- Behavioral changes:
  - *Irritability and aggression:* Increased frustration and anger outbursts.
  - *Apathy and social withdrawal:* Lack of motivation and reduced interest in social interactions.
  - *Impulsivity:* Difficulty in controlling impulses, leading to risky behaviors.

Initial psychiatric evaluation of TBI patients

- Obtain a detailed history of the TBI. Did it occur from a motor vehicle accident, a fall, or an assault? Find out about the severity and time since the injury to get a sense of the level of care the patient will likely require.
- Explore psychiatric symptoms, like mood disturbances, anxiety, psychosis, agitation, and aggression. Remember, some psychiatric symptoms may arise from the stress of living with the TBI, not solely from the injury itself.

- Conduct baseline cognitive assessments using instruments like the Mini-Mental State Examination (MMSE) or the Montreal Cognitive Assessment (MoCA). If available, refer the patient to a neuropsychologist for a comprehensive cognitive evaluation to identify specific deficits and recommend targeted interventions.

Treatment Options

Pharmacotherapy

- *Antidepressants:* Selective serotonin reuptake inhibitors (such as sertraline or fluoxetine) and serotonin/norephinephrine reuptake inhibitors (such as venlafaxine) for depression and anxiety.
- *Mood stabilizers:* Lamotrigine or valproate for mood swings and irritability.
- *Antipsychotics:* Low-dose second-generation antipsychotics (eg, quetiapine) for severe agitation or aggression.
- *Cognitive enhancers:* Stimulants (eg, methylphenidate) or cholinesterase inhibitors (eg, donepezil) for patients with severe attention and executive function deficits, like difficulties with planning and problem solving.
- *Benzodiazepines:* Use with caution, since they can paradoxically increase agitation and worsen cognitive deficits.

Behavioral and cognitive interventions

- *Cognitive behavioral therapy:* Effective for depression, anxiety, and PTSD. Focus on restructuring negative thoughts and developing coping strategies.
- *Behavioral therapy:* Establish a behavior modification plan to manage aggression and impulsivity. Set clear, consistent rules and expectations, and use positive reinforcement to encourage desired behaviors (see the "Sample Behavior Management Plan" fact sheet in the Psychotherapy on the Inpatient Unit section).
- *Trauma-focused therapies:* Eye movement desensitization and reprocessing and prolonged exposure therapy for PTSD.
- *Cognitive rehabilitation therapy:* Refer patients to occupational therapists for interventions such as memory drills, attention training, and other activities tailored to the patient's cognitive deficits identified in the neuropsychological evaluation.

Environmental modifications

Work with unit staff to establish a predictable daily routine for the patient. Place them in a quiet room with calm roommates and minimal clutter whenever possible.

Therapeutic approaches

- *Individual therapy:* Focus on coping strategies and emotional regulation. For example, you might say to the patient, "When you feel overwhelmed, try taking deep breaths or stepping away from the situation to regain your composure."
- *Group therapy:* Encourage the patient to join the unit's support groups to help develop a sense of community and learn from others facing similar challenges.
- *Family involvement:* Although family therapy is not typically conducted on inpatient units, consider scheduling one or two sessions with family members to educate them on managing TBI-related symptoms so they'll be better prepared when the patient returns home.

COMMON PSYCHIATRIC CONDITIONS

Personality Disorders

Overview of Personality Disorders

Personality disorders (PDs) are enduring patterns of behavior, cognition, and emotional regulation that can complicate treatment and disrupt the therapeutic environment of the unit. Here we outline each disorder's distinct features and review management strategies. Since patients with borderline personality disorder can be particularly challenging, we cover this topic in more detail in the following fact sheet.

Common Presentations

- *Antisocial personality disorder (ASPD):* Disregard for others' rights, deceitfulness, impulsivity, aggression, and lack of remorse. Patients may manipulate or engage in criminal behavior.
- *Avoidant personality disorder (AvPD):* Social inhibition, feelings of inadequacy, and hypersensitivity to negative evaluation. Patients may avoid social interactions and are often extremely self-critical.
- *Borderline personality disorder (BPD):* Intense mood swings, fear of abandonment, impulsivity, self-harm, and unstable relationships (see separate fact sheet for more details).
- *Dependent personality disorder (DPD):* Excessive need to be taken care of, leading to submissive and clinging behaviors, and fear of separation. Patients may have difficulty making decisions without reassurance from others.
- *Histrionic personality disorder (HPD):* Excessive emotionality, attention-seeking, superficial charm, and rapidly shifting emotions. Patients may dramatize situations and demand constant attention.
- *Narcissistic personality disorder (NPD):* Grandiosity, need for admiration, lack of empathy, and hypersensitivity to criticism. Patients may react with rage or withdrawal when self-esteem is threatened.
- *Obsessive-compulsive personality disorder (OCPD):* Preoccupation with orderliness, perfectionism, and control. Patients may be rigid, stubborn, and overly focused on details, interfering with treatment flexibility.
- *Schizotypal personality disorder (STPD):* Acute discomfort in close relationships, cognitive or perceptual distortions, and eccentric behavior. Patients may have odd beliefs, magical thinking, or social anxiety.

Management Strategies

- *Unit guidelines:* Establish and maintain clear, consistent guidelines for patient interactions to minimize manipulative behaviors and avoid staff being pitted against each other.
- Psychotherapy:
  - *Cognitive behavioral therapy (CBT):* Effective for most PDs, particularly NPD, OCPD, AvPD, and DPD, focusing on modifying maladaptive thoughts and behaviors.
  - *Supportive psychotherapy:* Provides emotional support and helps patients cope with stressors. Useful for HPD and STPD where emotional dysregulation or social anxiety is prominent.
  - *Dialectical behavior therapy (DBT):* While DBT is particularly effective for BPD, it can also be helpful in managing emotional regulation and impulsivity in other PDs.
  - *Social skills training:* Beneficial for AvPD and STPD, focusing on improving social interactions and reducing social anxiety.
- Medication management:
  - *Co-occurring conditions:* Treat co-occurring depression, anxiety, or psychotic symptoms with selective serotonin reuptake inhibitors, antipsychotics, or anxiolytics, as appropriate.
  - *Mood stabilizers:* Consider mood stabilizers for patients with impulsivity or emotional dysregulation, particularly in ASPD, HPD, and BPD.
  - *Avoid benzodiazepines:* Use caution or avoid benzodiazepines, especially in ASPD and BPD, due to the risk of misuse and disinhibition.
- Crisis intervention:
  - *De-escalation techniques:* Use calm, non-confrontational approaches for patients with ASPD, NPD, and BPD who may become aggressive or threatening (see the "How to Verbally De-Escalate an Aggressive Patient" fact sheet in the Agitation Management section).
  - *Safety planning:* Develop individualized safety plans, especially for patients at risk of self-harm or with severe anxiety (eg, AvPD, DPD, and BPD) (see the "Creating a Patient Safety Plan" fact sheet in the Suicide and Self-Injurious Behaviors section).
- Group therapy:
  - *Psychoeducation groups:* Offer psychoeducation on managing emotions, improving social interactions, and understanding the impact of personality disorders.
  - *Support groups:* Encourage participation in support groups to foster insight and peer support; particularly beneficial for HPD, AvPD, and BPD.

Borderline Personality Disorder

Patients with borderline personality disorder (BPD) account for about 20% of psychiatric inpatients and can often present challenges on the unit. In this fact sheet, we describe a systematic approach to diagnosis.

Overview

While the DSM-5 provides a helpful list of criteria, BPD is still often a confusing diagnosis for clinicians and patients. We recommend the following sequence for your evaluation:

- Start by reviewing the medical record for clues. Often there will be prior diagnoses of personality disorders along with comorbid issues like mood disorders, substance use disorders, and self-harm.
- Interview the patient, keeping the four key domains in mind (see below).
- If you believe that a BPD diagnosis is likely, review the nine DSM criteria with the patient, asking if these criteria describe their personality and requesting specific examples. This approach will help patients understand the reasons for their BPD diagnosis.
- Consider bipolar disorder, major depression, psychosis, or substance use disorder, all of which are often comorbid or may serve as alternative diagnoses to BPD.

Four Key Domains of Borderline Personality Disorder

As you evaluate your patient, consider these four domains:

1. *Unstable emotional responses:* Mood instability, inappropriate anger, and feelings of emptiness. Emotions can rapidly shift within minutes or hours, often in response to interpersonal distress.
2. *Inaccurate perceptions:* These often occur alongside emotional instability. A person's sense of identity can fluctuate, from feeling confident one day to experiencing profound worthlessness the next. Transient paranoia about others' intentions is also common.
3. *Impulsive behaviors:* The combination of unstable emotions and inaccurate perceptions can drive impulsive behaviors aimed at alleviating distress. This can include self-harm, substance use, sexual impulsivity, lashing out at others, etc.
4. *Unstable relationships:* All of the above emotions, perceptions, and behaviors contribute to unstable relationships, often leading to abandonment issues.

DSM-5-TR Diagnostic Criteria

A lifelong pattern of five of the following nine criteria:

1. Frantic efforts to avoid real or imagined abandonment.
   - "When you start a relationship, do you feel that you're going to be dumped from day one?"
2. A pattern of unstable and intense interpersonal relationships characterized by alternating between extremes of idealization and devaluation.
   - "Are you in a relationship? What happens to you in a relationship? Are there a lot of quarrels?"
3. Identity disturbance—markedly and persistently unstable self-image or sense of self.
   - "Do you have a sense of where you're going in life? What are your goals?"
4. Impulsivity in at least two areas that are potentially self-damaging (eg, spending, sex, substance abuse, reckless driving, binge eating).
   - "Have you engaged in reckless behavior involving money, sex, driving, drugs, alcohol, or eating?"
5. Recurrent suicidal behavior, gestures, threats, or self-mutilating behavior.
   - "Have you ever thought about suicide, and have you made an attempt?"
6. Affective instability due to a marked reactivity of mood (eg, intense episodic dysphoria, irritability, or anxiety usually lasting a few hours and only rarely more than a few days).
   - "Do you find that your mood changes a lot in the course of a day?"
7. Chronic feelings of emptiness.
   - "Do you feel empty inside, as if there's nothing there?"
8. Inappropriate, intense anger or difficulty controlling anger (eg, frequent displays of temper, constant anger, recurrent physical fights).
   - "Would people describe you as having a short temper? Do you lose control when you get mad?"
9. Transient, stress-related paranoid ideation or severe dissociative symptoms.
   - "When you're out in the world, do you feel like strangers are looking at you, commenting on you, and probably criticizing you?"

Defense Mechanisms in BPD

- Typical defense mechanisms that you may see in your patients include splitting (viewing people and situations as all good or all bad), idealization (overestimating someone's positive attributes), devaluation (undervaluing someone

after they disappoint), projection (attributing one's own unacceptable thoughts, feelings, or impulses to others), and acting out (expressing emotions impulsively).
- *Example:* Jordan idealizes his friend, praising him as the perfect companion. The next day, following a minor disagreement, Jordan abruptly shifts to devaluing him, labeling him as utterly untrustworthy. Acting impulsively, he sends a series of angry texts and leaves several irate voicemails.

Management Strategies

Disclose the diagnosis and educate about prognosis

- BPD is a difficult diagnosis to understand, and the label has acquired a stigma over the years, so you may feel tongue-tied when communicating the diagnosis to your patient. A good way to describe BPD is to simply repeat the symptoms and behaviors you hear from the patient. For example: "You described to me that your emotions are very unstable; you often lose control of your temper; you cut yourself; you have made suicide attempts; you use too many drugs; and your relationships are conflictual and don't work—that's borderline personality disorder."
- Emphasize that BPD is treatable, and that at the 10-year mark about 80% of patients no longer meet full criteria.

Psychotherapy

Numerous evidence-based therapies exist and are likely all equally effective for BPD if done competently. Many inpatient units offer groups with some component of dialectal behavior therapy or cognitive behavioral therapy. Given that inpatient admissions are typically brief, the therapeutic interventions you can realistically provide are limited; most of the in-depth therapy will occur in an outpatient setting. Nonetheless, you can still use a focused therapeutic strategy aimed at preventing suicidality, as follows:

- Discuss the typical cycle leading to self-harm in patients with BPD:
  - *Perceived rejection:* Patients often interpret certain actions as signs of rejection or abandonment.
  - *Isolation and dissociation:* The perceived rejection can intensify feelings of loneliness, leading to dissociation, detachment, and even greater isolation.
  - *Help-rejecting behavior:* Despite needing support, patients might refuse assistance and may lash out at those they perceive as rejecting them.
  - *Despair leading to self-harm:* These experiences often culminate in despair, driving patients toward seeing self-harm or suicidal thoughts as a way to cope with their overwhelming pain.
- Discuss strategies to disrupt the harmful pattern:
  - *Develop a crisis plan:* Create a plan that identifies early warning signs of a crisis and outlines steps they can take, including whom to contact.
  - *Teach emotional regulation skills:* These include mindfulness, deep breathing, listening to music, flicking a rubber band on the wrist, holding ice, and grounding exercises.
  - *Build interpersonal effectiveness skills:* Help patients develop skills to communicate their needs and boundaries more effectively and to manage interpersonal conflicts without damaging important relationships.

Psychopharmacology

- No medication is FDA approved for BPD, but medications can be helpful when targeted to specific symptom domains. Doses used for BPD are typically lower than those you might prescribe for conditions like bipolar disorder or a primary psychotic disorder.
- Second-generation antipsychotics are generally first line; they reduce mood swings, anxiety, anger, and impulsivity. Examples include risperidone 1 mg daily, aripiprazole 2.5–5 mg daily, and quetiapine 25–200 mg at night.
- Antidepressants help comorbid depression/anxiety. Examples include sertraline 50 mg daily and escitalopram 10 mg daily.
- Mood stabilizers can target anger and impulsivity. Examples include lithium 300–600 mg daily, valproic acid 500–1000 mg daily, and lamotrigine up to 200 mg daily.
- Be careful with benzodiazepines as they can be disinhibiting and potentially lead to more impulsivity. However, patients with panic attacks may benefit from as-needed lorazepam or clonazepam.

COMMON PSYCHIATRIC CONDITIONS

Schizophrenia and Other Psychotic Disorders

Interviewing Patients with Psychosis

When interviewing patients who are experiencing psychotic symptoms, strike a balance between providing support and empathy without reinforcing their delusional beliefs. Once you establish rapport, you can begin to gently guide the conversation to help patients gain insight into their delusions. Here are some tips for these interviews.

Interviewing Tips

Ask open-ended questions

Start with open-ended questions and progress to more structured ones if needed. For example:

- "Can you tell me more about your experiences recently?"
- "What has been on your mind lately?"

Use normalizing questions

Help the patient feel comfortable discussing their experiences by using normalizing questions:

- "I often hear from people that they hear unusual voices. Has this happened to you?"
- "Often when people are under a lot of stress, they have scary thoughts about people wanting to harm them. Has that happened to you?"

Avoid challenging delusions at the start

Don't start by questioning the validity of the patient's delusions. Instead, use neutral questions to explore their beliefs, such as:

- "Can you share more details about X?"
- "What events led you to believe Y?"

Validate emotions, not delusions

- Empathize with the patient's emotions, which are often rooted in fear.
- Phrases to use: "That sounds very upsetting." "How did that experience make you feel?"

Reflect patient's own words

- Build rapport by using the patient's exact words to describe their experiences. For example, ask, "When you heard whispers through the wall, what were they saying?"
- Avoid jargon: Steer clear of clinical terms like "delusion" or "hallucination."

Guide insight gently

Once rapport is established, gently help the patient explore discrepancies in their delusions to gain insight. Use questions that encourage reflection without direct confrontation:

- "What do you think others might say about that experience?"
- "Have you noticed any differences in how you see things compared to others?"

Patience and persistence

- Building trust can take time, often requiring several sessions. Be patient and persistent.
- Regular follow-ups and demonstrating a genuine interest in the patient's well-being can foster a stronger therapeutic relationship.

Safety considerations

- Ensure the interview space is free from objects that could be used to cause harm. Position yourself in a way that maintains a safe distance from the patient and ensures easy access to an exit if needed.
- Be familiar with de-escalation techniques and know how to quickly contact security or other staff members if necessary.

DSM-5 Diagnosis for Psychotic Disorders

Psychosis is common, and there are many varieties. This fact sheet guides you through the process of thinking through the main DSM-5 diagnoses that apply to psychotic disorders. For help with how to ask the right questions to discover psychosis in patients, see the "Interviewing Patients with Psychosis" fact sheet in this subsection.

Assess for the Presence of the Big Five Key Psychotic Symptoms

Mnemonic: **D**elusions **H**erald **S**chizophrenic's **B**ad **N**ews:

- **D**elusions (fixed false beliefs).
- **H**allucinations (usually auditory, but can be visual, tactile, or olfactory).
- Disorganized **S**peech (looseness of associations, tangential).
- Disorganized **B**ehavior (Illogical, irrational, odd behaviors).
- **N**egative symptoms (paucity of speech, isolation, lack of activities, lack of thought).

Based on Presence and Time Course of the Big Five, Sort Through the Differential Diagnosis

Psychosis without significant depression or mania

- *Schizophrenia:* One month of at least two major symptoms (one of which must be delusions, hallucinations, or disorganized speech), plus five months of prodrome (total duration at least six months).
- *Schizophreniform disorder:* Like schizophrenia, except the total duration is less (one to six months). About two-thirds of these patients eventually develop schizophrenia.
- *Brief psychotic disorder:* At least one major psychotic symptom lasting from one day to one month. About 50% of these patients will have another psychotic episode within three years.
- *Delusional disorder:* At least one delusion for one month or more, but without schizophrenia, without markedly impaired functioning, and without obviously odd or bizarre behavior. Subtypes include erotomanic, grandiose, jealous, persecutory, somatic, mixed, and unspecified.
- *Unspecified psychotic disorder:* Psychosis is present, but the patient's symptoms or time course don't quite fit into the above categories, or you just don't have enough information to decide yet.

Psychosis with a major mood component

- *Schizoaffective disorder* (specify either depressed type or bipolar type—use bipolar type if there is a history of mania):
  - Depression or mania in addition to two or more of the Big Five psychotic symptoms.
  - At least a two-week period of only psychotic symptoms without mood symptoms.
  - Mood symptoms are present a majority of the time.
- *Bipolar disorder:*
  - A history of at least one lifetime episode of mania, in addition to one or more episodes of depression.
  - Psychosis is present only during mood episodes.
- *Major depression with psychotic features:*
  - An episode of major depression with psychosis.
  - Psychosis is present only during the depression (disappears completely once the depression resolves).
- *Schizophrenia with comorbid depression:*
  - An established diagnosis of schizophrenia.
  - Discrete episodes of major depression that come and go.

Algorithm for Deciding on a Diagnosis

- Is there more than one psychotic symptom?
  - If no: Cannot be schizophrenia, schizoaffective, or schizophreniform.
  - If yes: Can be any psychotic disorder.
- Is the patient having a significant mood episode?
  - If yes, is there mania?
    - If yes, can be bipolar or schizoaffective.
    - Is psychosis present only during mania?
      - If yes, then bipolar disorder.
      - If psychosis is present for two weeks without mania, then schizoaffective disorder, bipolar type.

Schizophrenia: Assessment and Management

You will often encounter patients with schizophrenia, particularly during exacerbations that lead to psychiatric holds and inpatient hospitalizations. Schizophrenia is a chronic and severe mental disorder, but with the right treatment, many individuals experience significant improvement in their quality of life. Here we provide an overview of this illness.

Key Symptoms

Positive symptoms

- *Hallucinations:* Hearing voices or seeing things that aren't there.
- *Delusions:* Strongly held false beliefs, such as thinking one has special powers.

Negative symptoms

- *Affective flattening:* Reduced expression of emotions.
- *Anhedonia:* Lack of pleasure in everyday life.
- *Alogia:* Decreased speech.
- *Avolition:* Reduced motivation to initiate and sustain activities.
- *Asociality:* Reduced motivation for social contact.

Disorganized symptoms

- *Speech:* Loose associations, tangential, incoherent, or nonsensical.
- *Behavior:* Disorganized, irrational, or bizarre.

Diagnosis

- Symptoms must be present for at least six months, including at least one month of two or more major symptoms, with at least one being delusions, hallucinations, or disorganized speech.
- Schizophrenia usually shows up in late adolescence or early adulthood for men, and in early 20s to early 30s for women.
- When diagnosing schizophrenia, look for significant impairment in major areas of life, like work, relationships, or self-care.
- Often, subtle changes in thinking and social relationships precede the full-blown illness by years.

Differential Diagnosis

- *Schizophreniform disorder:* Symptoms last at least a month but less than six months. Many of these people go on to have schizophrenia, but for about one-third, the symptoms will resolve on their own.
- *Other conditions:* Rule out conditions like depressive or bipolar disorder with psychotic features and substance-induced psychosis.

Risk Factors

- *Genetic factors:* Family history increases the risk. For instance, if both parents have schizophrenia, the risk in their child is 40%.
- *Perinatal factors:* Malnutrition, viral infections during pregnancy, and obstetric complications can elevate risk.
- *Environmental factors:* Higher latitudes of birth, winter births, and urban upbringing are associated with higher risk.
- *Substance use:* Heavy marijuana use in adolescence is linked to an earlier onset of psychosis.

Prognosis

While schizophrenia is a chronic condition, many patients manage their symptoms effectively with treatment.

Factors predicting better outcomes

- Predominantly positive symptoms.
- Rapid onset.
- Prompt treatment intervention.
- Short duration of untreated psychosis.

Factors predicting worse outcomes

- Early onset.
- Family history of schizophrenia.
- Prominent negative symptoms.
- Comorbid substance use disorder.

Treatment

See the "Medication Strategies for Schizophrenia" fact sheet in this subsection, as well as the "Psychotherapy for Psychotic Disorders" fact sheet in the Psychotherapy on the Inpatient Unit section.

Post-Discharge Treatment and Support

Psychiatric hospitalizations provide an opportunity to connect patients with ongoing support and resources following discharge. Your team's social worker can facilitate these connections:

- *Coordinated specialty care:* Recovery-focused programs that include psychotherapy, medication, case management, psychoeducation, and family support.
- *Assertive community treatment (ACT):* Designed for individuals with a history of frequent hospitalizations or difficulty adhering to treatment. ACT teams are available 24/7 and provide intensive care in real-world settings like patients' homes or workplaces.
- *Dual diagnosis programs:* Many patients with schizophrenia also have substance use disorders, and integrated dual diagnosis programs address both conditions simultaneously. They are usually residential programs that last three to six months.

Additional Considerations

- People with schizophrenia have a 5% lifetime risk of suicide. Regularly screen for depression and suicidal ideation, offer treatment for depression if needed, and provide information about crisis intervention services and hotlines.
- Lifespans are up to 20 years shorter in people with schizophrenia. Contributing factors include cigarette smoking, poor nutrition, lack of exercise, obesity, chronic illnesses like diabetes, and substance abuse. Encourage patients to accept nicotine replacement therapies, educate them about healthy eating and exercise, ensure they have access to medical care, and refer them to substance use programs if indicated.
- Patients often face difficulty finding employment and are at elevated risk of poverty and homelessness. Work with your team's social worker to connect patients with vocational rehabilitation services, Social Security benefits, and supportive housing programs.

Resources for Patients and Families

- National Alliance on Mental Illness: www.nami.org
- Schizophrenia and Psychosis Action Alliance: https://sczaction.org
- National Institute of Mental Health (NIMH)'s webpage on schizophrenia: www.nimh.nih.gov/health/topics/schizophrenia
- Early Psychosis Intervention Network: www.nationalepinet.org
- NIMH's webpage on the Recovery After an Initial Schizophrenia Episode (RAISE) initiative: www.tinyurl.com/8by22t43
- NIMH's clinical trials webpage: www.nimh.nih.gov/health/trials
- Clinicaltrials.gov's current studies (can filter for schizophrenia): www.clinicaltrials.gov

Medication Strategies for Schizophrenia

Your patients with schizophrenia won't all be alike—some will have prominent delusions and hallucinations, while others might primarily display disorganized thinking and impaired social functioning. Regardless of a patient's presentation, medications help manage symptoms and improve their quality of life. Here we provide guidance on using medications to treat patients with schizophrenia.

Identify Target Symptoms and Goals

Key therapeutic goals in treating schizophrenia include reducing or eliminating hallucinations and delusions; improving thought coherence and organization; enhancing emotional expression and social engagement; and increasing motivation and daily functioning.

Medication Treatment

Antipsychotics

- Choice will depend on a variety of factors, including what meds your patient has responded to or failed in the past. There are dozens of options, and all can be effective; below are some of our top recommendations.
- Start with medications that are affordable and have low side effect profiles. These will usually be second-generation antipsychotics (SGAs), eg:
  - *Aripiprazole* (10–30 mg daily)—generally the most benign side effect profile, though anecdotally less effective for some patients.
  - *Risperidone* (2–6 mg daily)—long track record, high risk of extrapyramidal symptoms (EPS), moderate metabolic side effects, and long track record in schizophrenia treatment.
  - *Paliperidone* (6–12 mg daily)—similar profile as risperidone, but often chosen as an initial agent because there are many long-acting injectable (LAI) versions available (eg, Invega Sustenna).
  - *Lurasidone* (40–160 mg daily)—very well tolerated and has FDA approval for bipolar depression.
- Other SGAs to consider:
  - *Olanzapine* (5–20 mg daily)—high metabolic side effect burden, but anecdotally more effective for treatment-refractory patients.
  - *Quetiapine* (50–100 mg nightly; increase rapidly up to 600–800 mg daily)—high metabolic and sedation side effect burden, but often helpful for agitation and insomnia; FDA approved for depression.
- First-generation antipsychotics (FGAs):
  - *Haloperidol* (2–20 mg daily)—high risk of EPS, but good metabolic side effect profile, very inexpensive, and easily converted to LAI form.
  - *Chlorpromazine* (50–600 mg daily)—high risk of metabolic side effects, but anecdotally very effective for agitated psychotic patients.

Adjunctive medications

Adding other medications can help treat concurrent symptoms, like:

- *Mood stabilizers* (eg, valproic acid 1500–3000 mg daily) for poor impulse control.
- *Benzodiazepines* (eg, clonazepam 0.5–3 mg BID) for agitation or anxiety.
- *Antidepressants* (eg, sertraline 50–200 mg daily) for depressive symptoms.

Treatment-resistant schizophrenia options

- *Clozapine:* Consider using it for patients who have failed to respond to two different antipsychotics. Start with a low dose and titrate up; monitor for agranulocytosis.
- *Combination treatment* (eg, clozapine + aripiprazole, or Invega Sustenna + quetiapine).

Tips on choosing meds for specific patients

- Obesity or diabetes? Avoid olanzapine, quetiapine, and clozapine.
- History of EPS? Avoid aripiprazole and risperidone.
- At risk of osteoporosis (eg, underweight, female, older than 50, smoker)? Avoid prolactin-elevating meds like risperidone, paliperidone, and haloperidol; aripiprazole is a good choice.
- History of medication nonadherence? Choose an LAI.
- Ask about response of family members to specific drugs.

Tips on convincing patients to take meds

- Many patients with schizophrenia have poor insight into their condition and will tell you they don't need psychiatric medications. Refrain from challenging their delusions and try to validate their perspective while gently steering them toward accepting treatment:
  - "It sounds like you experience times that are really distressing. This medication can help lessen those times, making each day a bit easier to get through."
  - "I see that it's really important for you to maintain your independence and make sense of the world around you. This medication can help clear the fog, making it easier for you to think clearly."

Schizoaffective Disorder: Diagnosis and Treatment

Schizoaffective disorder presents significant diagnostic challenges due to its overlap with both bipolar disorder and schizophrenia. It's crucial to obtain as meticulous and reliable a history as possible, although this can be difficult with patients experiencing active psychosis. Ideally, you'll establish the timing of mood and psychotic symptoms, which is essential for ensuring an accurate diagnosis.

Diagnosis

Patients with schizoaffective disorder have symptoms of both psychosis and major mood issues—either mania or depression or both. There are two subtypes of schizoaffective disorder—depressed type and bipolar type—and you have to specify the type in the medical record. Just writing "schizoaffective disorder" is not enough.

Diagnosing schizoaffective disorder can be tricky, because you have to distinguish it from other disorders that can also blend psychosis with mood symptoms, such as bipolar disorder, depression with psychosis, or schizophrenia with depression. For a comprehensive look at the differential diagnosis of psychosis, see the "DSM-5 Diagnosis for Psychotic Disorders" fact sheet in this subsection.

Diagnostic Criteria for Schizoaffective Disorder

- *Concurrent psychotic and mood symptoms:* A significant period where psychotic symptoms occur alongside mood symptoms. (See below for what qualifies as psychotic and mood symptoms.)
- *Psychotic symptoms:* Presence of at least two of the following five major symptoms of psychosis—delusions, hallucinations, disorganized speech, disorganized behavior, or negative symptoms. At least one of the two qualifying psychotic symptoms must be delusions, hallucinations, or disorganized speech. (This is the same as the requirement for diagnosing schizophrenia.)
- *Major mood episode:* A major mood episode must be present for a majority of the total duration of the illness. This can be a major depressive episode, a full-blown manic episode, or a mixed manic episode.
  - Note: A hypomanic episode or dysthymia does not meet the criteria.
- *Delusions or hallucinations for at least two weeks without prominent mood symptoms:* This is a difficult criterion to ascertain. Often you will have to check in with collaterals like outpatient providers or family members to confidently confirm that at some point in the patient's life, they have been psychotic for two weeks without either mania or depression. This requirement helps distinguish it from conditions like bipolar disorder with psychosis or major depressive disorder with psychosis, where psychotic symptoms occur exclusively during mood episodes.

Treatment

Pharmacological management

- *Antipsychotics:*
  - The only FDA-approved medication for schizoaffective disorder is paliperidone (Invega), though risperidone (from which paliperidone is derived) also has good efficacy data.
  - It's likely that most, if not all, other antipsychotics are just as effective as the above medications, but the studies have not yet been published to prove this. A reasonable approach is to review the patient's history of medications, and if there is no documented trial of either paliperidone or risperidone, give these a try. But if they have already failed these agents, choose any other antipsychotic in the same way that you choose medications for schizophrenia (ie, based on side effect potential and patient preference).
- *Mood stabilizers:* For patients with bipolar-type schizoaffective disorder, add a mood stabilizer such as lithium, valproate, or lamotrigine.
- *Antidepressants:* For depressive-type schizoaffective disorder, add your antidepressant of choice.

Psychosocial interventions

- *Cognitive behavioral therapy:* This therapy targets delusional beliefs and hallucinations while also focusing on mood symptom improvement.
- *Family therapy:* Just a few sessions on the inpatient unit will help to educate family members and, post-discharge, will bolster treatment adherence and reduce relapse rates.
- *Psychoeducation:* This helps patients develop a better understanding of the disorder; it also promotes adherence to treatment and will help patients identify early signs of a potential relapse post-discharge.
- *Social skills training and supported employment/education programs:* While these long-term interventions might not be initiated in the hospital, they are crucial for long-term success because schizoaffective disorder is a chronic and disabling condition. Collaborate with your social worker in referring patients to these kinds of community programs.

Delusional Disorder

Delusional disorder is a psychiatric condition where individuals have persistent delusions but, unlike patients with schizophrenia, they can generally function normally in daily life. Here's a practical look at this condition.

Patient Profile

Jane, a 45-year-old woman, has been increasingly convinced that her neighbor is spying on her and trying to harm her. She believes her phone is tapped and that there are hidden cameras in her house. Despite these intense persecutory delusions, Jane continues to work effectively as a schoolteacher and maintains a relatively normal daily routine. She has no history of hallucinations or disorganized thinking. Her family is worried but finds it challenging to discuss her beliefs as Jane becomes defensive and insists on the truth of her experiences.

DSM-5-TR Diagnostic Criteria

- *Presence of delusions:* One or more delusions for at least one month.
- *Functioning:* Apart from delusions, functioning not markedly impaired, and behavior not obviously bizarre or odd.
- *Exclusion of schizophrenia:* Criteria for schizophrenia have never been met.
- *Mood episodes:* If mood episodes occur, they are brief relative to the duration of the delusional periods.
- *Not substance-induced:* Disturbance not attributable to the physiological effects of a substance/another medical condition.

Common Types of Delusions in Delusional Disorder

- *Persecutory:* Belief that they are being targeted or harassed.
- *Erotomanic:* Belief that someone, often of higher status, is in love with them.
- *Grandiose:* Belief in having exceptional abilities, wealth, or fame.
- *Jealous:* Belief that a partner is unfaithful without evidence.
- *Somatic:* Belief in having a physical defect or medical condition.

Symptom Picture

Patients with delusional disorder often present with well-systematized delusions that are nonbizarre and could conceivably occur in real life. They typically exhibit:

- Intact cognition, affect outside the delusion.
- Relatively preserved social, occupational functioning.
- Lack of insight into irrationality of their delusions.
- Possible irritability, aggression when delusions are challenged.

Treatment Options

Medications

- *Antipsychotics:* Risperidone and aripiprazole are commonly used. Can help reduce the intensity of delusional beliefs and improve overall functioning. Start with low doses and titrate slowly to monitor for side effects and efficacy.

Therapies

- *Cognitive behavioral therapy:* Helps the patient challenge/reframe delusional beliefs, promoting adaptive thinking.
- *Supportive therapy:* Focuses on improving the patient's overall functioning and coping strategies without directly confronting their delusional beliefs.
- *Psychoeducation:* Educates the patient and family about the disorder, treatment options, and coping mechanisms.

Management Tips

- *Build rapport:* Establishing trust is critical as patients are often wary of treatment.
- *Take a nonconfrontational approach:* Avoid directly challenging delusions; focus on managing symptoms and improving quality of life. Validate the patient's emotions without endorsing their delusions.
- *Monitor adherence:* Ensure regular follow-up to assess medication adherence and therapeutic engagement. Noncompliance is common due to poor insight.
- *Engage in safety planning:* Assess and manage any potential risks related to the delusions, such as harm to self or others, particularly in cases of persecutory or jealous delusions.

Prognosis

The prognosis for delusional disorder varies. Factors influencing prognosis include:

- *Duration of disorder:* Longer duration before treatment typically indicates a more chronic course.
- *Type of delusions:* Nonbizarre, situationally plausible delusions tend to respond better to treatment.
- *Insight:* Patients with some level of insight may have better outcomes.
- *Comorbid conditions:* Presence of other psychiatric or medical conditions can complicate treatment.

Many patients achieve significant symptom reduction and functional improvement with consistent treatment. However, some may experience persistent delusional beliefs that require long-term management.

Brief Psychotic Disorder

Brief psychotic disorder (BPD), also known as brief reactive psychosis, looks just like schizophrenia but is short-lived and typically presents with a much more favorable prognosis. Here we review the diagnosis and management of this condition.

Diagnosis

- *Onset:* Symptoms appear suddenly, often triggered by a significant stressor.
- *Symptoms:* Delusions, hallucinations, disorganized speech, or severely disorganized or catatonic behavior.
- *Duration:* Symptoms last for more than one day but less than one month, and then the patient returns to their normal level of functioning.
- *Exclusion:* Symptoms cannot be due to another psychiatric disorder, like substance use or a medical condition.

Specifiers

- With marked stressors (common examples include death, natural disasters, and major life changes like immigration).
- Without marked stressors.
- With postpartum onset (symptoms start within four weeks postpartum).
- With catatonia (if the patient shows signs of catatonia).

Evaluation

Rule out other causes by:

- Checking urine toxicology.
- Obtaining basic admission labs.
- Obtaining brain imaging to rule out neurological causes (eg, tumors, stroke).

Treatment Plan

- Medications:
  - *Antipsychotics:* For managing acute symptoms. Treat for one to three months, with a gradual taper as the patient's symptoms resolve.
  - *Benzodiazepines:* Use short term for agitation or anxiety.
- As the patient recovers, provide supportive psychotherapy to help them process the event and develop coping strategies.
- Arrange close outpatient follow-up after discharge to ensure there is no progression to a more chronic psychotic disorder.
- Educate patients and families about early warning signs of psychosis and the importance of sticking to the treatment plan.

Prognosis

- BPD generally has a favorable prognosis, with most patients returning to their baseline level of functioning.
- However, some individuals may experience recurrent episodes, especially if the original stressor recurs or if new significant stressors arise.

Antipsychotic Comparison: Quick Reference

Note: Information is accurate as of September 2024. Listing is alphabetical by brand name. Abbreviations used: EPS (extrapyramidal symptoms); FGA (first-generation antipsychotic); IM (intramuscular); LAI (long-acting injectable); ODT (orally disintegrating tablet); SGA (second-generation antipsychotic); TD (tardive dyskinesia).

Abilify (Aripiprazole)
- *Starting dose:* 2–5 mg/day.
- *Target dose:* 10–30 mg/day.
- *LAI:* Available. Abilify Maintena: 300–400 mg Q4 weeks; Aristada Initio: 675 mg; Aristada: 441–1064 mg Q4–6 weeks, 300–724 mg Q6 weeks.
- *IM for agitation:* Not available.
- *ODT:* Available.
- *Advantages:* Low risk of weight gain and metabolic side effects; approved for depression augmentation.
- *Disadvantages:* Akathisia is a common side effect.

Caplyta (Lumateperone)
- *Starting dose:* 42 mg/day.
- *Target dose:* 42 mg/day.
- *LAI:* Not available.
- *IM for agitation:* Not available.
- *ODT:* Not available.
- *Advantages:* Low risk of EPS, metabolic side effects, and prolactin elevation; approved for schizophrenia and bipolar depression.
- *Disadvantages:* Limited long-term data; expensive due to lack of generic options.

Clozapine
- *Starting dose:* 12.5–25 mg/day.
- *Target dose:* 300–900 mg/day.
- *LAI:* Not available.
- *IM for agitation:* Not available.
- *ODT:* Available: FazaClo.
- *Advantages:* Gold standard for treatment-resistant schizophrenia; effective for positive and negative symptoms; low risk of EPS and TD.
- *Disadvantages:* Agranulocytosis risk requiring regular blood monitoring; significant metabolic side effects; sedation; anticholinergic effects; increased risk of seizures.

Fanapt (Iloperidone)
- *Starting dose:* 1 mg twice daily.
- *Target dose:* 12–24 mg/day.
- *LAI:* Not available.
- *IM for agitation:* Not available.
- *ODT:* Not available.
- *Advantages:* Lower risk of weight gain and metabolic side effects; lower risk of EPS and TD.
- *Disadvantages:* Requires slow titration due to the risk of orthostatic hypotension; limited data compared to other SGAs.

Geodon (Ziprasidone)
- *Starting dose:* 20–40 mg/day.
- *Target dose:* 40–160 mg/day.
- *LAI:* Not available.
- *IM for agitation:* Available. 10–20 mg IM for agitation; may be used for acute agitation.
- *ODT:* Not available.
- *Advantages:* Low risk of metabolic side effects; low risk of EPS and TD.
- *Disadvantages:* QT prolongation risk; must take with food for adequate absorption.

Haldol (Haloperidol)
- *Starting dose:* 0.5–2 mg/day.
- *Target dose:* 5–20 mg/day.
- *LAI:* Available. 50–100 mg Q4 weeks.

- *IM for agitation:* Available. 5 mg IM for agitation, often combined as "B-52" cocktail with lorazepam (Ativan) and diphenhydramine (Benadryl).
- *IV for agitation:* Only antipsychotic available as an IV formulation, often used in ICUs for agitation.
- *ODT:* Not available, but oral liquid concentrate is available (2 mg/mL).
- *Advantages:* Inexpensive; long track record; anecdotally unusually effective for severe psychosis with agitation.
- *Disadvantages:* Higher risk of EPS and TD.

Invega (Paliperidone)

- *Starting dose:* 3–6 mg/day.
- *Target dose:* 3–12 mg/day.
- *LAI:*
  - Invega Sustenna: Loading 234 mg, 156 mg one week later, 117 mg three weeks later, then monthly.
  - Invega Trinza: 234–819 mg Q12 weeks.
  - Invega Hafyera: 1092–1560 mg Q6 months.
- *IM for agitation:* Not available.
- *ODT:* Not available.
- *Advantages:* Moderate weight gain potential; available in several LAI formulations.
- *Disadvantages:* Risk of prolactin elevation.

Latuda (Lurasidone)

- *Starting dose:* 20–40 mg/day.
- *Target dose:* 40–160 mg/day.
- *LAI:* Not available.
- *IM for agitation:* Not available.
- *ODT:* Not available.
- *Advantages:* Low risk of metabolic side effects; low risk of EPS and TD; approved for bipolar depression.
- *Disadvantages:* Must be taken with food for adequate absorption; some risk of akathisia.

Nuplazid (Pimavanserin)

- *Starting dose:* 34 mg/day.
- *Target dose:* 34 mg/day.
- *LAI:* Not available.
- *IM for agitation:* Not available.
- *ODT:* Not available.
- *Advantages:* Specifically approved for Parkinson's disease psychosis; no known risk of worsening motor symptoms in Parkinson's patients; low risk of EPS and TD.
- *Disadvantages:* Not generic, so expensive; limited use outside of Parkinson's disease psychosis; less studied for other indications.

Prolixin (Fluphenazine)

- *Starting dose:* 2.5–5 mg/day.
- *Target dose:* 5–20 mg/day.
- *LAI:* Available. 12.5–50 mg Q2–4 weeks.
- *IM for agitation:* Available. 2.5–10 mg IM for acute agitation.
- *ODT:* Not available.
- *Advantages:* Long track record; LAI formulation available.
- *Disadvantages:* Higher risk of EPS and TD compared to SGAs.

Rexulti (Brexpiprazole)

- *Starting dose:* 1–2 mg/day.
- *Target dose:* 2–4 mg/day.
- *LAI:* Not available.
- *IM for agitation:* Not available.
- *ODT:* Not available.
- *Advantages:* Low risk of metabolic side effects; low risk of EPS and TD.
- *Disadvantages:* Not generic, so very expensive.

Risperdal (Risperidone)

- *Starting dose:* 1–2 mg/day.
- *Target dose:* 4–6 mg/day.
- *LAI:* Available. Risperdal Consta: 25–50 mg Q2 weeks; Perseris: 90–120 mg Q4 weeks.

- *IM for agitation:* Not available.
- *ODT:* Available. Risperdal M-Tab.
- *Advantages:* Often considered a first-line treatment due to efficacy and moderate side effects.
- *Disadvantages:* Higher risk of EPS and prolactin elevation compared to other SGAs.

Saphris (Asenapine)

- *Starting dose:* 5 mg sublingually twice daily.
- *Target dose:* 10 mg sublingually twice daily.
- *LAI:* Not available.
- *IM for agitation:* Not available.
- *ODT:* Not available.
- *Advantages:* Low risk of weight gain and metabolic side effects; sublingual administration may be advantageous for some patients.
- *Disadvantages:* Sublingual administration can be inconvenient; may cause oral hypoesthesia (numbness of the mouth).

Seroquel (Quetiapine)

- *Starting dose:* 25–50 mg/day (immediate release) or 300 mg/day (extended release).
- *Target dose:* 150–800 mg/day.
- *LAI:* Not available.
- *IM for agitation:* Not available.
- *ODT:* Not available.
- *Advantages:* Low risk of EPS and TD; useful for patients with insomnia; approved for bipolar depression.
- *Disadvantages:* Higher risk of sedation, orthostatic hypotension, and metabolic side effects compared to other SGAs.

Thorazine (Chlorpromazine)

- *Starting dose:* 25–50 mg/day.
- *Target dose:* 100–800 mg/day.
- *LAI:* Not available.
- *IM for agitation:* Available. 25–50 mg.
- *ODT:* Not available.
- *Advantages:* Inexpensive; long track record; useful for severe agitation.
- *Disadvantages:* Higher risk of EPS and TD compared to SGAs; sedation; anticholinergic effects.

Trilafon (Perphenazine)

- *Starting dose:* 4–8 mg/day.
- *Target dose:* 8–64 mg/day.
- *LAI:* Not available.
- *IM for agitation:* Not available.
- *ODT:* Not available.
- *Advantages:* Good choice among FGAs; minimal weight gain; well tolerated overall.
- *Disadvantages:* Higher risk of EPS and TD compared to most SGAs.

Vraylar (Cariprazine)

- *Starting dose:* 1.5 mg/day.
- *Target dose:* 3–6 mg/day.
- *LAI:* Not available.
- *IM for agitation:* Not available.
- *ODT:* Not available.
- *Advantages:* Low risk of metabolic side effects; low risk of EPS and TD.
- *Disadvantages:* No generic, so very expensive; akathisia is a common side effect.

Zyprexa (Olanzapine)

- *Starting dose:* 5–10 mg/day.
- *Target dose:* 10–20 mg/day.
- *LAI:* Available. Zyprexa Relprevv: 210–405 mg Q2–4 weeks.
- *IM for agitation:* Available. 10 mg IM.
- *ODT:* Available. Zyprexa Zydis.
- *Advantages:* Possibly more effective than other antipsychotics; olanzapine + samidorphan combination (Lybalvi) decreases weight gain.
- *Disadvantages:* Very significant metabolic side effects, including weight gain and increased risk of diabetes.

Clozapine: Guidelines for Use and Monitoring

Clozapine is an important option for your patients with treatment-resistant schizophrenia. It's also particularly effective in reducing suicide risk for those with schizophrenia or schizoaffective disorder. However, due to its potential serious side effects, you'll need to be diligent with dosing and rigorous in monitoring. Here's a rundown of the current guidelines for prescribing clozapine and managing its risks.

Before initiating clozapine, you'll need to enroll in the Clozapine Risk Evaluation and Mitigation Strategy (REMS) program. Visit the Clozapine REMS website to create an account: https://www.newclozapinerems.com/home.

Clozapine-Induced Agranulocytosis

Clozapine-induced agranulocytosis, where the absolute neutrophil count (ANC) drops below 500/µL, is a serious side effect, occurring in approximately 0.8% of patients. The highest risk is within the first six months of treatment.

Before starting clozapine, the patient's initial ANC must be at least 1500/µL, or 1000/µL for those with benign ethnic neutropenia (BEN).

Start with a low dose, typically 12.5 mg once or twice daily, and gradually titrate upward to avoid hypotension, bradycardia, and sedation. You can increase by 25–50 mg per day, aiming for a therapeutic dose range of 300–600 mg per day, though some patients may require doses up to 900 mg per day. If a patient misses two or more days of clozapine, restart the dosing titration from the beginning (although you can increase it more rapidly).

Monitoring for Agranulocytosis

- *Weekly monitoring:* Perform weekly complete blood counts for the first six months of treatment.
- *Biweekly monitoring:* After six months of stable ANC levels, reduce monitoring to every two weeks.
- *Monthly monitoring:* After one year of stable ANC levels, reduce monitoring to once monthly.

Therapeutic Drug Monitoring

Check clozapine serum levels five to seven days after reaching the target dose. Obtain a trough level (10–12 hours post-dose) to ensure it falls within the therapeutic range of 350–600 ng/mL.

What to Do in Cases of Neutropenia (Low ANC)

Mild neutropenia (ANC 1,000–1,499/µL, or 500–999/µL for patients with BEN)

- Continue clozapine treatment but increase ANC monitoring to three times weekly until ANC returns to ≥1,500/µL (or ≥1,000/µL for BEN patients).

Moderate neutropenia (ANC 500–999/µL; same for patients with BEN)

- Interrupt clozapine treatment.
- Monitor ANC daily.
- If ANC recovers to ≥1,000/µL within one week (or to ≥500/µL for BEN patients), cautiously reinitiate clozapine at a lower dose with close monitoring.
- Once the ANC fully recovers to ≥1,500/µL (or to ≥1,000/µL for BEN patients), you can resume the standard clozapine dose and monitoring schedule.

Severe neutropenia (ANC <500/µL for all patients including BEN)

- Immediately stop clozapine and transfer the patient to a medical ward for hematological evaluation and treatment, potentially with granulocyte colony-stimulating factor.
- Clozapine should generally be permanently discontinued in cases of severe neutropenia.

Other Adverse Effects

- *Myocarditis and cardiomyopathy:* Monitor for signs of myocarditis, especially during the first eight weeks of treatment. Symptoms include chest pain, dyspnea, and palpitations. Get a baseline ECG and check troponin levels weekly for at least the first four weeks.
- *Seizures:* Clozapine lowers the seizure threshold, particularly at higher doses or with clozapine blood levels that exceed 600 mcg/L. Consider dose reduction or the addition of an anticonvulsant in patients at risk.
- *Metabolic syndrome:* Monitor for weight gain, hyperglycemia, and lipid abnormalities, with regular checks on weight, fasting glucose, HbA1c, and lipid profile.
- *Sialorrhea:* Excessive salivation is a common side effect. You can manage it with anticholinergic meds or nonpharmacological options, like chewing gum or adjusting the patient's sleeping position.
- *Constipation:* Very common side effect. Encourage patients to increase their fiber and fluid intake and prescribe a stool softener or laxative if needed. Manage this early; constipation can be so severe as to lead to bowel obstruction in some cases.

Patient Education

Educate patients and their families on the importance of adherence to the medication regimen and the blood monitoring schedule. Inform them about potential side effects and instruct them to report symptoms like fever, sore throat, or signs of infection immediately.

Long-Acting Injectable Antipsychotics

You've probably encountered patients who are reluctant about receiving regular injections of medications, but it's important to stress the significant benefits of long-acting injectables (LAIs). Their ability to maintain consistent antipsychotic blood levels makes them advantageous not only for those struggling with pill adherence, but also for anyone requiring antipsychotic treatment. In this fact sheet, we start with practical tips on how to choose an LAI, followed by basic prescribing information for each of the LAIs currently available.

Tips on Prescribing LAIs

- The following types of patients are the best candidates for LAIs:
  - Patients who have been nonadherent with antipsychotics due to factors like forgetfulness or difficulty managing daily medications.
  - Patients with a history of recurrent relapses, often linked to medication nonadherence.
  - Patients who prefer the convenience of LAIs over daily medication.
- Choose an LAI version of a medication your patient has previously taken orally to make sure it's effective and well tolerated.
- If you have a patient who is starting a new oral antipsychotic, consider whether they are a good candidate for an LAI—and if they are, choose an oral med with this in mind, eg:
  - Risperidone or paliperidone oral: You can then switch to Invega Sustenna, Invega Trinza, Invega Hafyera, Perseris, Risperdal Consta, Rykindo, or Uzedy.
  - Aripiprazole oral: You can then switch to Abilify Maintena, Asimtufii, or Aristada.
- For patients who prefer less frequent dosing, Invega Trinza (Q3 months), Invega Hafyera (Q6 months), Aristada (up to Q8 weeks), and Uzedy (Q2 months) are good choices.
- If your patient is unlikely to be adherent to oral medications, even for a short while, consider LAIs that don't require an oral overlap: Invega Hafyera or Sustenna, Perseris, Relprevv, or Uzedy.
- Never start an LAI in patients with a history of neuroleptic malignant syndrome.
- LAIs may take longer to show full effects compared to oral medications. Avoid adjusting the LAI dosage too soon.

LAI Options

First-generation antipsychotics

- *Fluphenazine (Prolixin Decanoate):* Administered every two to three weeks; painful injections; high risk of extrapyramidal symptoms and tardive dyskinesia. Oral overlap necessary.
- *Haloperidol (Haldol Decanoate):* Dosed monthly. Oral overlap required, although you can use a "loading dose" method (20 times oral dose, followed by 10–15 times oral dose in subsequent months) that requires no oral overlap.

Second-generation antipsychotics

- *Abilify Maintena:* Dosed monthly. Requires 14-day oral overlap. Good side effect profile.
- *Abilify Asimtufii:* Dosed every two months. Requires 14-day oral overlap. Good side effect profile.
- *Aristada:* Dosed monthly, every six weeks, or every two months. Requires 21-day oral overlap unless you give your patient a dose of Aristada Initio 675 mg plus 30 mg oral aripiprazole on the same day as your first dose of Aristada. The first dose of Aristada may be delayed up to 10 days after Initio. Good side effect profile.
- *Zyprexa Relprevv:* Biweekly or monthly dosing. No oral overlap. There's a small risk (less than 1%) of a postinjection delirium/sedation syndrome caused by accidental intravascular injection, so you must give the injection at a registered health care facility where patients can be continuously monitored for at least three hours after the injection.
- *Invega Sustenna:* Monthly dosing. No oral overlap and has the potential to transition to every-three-month and every-six-month formulations.
- *Invega Trinza:* Dosed every three months, but your patient must have done well on monthly injections of Sustenna for at least four months before switching to Trinza.
- *Invega Hafyera:* Dosed every six months, but your patient must have done well on monthly injections of Sustenna for at least four months or on Trinza for at least one three-month cycle.
- *Risperdal Consta:* Dosed every two weeks. Requires a three-week oral overlap. Painful injection.
- *Rykindo:* Dosed every two weeks. One-week oral overlap.
- *Perseris:* Dosed monthly. No oral overlap. Dosed subcutaneously rather than a deep and more painful IM injection. The highest dose of Perseris is equivalent to 4 mg/day of oral risperidone.
- *Uzedy:* Dosed monthly or every two months. No oral overlap. Subcutaneous dosing like Perseris.

Table 3: **Long-Acting Injectable Antipsychotics**

Generic Name (Brand Name) Year FDA Approved *[G] denotes generic availability*	Relevant FDA Indication(s)	Available Strengths	Oral Overlap	Dosing Interval	Initial Dosing	Maintenance Dose*	Cost for Monthly Supply at Average Dose (September 2023)
First-Generation Antipsychotics							
Fluphenazine decanoate [G] (Prolixin Decanoate [brand discontinued]) 1972	Schizophrenia	25 mg/mL	Continue total oral dose for 2–3 days, then ↓ by 50% increments every 2–3 days until discontinued (by next injection)	2–3 weeks	1.25× total daily oral dose Q2–3 weeks (eg, 10 mg/day oral ~ 12.5 mg IM Q2–3 weeks)	Increase in increments of 12.5 mg; do not exceed 100 mg per dose; usual dose 6.25–25 mg Q2–3 weeks	$ [G]
Haloperidol decanoate [G] (Haldol Decanoate) 1986	Schizophrenia	50 mg/mL and 100 mg/mL	Decrease oral dose by 50% after first injection, then discontinue after second injection (third for some patients); alternatively, no oral overlap if loading dose of 20× oral given	4 weeks	10–15× total oral daily dose (eg, 10 mg/day oral ~ 100–150 mg IM). Alternatively, 20× total oral daily dose if loading dose with no oral overlap (eg, 10 mg/day oral ~ 200 mg IM). First dose should be ≤100 mg; if higher dose needed, give remainder in 1–2 weeks	Continue 10–15× total oral daily dose Q4 weeks with either method (eg, 10 mg/day ~ 100–150 mg IM Q4 weeks)	$ [G] $$$$ Haldol Dec
Second-Generation Antipsychotics							
Aripiprazole (Abilify Maintena) 2013	Schizophrenia Bipolar disorder	300 mg and 400 mg vials and prefilled syringes	For 14 days	4 weeks	400 mg Q4 weeks (estimated equivalence is 15–20 mg/day oral ~ 300 mg IM monthly and 20–30 mg/day oral ~ 400 mg IM monthly)	400 mg Q4 weeks; decrease to 300 mg Q4 weeks if side effects	$$$$$
Aripiprazole (Abilify Asimtufii) 2023	Schizophrenia Bipolar disorder	720, 960 mg syringes	For 14 days	2 months	960 mg every two months; give 720 mg if 2D6 poor metabolizer or taking 2D6 or 3A4 inhibitor	Continue initial dosing every two months or reduce dose to 720 mg if adverse effects at higher dose	$$$$$
Aripiprazole lauroxil (Aristada) 2015	Schizophrenia	441, 662, 882, 1064 mg	For 21 days	Monthly, every 6 weeks, or every 2 months	441, 662, or 882 mg monthly (equivalent to 10, 15, and 20 mg/ day); or 882 mg every 6 weeks (15 mg/day); or 1064 mg every 2 months (15 mg/day)	Continue initial dosing or adjust based on clinical response	$$$$$
Aripiprazole lauroxil (Aristada Initio) 2018	Schizophrenia	675 mg syringes	Aripiprazole 30 mg PO ×1 dose	See Aristada above	To be given as single initial dose, in conjunction with Aristada as above (on same day or within 10 days of Initio)	See above	$$$$$
Olanzapine (Zyprexa Relprevv) 2009	Schizophrenia	210, 300, 405 mg vials	No overlap	2–4 weeks	• 10 mg/day oral: 210 mg Q2 weeks ×4 doses or 405 mg Q4 weeks • ×2 doses • 15 mg/day oral: 300 mg Q2 weeks ×4 doses • 20 mg/day oral: 300 mg Q2 weeks	• 10 mg/day oral: 150 mg Q2 weeks or 300 mg Q4 weeks • 15 mg/day oral: 210 mg Q2 weeks or 405 mg Q4 weeks • 20 mg/day oral: 300 mg Q2 weeks • Maximum dose: 300 mg Q2 weeks or 405 mg Q4 weeks	$$$$$

Generic Name (Brand Name) Year FDA Approved *[G] denotes generic availability*	Relevant FDA Indication(s)	Available Strengths	Oral Overlap	Dosing Interval	Initial Dosing	Maintenance Dose*	Cost for Monthly Supply at Average Dose (September 2023)
Paliperidone palmitate (Invega Sustenna) 2009	Schizophrenia Schizoaffective disorder (monotherapy or adjunct)	39, 78, 117, 156, 234 mg in prefilled syringes	No overlap	4 weeks	234 mg IM in deltoid, then 156 mg 1 week later	117 mg 3 weeks after second dose then Qmonth; may adjust monthly dose (maintenance given deltoid or gluteal) Approx. equivalence: • 3 mg oral: 39–78 mg • 6 mg oral: 117 mg • 12 mg oral: 234 mg	$$$$$
Paliperidone palmitate (Invega Trinza) 2015	Schizophrenia (only after at least 4 months of adequate treatment on Invega Sustenna)	273, 410, 546, 819 mg in prefilled syringes	No overlap	3 months	Based on previous monthly Invega Sustenna dose: • For 78 mg, give 273 mg Trinza • For 117 mg, give 410 mg Trinza • For 156 mg, give 546 mg Trinza • For 234 mg, give 819 mg Trinza	Give same conversion dose of Trinza every 3 months; adjust if necessary per patient response	$$$$$
Paliperidone palmitate (Invega Hafyera) 2021	Schizophrenia (only after at least 4 months of adequate treatment on Sustenna or 3 months on Trinza)	1,092, 1,560 mg in prefilled syringes	No overlap	6 months	Based on previous monthly Sustenna dose: • For 156 mg, give 1,092 mg Hafyera • For 234 mg, give 1,560 mg Hafyera Or 3-month Trinza dose: • For 546 mg, give 1,092 mg Hafyera • For 819 mg, give 1,560 mg Hafyera	Give same conversion dose of Hafyera every 6 months; adjust if necessary per patient response	$$$$$
Risperidone (Perseris) 2018	Schizophrenia	90, 120 mg	No overlap	Monthly	Start 90 or 120 mg SQ to abdomen monthly	Approx. equivalence: 90 mg monthly: 3 mg/day oral 120 mg monthly: 4 mg/day oral	$$$$$
Risperidone (Uzedy) 2023	Schizophrenia	50, 75, 100, 125, 150, 200, 250 mg syringes	No overlap	Monthly or every 2 months	Start equivalent monthly or every-2-month dose the day after last oral dose, given SQ to abdomen or upper arm: • For 2 mg/day oral, give 50 mg monthly or 100 mg Q2 months Uzedy • For 3 mg/day oral, give 75 mg monthly or 150 mg Q2 months Uzedy • For 4 mg/day oral, give 100 mg monthly or 200 mg Q2 months Uzedy • For 5 mg/day oral, give 125 mg monthly or 250 mg Q2 months Uzedy	Continue initial dosing or adjust based on clinical response	$$$$$

Generic Name (Brand Name) Year FDA Approved *[C] denotes generic availability*	Relevant FDA Indication(s)	Available Strengths	Oral Overlap	Dosing Interval	Initial Dosing	Maintenance Dose*	Cost for Monthly Supply at Average Dose (September 2023)
Risperidone (Risperdal Consta) 2003	Schizophrenia Bipolar, manic/mixed (monotherapy or adjunct)	12.5, 25, 37.5, 50 mg vials	With usual oral dose for 21 days	2 weeks	Start at 25 mg Q2 weeks; adjust dose no more frequently than Q4 weeks as needed for response	Approx. equivalence: • <4 mg/day oral: 25 mg • 4–6 mg/day oral: 37.5 mg • >6 mg/day oral: 50 mg • Maximum dose: 50 mg Q2 weeks	$$$$$
Risperidone (Rykindo) 2023	Schizophrenia Bipolar disorder	12.5, 25, 37.5, 50	For 7 days	2 weeks	Start at 25 mg Q2 weeks; adjust dose no more frequently than Q4 weeks as needed for response	Approx. equivalence: • <4 mg/day oral: 25 mg • 4–6 mg/day oral: 37.5 mg • >6 mg/day oral: 50 mg • Maximum dose: 50 mg Q2 weeks	$$$$$

Discontinuing and Switching Antipsychotics

We often switch antipsychotics due to side effects or lack of efficacy. There are two types of switches: immediate and cross-tapering. You can use either one, though cross-tapering is more standard.

Cross-Tapering

- Ideally, cross-tapering involves gradually tapering the old drug while gradually titrating up the dose of the new drug. Of course, we've likely all seen cases in which an intended cross-taper stalled and resulted in unintended long-term polypharmacy.
- Anecdotally, it appears that most clinicians use the cross-tapering strategy, because it seems like the more cautious and reasonable approach. It minimizes the risk of withdrawal symptoms from the original medication and adverse reactions to the new drug.
- While there's not much evidence that this approach is any better than immediate switching, we recommend it when time allows.

Example of a Cross-Tapering Schedule: Risperidone to Aripiprazole

Initial conditions:

- Patient is currently on risperidone 4 mg/day.

Week 1:

- Reduce risperidone to 3 mg/day.
- Start aripiprazole at a low dose (eg, 5 mg/day).

Week 2:

- Reduce risperidone to 2 mg/day.
- Increase aripiprazole to 10 mg/day.

Week 3:

- Reduce risperidone to 1 mg/day.
- Increase aripiprazole to 15 mg/day.

Week 4:

- Discontinue risperidone.
- Continue aripiprazole 15 mg/day or adjust up to 15 mg BID based on response and tolerability.

Immediate Switching

- Immediate switching involves beginning the new medication on the same day that you discontinue the old one.
- This method appears just as effective as cross-tapering in preventing relapse, and there is no evidence of more side effects.

Special Considerations

- *Cholinergic rebound:* Antipsychotics like clozapine and olanzapine are particularly anticholinergic. This can lead to cholinergic supersensitivity: When these meds are stopped (or when you switch a patient to a less anticholinergic drug), symptoms of the parasympathetic nervous system can result, including nausea, vomiting, diarrhea, headache, sweating, and insomnia. Taper these anticholinergic medications gradually, such as over the course of two to four weeks, to minimize this risk.
- *Withdrawal from long-acting injectables (LAIs):* When switching from LAI antipsychotics (eg, Invega Sustenna, Abilify Maintena), withdrawal symptoms might not show up for several weeks due to the long half-life of these medications.
- *Supersensitivity psychosis:* Relapse to mood or psychotic symptoms is more likely when patients abruptly stop antipsychotic medications. Taper meds over two to four weeks to minimize this risk.
- *Withdrawal dyskinesia:* This can occur after stopping or reducing the dose of an antipsychotic. Symptoms look like tardive dyskinesia (lip puckering, tongue movements, etc). If it persists, reintroduce an antipsychotic at low doses (eg, quetiapine 100 mg BID) that you can then taper gradually.

COMMON PSYCHIATRIC CONDITIONS

Substance Use Disorders

Managing Alcohol Withdrawal

Psychiatric patients often have comorbid alcohol use disorders. While mild to moderate alcohol withdrawal can be managed on the psychiatric unit, cases with severe autonomic instability, seizure history, or significant medical issues require transfer to the medical floor. This article provides practical guidance on the management of mild to moderate alcohol withdrawal on psych units.

Time Course

Alcohol withdrawal symptoms typically appear six to eight hours after the last drink and can persist for up to 72 hours. However, heavy drinkers may experience delayed onset (around 24 hours after the last drink), and their withdrawal symptoms may last a week or longer.

Symptoms

- Insomnia, anxiety, tremors, sweating, palpitations, headache, GI upset, irritability, elevated blood pressure, tachycardia, hyperthermia, diaphoresis, hyperarousal, and disorientation.
- Severe cases may lead to withdrawal seizures (six to 48 hours following the last drink) or alcoholic hallucinosis (12–48 hours following the last drink).
- Delirium tremens (DT) can occur 48–96 hours after the last drink and is characterized by disorientation, hallucinations, tremors, tachycardia, hypertension, hyperthermia, anxiety, and diaphoresis. DT has a 5%–8% mortality rate.

Symptom-Triggered Withdrawal Protocol (CIWA Protocol)

The CIWA Protocol is the primary method for managing inpatient alcohol withdrawal. It involves assessing withdrawal symptoms using the Clinical Institute Withdrawal Assessment for Alcohol Scale (CIWA) on admission and every two to six hours, dosing medications based on symptom severity:

1. Initial loading dose of benzodiazepine administered upon admission (eg, chlordiazepoxide 50 mg or diazepam 20 mg PO; or oxazepam 30 mg or lorazepam 2 mg for patients with liver disease).
2. Medication dosing based on CIWA scores:
    - 0–4: No withdrawal; no medication.
    - 5–11: Mild withdrawal; chlordiazepoxide 25 mg or lorazepam 1 mg.
    - 12–20: Moderate withdrawal; chlordiazepoxide 50 mg or lorazepam 2 mg.
    - >20: Severe withdrawal; chlordiazepoxide 75–100 mg or lorazepam 3–4 mg.
3. CIWA assessments are discontinued when the patient scores below 5 for 24 hours.
4. Typical detox duration is three to four days.

Scheduled Dosing and Comfort Medications for Alcohol Withdrawal

Scheduled tapers can be beneficial for certain inpatients, particularly those who may be exaggerating symptoms or have underlying anxiety disorders. Here's a typical five-day chlordiazepoxide protocol (substitute diazepam, lorazepam, oxazepam, or other benzodiazepines depending on your hospital's protocol and the needs of the patient):

- Day 1: Loading dose of chlordiazepoxide 50 mg on admission.
- Day 1: Chlordiazepoxide 50 mg every six hours (QID).
- Days 2–3: Chlordiazepoxide 50 mg three times daily (TID).
- Day 4: Chlordiazepoxide 50 mg twice daily (BID).
- Day 5: Chlordiazepoxide 50 mg at bedtime (last day of chlordiazepoxide).

Hybrid Management (Scheduled Plus CIWA)

Initially use scheduled dosing but also order CIWA assessments. This approach allows for dose adjustments based on CIWA scores.

Managing Opioid Withdrawal

Who Is Likely to Experience Withdrawal Symptoms?

- Risk group: Anyone consistently taking opioids for two weeks or more.
- Predictors of severe withdrawal: Daily use, high dosage, and use of short-acting opioids.

Common Symptoms of Opioid Withdrawal: FLU OPRS Mnemonic

- **F**lu-like: Fever, sweating, chills.
- **L**eg movements: Restlessness, kicking.
- **U**nwell: General malaise.
- **O**veractive reflexes: Twitches, spasms.
- **P**ain: Muscles, stomach, bones.
- **R**uns: Diarrhea.
- **S**leep: Insomnia.

Withdrawal Time Course

- *Fentanyl:* Onset 3–12 hours, peak 12–36 hours, duration 5–7 days.
- *Heroin:* Onset 8–24 hours, peak 36–72 hours, duration 7–10 days.
- *Short-acting analgesics (eg, hydrocodone, oxycodone):* Onset 6–12 hours, peak 12–36 hours, duration 5–7 days.
- *Long-acting analgesics (eg, morphine):* Onset 8–24 hours, peak 36–72 hours, duration 7–10 days.
- *Methadone:* Onset 1–3 days, peak 4–7 days, duration 2–4 weeks.

Severity Measurement

Severity is measured with the Clinical Opiate Withdrawal Scale (COWS), which is clinician-administered (for the scale and instructions, visit www.thecarlatreport.com/AdministeringCOWS.

Management of Withdrawal Symptoms

Opioid-assisted: Can use either buprenorphine or methadone (though buprenorphine is most common).

Buprenorphine

- Start when the patient is in mild/moderate withdrawal (COWS score 8–12).
- Prescribe 4 mg SL buprenorphine; reevaluate the patient after 30–45 minutes to assess withdrawal symptoms and determine if another 4 mg SL buprenorphine is necessary.
- Reevaluate the patient after another 30–45 minutes and administer another 4 mg SL buprenorphine if the patient still has a COWS score of 8–12.
- A total of 12 mg SL buprenorphine is usually sufficient.
- Once you know the total dose needed, administer it once daily.
- Encourage patients to remain on buprenorphine long term, even after withdrawal symptoms subside, as they'll otherwise face a high risk of relapse/overdose after discharge. Remember to refer them for outpatient buprenorphine treatment.

Methadone

- Methadone can also be used to treat opioid withdrawal. Consider methadone for patients who have difficulty tolerating the mild withdrawal symptoms needed for treatment with buprenorphine, or those who refuse buprenorphine.
- Start with a single 20–30 mg dose of methadone. You can give small additional doses of 5–10 mg at a time if the patient is still experiencing withdrawal symptoms. Maximum dose in 24 hours is 40 mg.
- Again, encourage patients to remain on methadone long term. Patients who elect to stay on methadone will need to be referred to a federally regulated opioid treatment program (aka "methadone clinic"). Typical daily doses of methadone in these programs are 40–120 mg, though some patients may require higher doses.
- For patients who refuse longer-term treatment, maintain 40 mg daily for two to three days, and then taper off as tolerated over the course of a week or so.

Symptom-based treatment (when opioid detox is not available)

- Autonomic symptoms (GI distress, anxiety, sweating, cramping): Clonidine 0.1–0.2 mg Q1 hour; max 0.8 mg/day. Check blood pressure before each dose.
- Nausea: Ondansetron 4 mg Q4–6 hours; max 16 mg/day.
- Diarrhea: Loperamide 4 mg, then 2 mg after each loose stool; max 16 mg/day.
- Cramps: Dicyclomine 10–20 mg Q6 hours.
- Muscle spasm: Methocarbamol 750–1500 mg Q8 hours or cyclobenzaprine 5–10 mg Q8 hours; max 30 mg/day.

Treatment of Stimulant Use Disorders

Stimulant use disorders are all too common among patients in psychiatric units. They exacerbate underlying psychiatric symptoms and can lead to serious medical complications. Plus, they're notoriously tricky to distinguish from primary psychiatric disorders. Here we review how to manage stimulant use disorders on the psychiatric unit.

Overview of Psychostimulants

- *Prescription stimulants:* Used for ADHD but misused when taken without a prescription. Examples include methylphenidate and amphetamine-based medications like lisdexamfetamine and dextroamphetamine. Their onset and duration vary based on the formulation.
- *Methamphetamine:* Known for its rapid onset and long duration (12–15 hours). Use is more prevalent in the Midwest and West Coast.
- *Cocaine:* Rapidly absorbed and short-acting (20–30 minutes), leading to frequent, successive use.

Distinguishing Stimulant-Induced Symptoms from Primary Psychiatric Diagnoses

Stimulant use can mimic primary psychiatric conditions, making it difficult to differentiate between the two. It's important to consider whether the symptoms are acute (intoxication), chronic (long-term use), or related to withdrawal. Here are symptoms to watch for in each category.

Acute symptoms (intoxication)

- *Hallucinations and paranoia:* Auditory, visual, and even tactile hallucinations (such as formication, the sensation of insects crawling on or under the skin) can occur during acute intoxication.
- *Mood disturbances:* Rapid mood changes, ranging from euphoria and hyperactivity to irritability and agitation.
- *Cognitive impairment:* Increased alertness and concentration in the short term, but often accompanied by confusion and disorganized thinking.

Chronic symptoms (long-term use)

- *Hallucinations and paranoia:* Persistent hallucinations and delusional thinking can develop with chronic use.
- *Mood disturbances:* Prolonged use can lead to chronic mood instability, including persistent irritability, anxiety, and depression.
- *Cognitive impairment:* Long-term use is associated with attention deficits, memory problems, and slowed cognitive processing.

Withdrawal symptoms (detox)

- *Mood disturbances:* Depression, fatigue, and anhedonia (inability to feel pleasure) are common during withdrawal.
- *Cognitive impairment:* Difficulty concentrating and memory issues may persist during the detox period.
- *Physical symptoms:* Increased appetite, sleep disturbances, and general malaise.

Diagnostic Steps

1. Gather detailed collateral information to identify the temporal relationship between substance use and psychiatric symptoms. Do hallucinations occur only when the patient is using stimulants, or do they persist even during periods of abstinence?
2. Obtain a urine drug screen (UDS). Keep in mind that a negative test does not rule out stimulant use. Methamphetamine, cocaine, and prescription stimulants can only be detected in a UDS for two to four days.
3. Watch the patient over the first few days on the unit; stimulant-induced psychosis typically resolves much more quickly (within two to seven days) compared to primary psychotic disorders.

Management

Pharmacological treatments

While there are no FDA-approved treatments for stimulant use disorder, the following can be tried:

- *Naltrexone plus bupropion:* This combination treatment can help reduce methamphetamine cravings.
  - Dosage: Injectable naltrexone 380 mg every three weeks plus bupropion 450 mg daily, or naltrexone oral 50 mg daily plus bupropion 150 mg twice daily.
  - Efficacy: The response rate was 13.6% in one study, compared to 2.5% for placebo (Trivedi MH et al, *NEJM* 2021;384:140–153). That's a relatively low response rate, but still significantly better than placebo. Given the severe functional impairment and frequent relapses associated with methamphetamine use, this intervention may be worth considering.
- *Topiramate (25–200 mg daily) and mirtazapine (15–45 mg):* Some evidence for stimulant use disorder.
- *Stimulant substitution:* In certain cases, prescription stimulants (eg, methylphenidate for cocaine, mixed amphetamine salts for methamphetamine) have been used under very careful monitoring. This approach is based on the principle of harm reduction, replacing a dangerous unregulated drug with a safer prescription medication. An addiction specialist should be closely involved to minimize the risk of misuse after discharge.

Nonpharmacological treatments

- *Cognitive behavioral therapy:* To help patients recognize and change maladaptive behaviors.
- *12-step programs and peer support groups:* Encourage participation in the unit's support groups and, if available, the unit's 12-step programs.

Referral to substance use programs

A frustration among clinicians working with patients who use stimulants is that they often are "frequent fliers" and return to the unit multiple times due to relapsing back to stimulant use. Here are tips to engage these patients in treatment:

- *Build rapport:* Work to establish trust using a nonjudgmental and empathic approach.
- *Emphasize the positive outcomes of treatment:* These include improved mental health, better relationships, and higher quality of life.
- *Employ motivational interviewing:* Use open-ended questions and reflective listening to highlight the impact of substance use (see the "Motivational Interviewing Techniques" fact sheet in the Psychotherapy on the Inpatient Unit section).

Possible medical complications to watch for

- *Infectious diseases:* Increased risk of HIV and hepatitis C due to risky behaviors. Provide testing and involve the medical team as needed.
- *"Meth mouth":* Severe dental decay and gum disease associated with methamphetamine use. Encourage dental hygiene on the unit and refer to dental services post-discharge.
- *Cardiovascular issues:* Hypertension, tachycardia, arrhythmias, myocardial infarction. These can occur even days after the last use of stimulants. Monitor vital signs regularly and consider cardiology consultation if needed.
- *Neurological complications:* Seizures, stroke. These risks persist even days after the last use of stimulants. Watch for focal neurological deficits and obtain imaging or EEG if indicated.

Incorporate harm reduction principles

- *Encourage safer methods of administration:* Advise patients to smoke instead of injecting to reduce the risk of infections and other complications.
- *Take steps to reduce the risk of accidental overdose of opioids:* Accidental fentanyl contamination in stimulants poses a risk for opioid overdose, even for those who do not primarily use opioids. At discharge, offer naloxone and provide fentanyl testing supplies. If your hospital does not offer fentanyl test strips, direct patients to resources where they can obtain these supplies, like:
  - Next Distro: A national mail-based harm reduction service that provides fentanyl test strips and other harm reduction supplies (www.nextdistro.org).
  - DanceSafe: A nonprofit organization that provides drug checking kits, including fentanyl test strips, and educational resources (www.dancesafe.org).
  - National Harm Reduction Coalition: A group that offers resources and information on harm reduction services across the US (www.harmreduction.org).
  - BTNX Inc.: A company that manufactures and sells fentanyl test strips online (www.btnx.com).

Wernicke's Encephalopathy

Wernicke's encephalopathy (WE) is an acute neurologic disorder arising from thiamine deficiency. It's more common than you might think, and if untreated it can progress to Korsakoff syndrome—an irreversible neuropsychiatric disorder characterized by global memory deficits and behavioral changes. If there's any chance your patient has WE, administer thiamine! It's safe and well tolerated, and it may well protect your patient from permanent brain damage and disability.

Etiology

Though classically linked to chronic alcoholism, thiamine deficiency can also result from malnutrition, restrictive eating disorders, hyperemesis gravidarum, gastric bypass surgery, and other conditions that result in inadequate nutrient absorption.

Epidemiology

Prevalence is 1%–3% according to autopsy studies.

Clinical Presentation

In patients with a history of malnutrition or chronic alcohol abuse, suspect WE if you notice any of the following—keeping in mind that all three symptoms occur in only 10% of cases:

- Altered mental status (AMS).
- Ocular signs: Ophthalmoplegia (difficulty in moving the eyes side to side or up and down), horizontal nystagmus, ptosis, constricted pupils.
- Ataxic or broad-based gait.

Evaluation

If you suspect WE, don't wait for test results before initiating thiamine treatment. Still, it's worth getting the following tests since they help confirm the diagnosis:

- Thiamine level (with overnight fasting): Will typically be low (<70 nmol/L if whole blood, <8 nmol/L if serum)—but normal levels don't exclude the condition, as serum levels might not accurately reflect brain levels.
- MRI: Expect to see volume loss in the mammillary bodies, but MRI will be normal in early or mild cases.

Treatment and Management

Rapid thiamine replenishment is essential.

- Administer 200–500 mg of thiamine (ideally IV, otherwise IM) one to three times daily for three to five days, followed by 100 mg oral thiamine three times daily until the AMS resolves.
- Correct magnesium deficiency if present, since thiamine activity requires adequate magnesium levels.
- Don't administer glucose until after you've initiated thiamine treatment, as glucose will deplete the patient's meager thiamine stores and you'll risk precipitating acute WE.

Prognosis

WE can result in significant disability. Though thiamine administration improves symptoms, neuropsychological deficits may persist, especially if thiamine treatment is not initiated early. A small percentage of patients with WE will progress to Korsakoff syndrome, characterized by severe and irreversible impairment in anterograde and retrograde memory. A hallmark of Korsakoff syndrome is confabulation, where patients fabricate stories to fill memory gaps.

COMMON PSYCHIATRIC CONDITIONS

Less Common Syndromes

Catatonia

Catatonia is a syndrome marked by an apparent lack of responsiveness to external stimuli, despite the individual appearing to be awake. While it's often linked with schizophrenia, you'll also see catatonia among patients with depression, bipolar disorder, schizoaffective disorder, and brief psychotic episodes.

Prevalence

- Occurs in about 10% of acute psychiatric inpatients.

Symptoms/Diagnosis

- Immobility, staring, mutism, waxy flexibility, posturing, echolalia, echopraxia, stupor, stereotypy, purposeless activity.
- Bush-Francis Catatonia Rating Scale (BFCRS): The gold standard for diagnosing catatonia. It's a 23-item scale for assessing symptoms and monitoring treatment response. See: www.thecarlatreport.com/BushFrancisCatatoniaRatingScale
- DSM-5 criteria: Requires at least three catatonic symptoms like stupor, catalepsy, mutism, etc.

Types of Catatonia

- *Retarded catatonia:* Patient stares and appears nonresponsive but is alert.
- *Excited catatonia:* Involves pointless, impulsive movements; may appear agitated or combative.
- *Malignant catatonia:* Dangerous and associated with autonomic instability; may evolve rapidly.

Differential Diagnosis

- Neuroleptic malignant syndrome.
- Encephalitis.
- Malignant hyperthermia.

Treatment

- Benzodiazepines:
  - Lorazepam (Ativan): First line, effective in 70% of cases.
    - Start with "Ativan challenge," with 1–2 mg IV or IM TID.
    - Most patients respond to 6–20 mg daily, usually within six to 10 days.
    - Monitor for respiratory depression, especially in high-risk populations like elderly patients, obese patients, or patients with cardiovascular or respiratory illnesses.
    - Once the patient is stabilized, continue benzodiazepines for three to six months before gradually tapering the dose; some patients may need long-term benzodiazepine therapy to avoid relapse.
  - Valproic acid: 500–1500 mg/day.
- N-methyl-D-aspartate (NMDA) receptor antagonists: Case reports have been promising.
  - Memantine: Start at a low dose (5 mg/day) and titrate up as tolerated and as symptoms require, to a maximum of 20 mg/day.
  - Amantadine: Typical doses are 100–400 mg/day.
- Antipsychotics: Used rarely as they can exacerbate catatonia.
- Electroconvulsive therapy: Used if no response to pharmacological interventions.

Monitoring and Follow-Up

- Use a scale like the BFCRS to monitor progress.

Dissociative Identity Disorder

Occasionally you will encounter patients who report having multiple personalities or distinct identities, also called alters. Formerly called "multiple personality disorder," this condition is now termed dissociative identity disorder (DID). Here are the essential points to know about this disorder.

DSM-5 Diagnostic Criteria

- Two or more alters control the person's behavior at different times.
- Patients experience memory gaps, especially relating to experiences that occurred while a specific identity was controlling them.

Clinical Manifestations

- Patients with DID are usually admitted due to depression, suicidal ideation, and/or self-harm.
- Patients may have many alters with specific names, genders, and personalities; a patient's average number of reported alters has increased from about two in the 1970s to over 10 currently.
- It can be hard to distinguish alters from auditory hallucinations.
- Certain stimuli, or triggers, can prompt a switch between identities or lead to distressing dissociative symptoms. Triggers include sounds, sights, physical sensations, and specific situations or interpersonal interactions.
- Don't expect identity switches to be dramatic or obvious; they can be subtle.
- Different identities might have different allergies or even need different vision prescriptions.

Etiology

A history of trauma, especially childhood sexual or physical abuse, is very common in patients with DID (about 90%). Theoretically, DID serves as a way of coping with painful memories by transferring the experiences from the main personality to one of the alters, so that the emotional pain is walled off.

Comorbidities

Depression, anxiety, substance use disorders, eating disorders, and PTSD.

Differential Diagnosis

- *Bipolar disorder:* Patients may appear to have distinct personalities in different mood states.
- *Borderline personality disorder:* Patients often experience dissociative symptoms and engage in self-injurious behaviors.
- *Factitious disorder/malingering:* Watch out for exaggerated symptoms, inconsistent stories, and possible secondary gains like disability benefits or avoidance of criminal prosecution.

Sample Questions to Ask

- "Have others mentioned things you've done, but you can't recall them?"
- "Do you ever find yourself in places without remembering how you got there?"
- "Do you find new items in your home that you don't recall purchasing?"

Management Strategies for DID in an Inpatient Psychiatric Unit

- Sudden switches between alters can be disorienting not just for the patient, but also for the staff and other patients. Create a DID management plan specific to the patient, outlining triggers and preferred interventions for each identity.
- With frequent staff shifts and interactions with multiple health care professionals, patients with DID might struggle to establish consistent trust. Assign a primary staff member who interacts with the patient regularly.
- The controlled nature of inpatient settings can resemble abusive environments from the patient's past. Create a safe space where patients can retreat if feeling overwhelmed. Staff should be trained in trauma-informed care, emphasizing empathy, patience, and understanding.
- Different identities might have varied responses to medications. Maintain a detailed medication log noting responses of different identities.
- Group therapies, which are common on inpatient units, might expose DID patients to triggers. If available, prioritize individual therapy sessions for DID patients.

Treatment Approaches

- First, ensure safety by addressing self-injurious thoughts and behaviors, if any.
- *Psychotherapies:* Cognitive behavioral therapy, dialectical behavior therapy, insight-oriented therapy, hypnotherapy, and eye-movement desensitization and reprocessing can help. If these therapies aren't provided on your psychiatric unit, arrange for outpatient treatment.
- *Pharmacotherapy:* Consider prescribing antidepressants, anxiolytics, or antipsychotic medications to address comorbid symptoms.

Factitious Disorder

People with factitious disorder aren't merely "faking it"—they go to great lengths to make themselves or others appear ill. They may inflict significant self-harm or engage in other extreme behaviors to sustain the illusion of illness. Factitious disorder used to be known by the term "Munchausen disorder."

DSM-5 Diagnostic Criteria

- Deliberate falsification of physical or psychological symptoms, or induction of injury or disease.
- Presentation as ill, impaired, or injured.
- No apparent external rewards for the behavior.
- Behavior that isn't better explained by another mental disorder.

Differential Diagnosis

- *Somatic symptom disorder:* This condition is characterized by an extreme focus on physical symptoms—such as pain or fatigue—that causes significant distress and functional impairment. The symptoms aren't intentionally produced.
- *Illness anxiety disorder (formerly hypochondriasis):* Individuals are preoccupied with having or getting a serious disease, despite having no or only mild symptoms. They frequently seek medical reassurance.
- *Functional neurological disorder (formerly conversion disorder):* Patients show neurological symptoms like paralysis, blindness, or seizures that can't be traced back to a medical cause. The symptoms aren't under the patient's conscious control.
- *Malingering:* While both factitious disorder and malingering involve the exaggeration or fabrication of symptoms, malingering is motivated by external gains—like financial benefits or avoiding work. Factitious disorder, in contrast, is rooted in a complex emotional need to assume the "sick role."

Key Variant

- *Factitious disorder imposed on another (FDIA):* Formerly known as "Munchausen by proxy," this variant involves a caregiver inducing illness in another person, often a child.

Diagnostic Tips

- *Medical history:* Check for inconsistencies in medical records (eg, the patient may have presented with vastly different symptoms during recent visits to the ED, such as chest pain at one and seizures at another).
- *Specialist consultation:* Multiple perspectives can reveal inconsistencies (eg, records from a neurologist may reveal a negative workup for a patient's complaint of seizures).
- *Patient behavior:* The patient may seem unusually eager to undergo extensive workups and/or treatments and may appear to deteriorate when you raise the prospect of hospital discharge.
- *Lab tests:* Can reveal evidence contradicting reported symptoms (eg, stool samples in cases where patients claim to have chronic diarrhea might show traces of laxatives; tests in nondiabetic hypoglycemia cases might indicate externally administered insulin).

Management

- *Multidisciplinary team:* Include psychologists (to address the patient's underlying psychological needs and motivations), nurses (who spend more time with the patient and whose observations can be crucial in detecting factitious behaviors), and possibly legal advisors (especially important in FDIA).
- *Confrontation:* Confronting these patients is a pivotal part of treatment. When confronting, be prepared with concrete evidence of the deceptive behaviors, but also maintain a tactful, nonaccusatory approach, emphasizing your concern for their well-being.
- *Therapeutic intervention:* Cognitive behavioral therapy can be helpful, with a focus on identifying triggers for the deceptive behaviors, developing coping mechanisms, and building healthier ways to seek attention or cope with stress.

Risks and Complications

- *Self-harm:* Patients may go to extremes to appear ill, including taking harmful substances or causing physical injuries to themselves.
- *Harm to others:* In cases of FDIA, there is a risk of harm to the person being made to appear ill.
- *Resistance to psychiatric evaluation:* Patients are often in denial about their psychiatric needs.

Legal Aspects

You may need to consider legal action in severe cases, especially involving FDIA. It's also possible that patients could harm themselves significantly enough to necessitate legal interventions for their safety.

Functional Neurological Disorder

Functional neurological disorder (FND) refers to neurological symptoms that are inconsistent with or cannot be fully explained by medical or neurological conditions. Prior to DSM-5, it was known as "conversion disorder." The change in terminology emphasizes the neurological nature of the symptoms, focusing on their functional aspect rather than suggesting a psychological "conversion."

Clinical Presentation

- *Functional movement disorder:* A patient may present with abnormal movements, like tremor, dystonia, jerky or myoclonic-like movements, gait disorders, weakness, or paralysis. However, tests reveal no structural abnormalities. They might also display inconsistent weakness (eg, a patient might not be able to lift their arm but can still use it to push themselves out of a chair).
- *Functional seizures (psychogenic nonepileptic seizures [PNES]):* A patient might describe seizures that don't correlate with typical postictal (postseizure) signs like tongue biting or incontinence. The seizures might be longer and have atypical movements compared to epileptic seizures.
- *Persistent postural-perceptual dizziness (PPPD):* Chronic dizziness and unsteadiness.

Diagnosis

A thorough medical and neurologic evaluation is imperative to exclude organic causes.

- *EEG:* Crucial for distinguishing PNES from epileptic seizures. PNES won't show abnormal brain activity associated with epilepsy.
- *EMG:* Especially valuable when assessing a patient complaining of paralysis. A lack of electrical activity can help confirm the diagnosis.
- *Evoked potentials:* For example, a patient might claim blindness, but their pupils still respond to light stimulus, indicating brain activity.
- *CT/MRI:* In the context of a patient with seizures, normal scans can rule out lesions or structural causes.

Differential Diagnosis

- *Factitious disorder (formerly Munchausen syndrome):* In factitious disorder, symptoms are intentionally produced for various types of secondary gain. In FND, symptoms are involuntary and perceived as real.

Etiology

Though the exact causes remain unclear, individuals with FND often have a history of traumatic events, depression, or anxiety. In cultures where mental health is stigmatized, physical manifestations of emotional distress can be more prevalent.

Management

- *Psychoeducation:* Emphasize that the symptoms are real and legitimate. Say, "You have functional neurological disorder," and explain the symptoms in neurological terms. Emphasize that the condition is common and disabling. Excellent patient education resources include the website www.neurosymptoms.org and Jon Stone's article in *Practical Neurology* (Stone J, *Pract Neurol* 2016;16(1):7–17).
- *Rehabilitation/physiotherapy:* Focus on function, using specific activities as goals. For example, use visualization to imagine normal movement, or employ distraction techniques while practicing movements (eg, the patient can perform a cognitive task like counting backwards by sevens or tossing a ball between their hands).
- *Psychotherapy:* Cognitive behavioral therapy is especially helpful for functional seizures. Train the patient to identify triggers or emotions that precede a seizure; give them tools to intervene or seek a safe environment.
- *Mindfulness and relaxation:* A patient with functional pain might find symptom relief through guided progressive muscle relaxation.
- *Sensory grounding techniques:* These can help prevent symptom escalation and functional seizures. Use "5, 4, 3, 2, 1"—identifying five things in the environment that the patient can see, four things they can hear, three they can feel, two they can smell, and one they can taste.
- *Medication:* Consider prescribing selective serotonin reuptake inhibitors (SSRIs) to a patient whose FND symptoms worsen with their coexisting anxiety; SSRIs are most helpful with PPPD.
- *Medication reevaluation:* A patient mistakenly diagnosed with epilepsy and given antiepileptic drugs for PNES will need these medications gradually withdrawn. However, about 20% of patients with functional seizures also have comorbid epileptic seizures, so ensure that a seizure workup has been done before discontinuing these meds.
- *Emerging treatments:* For example, a patient might undergo hypnotherapy sessions where the therapist guides them in revisiting traumatic events to alter their emotional response.

Prognosis

FND is a chronic illness. Without treatment, only 20% go into remission after seven years.

Psychotherapy on the Inpatient Unit

Introduction to Inpatient Psychotherapy

As a psychiatric inpatient clinician, you are generally focused on doing a comprehensive assessment, coming up with the DSM-5 diagnoses, prescribing medications, and coordinating care with other disciplines. Psychotherapy may fall by the wayside given the volume of patients and the pace of the work. However, don't forget that psychotherapy is an effective depression treatment, and if you can combine some therapy with medications, your patients are likely to improve more and to be grateful for your efforts. In this fact sheet, we provide a quick overview of effective therapeutic tools that you can deploy during your work with depressed patients.

Cognitive Behavioral Therapy (CBT)

CBT focuses on identifying and changing negative thought patterns and behaviors that contribute to depression. Common CBT techniques used in inpatient settings include:

- *Cognitive restructuring:* Identifying distorted negative automatic thoughts, evaluating their accuracy, and replacing them with more realistic positive thoughts.
- *Behavioral activation:* Scheduling activities and tasks that provide a sense of pleasure and accomplishment, even when motivation is low. Hospital staff can assist with activity planning.
- *Relaxation training:* Learning breathing, imagery, and meditation techniques to reduce stress, anxiety, and depressive feelings. These can be practiced independently or with staff guidance.

Interpersonal Therapy (IPT)

IPT aims to improve interpersonal relationships and social skills. IPT topics commonly addressed during inpatient treatment include:

- *Grief:* Processing feelings of loss (relationships, jobs, health). Staff help patients experience grief openly.
- *Role disputes:* Resolving conflicts in relationships with family members, friends, or colleagues. Staff coach patients on effective communication.
- *Role transitions:* Adjusting to major life changes. Staff validate feelings and provide practical support.
- *Interpersonal deficits:* Improving assertiveness and relationship-building skills. Staff give feedback during group interactions.

Mindfulness-Based Cognitive Therapy

This integrates mindfulness meditation practices with cognitive therapy principles. Patients learn to pay purposeful, nonjudgmental attention to the present moment to reduce rumination on negative thoughts. Common techniques include:

- *Mindfulness meditation:* Focusing on breathing and observing thoughts/feelings without judgment. Done independently or with guidance.
- *Yoga:* Executing gentle stretches and poses while paying mindful attention to the body. Provides mild exercise and relaxation.
- *Body scan meditation:* Mentally scanning the body to notice areas of tension and release. Helps connect the mind and body.

Positive Psychology Interventions

Positive psychology aims to build positive emotions, character strengths, and a sense of meaning. Examples include:

- *Gratitude journaling:* Writing down two to three things the patient is thankful for each day. Helps reframe thinking.
- *Signature strengths:* Identifying top character strengths through assessment and intentionally applying them. Builds self-confidence.
- *Acts of kindness:* Doing small acts of kindness for others on the unit. Boosts mood through contribution.
- *Savoring:* Mindfully enjoying pleasant experiences, like savoring favorite foods. Can be scheduled into each day.
- *Hope therapy:* Envisioning and taking steps toward a positive future. Staff help patients articulate life goals.

Dialectical Behavior Therapy (DBT)

DBT provides coping skills to manage difficult emotions and self-destructive urges. Patients attend DBT groups and/or individual coaching on skills like:

- *Distress tolerance:* Crisis survival tactics to resist urges to self-harm when extremely upset.
- *Emotion regulation:* Strategies to understand emotions and reduce emotional reactivity.
- *Interpersonal effectiveness:* Assertiveness and relationship-building skills.
- *Mindfulness:* Staying present in the moment nonjudgmentally.

Helping patients build an inpatient psychiatrist treatment "toolbox" of research-backed approaches like CBT, IPT, mindfulness, and DBT provides a solid foundation for managing depressive symptoms initially and maintaining mental health after discharge. The supportive inpatient environment allows patients to practice new skills with staff feedback, enabling effective learning of therapeutic techniques to support the transition to outpatient treatment.

Motivational Interviewing Techniques

Motivational interviewing (MI) is a counseling approach designed to fortify patients' motivation to change, especially relevant in a psychiatric hospital setting where patients are often ambivalent about treatment. Initially rooted in substance abuse treatments, MI has evolved to address issues faced in psychiatric units such as medication nonadherence, social withdrawal, and self-injurious behaviors.

The Foundations of MI

- *Express empathy:* Understand and validate the patient's feelings and thoughts.
- *Develop discrepancy:* Highlight the difference between the patient's actions and their aspirations. Example: Point out a patient's desire for a more fulfilling life vs their self-injurious behaviors.
- *Roll with resistance:* Instead of countering resistance directly, try to understand the underlying fears or concerns. Example: When a patient resists group therapy and cites it as unhelpful, instead of insisting on attendance, ask, "What are your main concerns about group therapy?"
- *Support self-efficacy:* Encourage the patient's confidence in their potential to change.

Core Techniques of MI: OARS

- ***O**pen-ended questions:* Push the patient to delve deeper into their feelings and thoughts. Example: "Can you help me understand what you felt during that episode?"
- ***A**ffirmations:* Use positive feedback. Example: "It's commendable how you managed your anxiety during our last session."
- ***R**eflective listening:* Mirror back what the patient says to help them feel understood.
- ***S**ummaries:* Recount the main points, ensuring the patient and you are on the same page. Example: "From our talk, it seems you're most concerned about..."

Processes

These are the steps through which you'll apply the OARS techniques.

1. *Engaging:* Work to build trust, especially with psychiatric patients who may have past traumatic experiences. Set the agenda collaboratively and maintain a neutral, nonjudgmental tone.
2. *Focusing:* Narrow down the therapeutic goals so the patient won't feel overwhelmed.
3. *Evoking:* Elicit "change talk." For instance, if a patient says, "I wish I could manage my anxiety better," you might ask, "Why is managing your anxiety important to you? How do you envision doing that?" Change talk includes reasons to change and steps that can be taken.
4. *Planning:* Strategize around the challenges psychiatric patients might face, like managing triggers or obstacles.

Administration

- Session lengths can vary based on the patient's immediate needs, with durations of 15–45 minutes.
- Consistency and increased sessions tend to yield better results in the psychiatric context, ensuring patients feel supported throughout their hospital stay.

Cognitive Behavioral Therapy Techniques

Cognitive behavioral therapy (CBT) is an effective approach for patients with various mental health disorders, including anxiety, depression, PTSD, and obsessive-compulsive disorder (OCD)—but only if they demonstrate motivation and a commitment to complete therapeutic exercises and apply learned coping mechanisms.

Overall Strategy

Controlling our behaviors becomes challenging when we don't understand how our thoughts and emotions lead to them. CBT helps patients dismantle the chain of automatic negative thoughts (ANTs) that lead to distressing emotions and maladaptive behaviors. Your role will be to teach your patient strategies for challenging and changing these thoughts, reshaping their emotional responses, and adopting healthier behaviors.

Identify a Specific Distress-Inducing Incident to Begin Analysis

Begin by briefly explaining CBT to your patient. Then, ask them to detail a recent troubling event: "Let's try to figure out what we can learn from what happened. Tell me more about the situation that caused your distress."

For each situation, identify:

- ANTs.
- Emotions.
- Behavior.

Clinical vignettes

- A 30-year-old woman who has been struggling with social anxiety had a panic attack during a work presentation. During the session, you identify that the trigger was the fear of judgment from her colleagues. The ANT was, "Everyone will laugh at me. They'll think I'm incompetent." The emotion was fear and panic, and the behavior was declining to do any more presentations, which threatens her job security. You intervene to demonstrate how her thoughts about her coworkers led directly to her fear and panic, and then help her challenge the accuracy of those thoughts. She agrees that her colleagues are generally supportive and understanding, and this balanced thought might have led her to ask for support rather than isolating herself in fear.
- A 42-year-old man experiencing depressive symptoms avoids social interactions due to thoughts like, "No one enjoys my company. I'll just make things worse." This has led to self-isolation and feelings of loneliness. During the session, you focus on challenging these thoughts, considering evidence of past positive social interactions and encouraging small steps toward social engagement.

Common ANTs and Other Cognitive Distortions

- *Catastrophizing:* A patient might think, "I'm going to mess up this presentation, and then I'll lose my job." Encourage a replacement thought, such as: "I am well prepared for this presentation. Even if I stumble, it doesn't mean I'll lose my job."
- *Generalizing:* A person with OCD might believe, "If everything isn't perfect, it's a complete disaster." Teach them to see the spectrum between perfection and failure.
- *Worry and rumination:* Someone with PTSD might be plagued by thoughts like, "I'm never safe." Educate that persistent worrying does not prevent adverse events. Teach them coping strategies like deep breathing, grounding exercises, or distraction techniques to break the cycle of rumination.

Supportive Therapy in the Inpatient Setting

Supportive therapy is a psychotherapeutic approach focused on providing emotional and practical support and strengthening a patient's coping mechanisms. Here we share tips for how to implement supportive therapy in the inpatient unit.

Key Components

Active and empathic listening

- Provide a calm, focused presence, acknowledging the stress of the inpatient environment: "I know this environment can be overwhelming. Let's take this time to focus on your thoughts and feelings."
- Summarize and reflect back to ensure the patient feels heard: "It sounds like you've been going through a tough time and haven't felt like you've had much support. Is that right?"

Emotional support and encouragement

- Validate the patient's experiences: "You've been through a lot. It makes sense you're feeling this way."
- Offer words of encouragement and acknowledge progress, no matter how small: "You've shown a lot of strength in dealing with these challenges."
- Ensure you or someone else is available to provide support when needed: "If you start feeling overwhelmed again, you can reach out to me or nursing staff."

Development of coping and problem-solving skills

- Help the patient develop coping strategies that can be practiced in the inpatient environment, like deep breathing, art therapy, and journaling.
- Guide the patient in identifying their problems and brainstorming potential solutions: "Let's identify the main challenges you're facing and think of different ways you can approach them. What feels the most manageable to start with?"
- Encourage reframing of negative thoughts: "When you think, 'I can't handle this,' try telling yourself, 'I'm learning new ways to cope every day.'"
- Offer guidance on recognizing the early warning signs of a crisis and effective strategies for seeking help, like reaching out to nurses.

Mindfulness and relaxation techniques

- Integrate mindfulness practices like guided meditation, progressive muscle relaxation, and mindful breathing exercises to help the patient manage stress and anxiety. (See the "Relaxation and Deep Breathing Exercises" fact sheet in this section.)
- Teach relaxation techniques that the patient can easily practice, such as visualization, yoga, or tai chi.

Use of digital tools and apps

- Introduce the patient to digital tools and apps that can support mental health, such as meditation apps, mood trackers, or cognitive behavioral therapy–based apps.
- Highly rated apps include Calm, Happify, Headspace, MoodKit, Sanvello, and Worry Watch.

Group Programs

Group programs are an essential component of therapy in inpatient psychiatric units, providing structured settings where patients can participate in therapeutic activities, develop coping skills, and engage with peers for support. While you won't typically lead these groups, occasional participation can be helpful for gaining deeper insights into your patients' experiences and their responses to treatment. This fact sheet outlines various types of group programs available in inpatient psychiatric settings and provides strategies to enhance their effectiveness.

Types of Group Programs

Therapeutic groups

These groups focus on psychotherapy interventions, like cognitive behavioral therapy or dialectical behavior therapy, to help patients understand their behaviors and emotions and develop coping strategies.

- Patient-friendly description: These are talk therapy groups that help you understand your feelings and thoughts and develop tools to manage them. It's like learning a new way to deal with stress and painful emotions.

Skill-building groups

These groups concentrate on developing specific skills such as stress management, communication, or life skills like cooking, budgeting, and self-care.

- Patient-friendly description: Ever wish you were better at managing stress, talking to people, or taking care of yourself? These groups focus on practical skills to make life easier, like managing money, healthy cooking, or communication.

Support groups

These groups provide a platform for patients to share experiences, challenges, and achievements, and foster a sense of belonging and mutual support.

- Patient-friendly description: Sometimes people feel alone with their struggles—these groups help you share your experiences, get encouragement, and learn from others who are going through similar situations. It's basically a built-in support network.

Educational groups

These groups educate patients about their diagnoses, medication management, and the importance of adherence to treatment plans.

- Patient-friendly description: Do you want to know more about your diagnosis, your medications, or how to stay healthy? These groups will answer your questions.

Recreational groups

These groups include activities like art, music, exercise, and outdoor activities to encourage creativity and relaxation.

Pet therapy groups

While not universally available, pet therapy groups leverage the calming and therapeutic benefits of animals to enhance emotional and social well-being.

- Patient-friendly description: You can think of these as fun and relaxation groups. They can help you unwind, express yourself, and enjoy the company of animals.

Effective Delivery of Group Programs

Structure and scheduling

The unit establishes a consistent schedule for groups, typically around times that don't coincide with medication dispensing or meals. Ideally, groups are kept small (eight to 10 participants) to allow for individual attention and interaction. Posting the schedule visibly can help increase patient participation.

Facilitation

Group sessions are typically led by social workers, occupational therapists, and recreation therapists, who are skilled in managing group dynamics, including conflict resolution.

Discussing Groups with Your Patients

Highlight the benefits

Tell patients how group programs will help them develop coping mechanisms, enhance social skills, and reduce feelings of isolation. Mention that many patients regard groups as one of the most beneficial aspects of their inpatient experience.

- Script: "Group programs can help you develop coping skills, connect with others, and feel less isolated. Many patients tell me that the groups are one of the most helpful aspects of being in the hospital."

Encourage consistent participation

Stress the importance of regular attendance to maximize the therapeutic benefits.

- Script: "The more you participate, the more you'll get out of it. Regular attendance helps build a supportive community and allows you to learn from others and solidify new skills."

Set expectations

For patients dealing with significant depression or social isolation, make it clear that regular group attendance may be a prerequisite for discharge.

Address reluctance

Some patients may feel hesitant to share their experiences in a group setting. Offer reassurance about the confidentiality of the sessions and note that even passive participation can be helpful.

- Script: "Sharing in a group can feel scary, but these sessions are confidential and led by professionals trained to create a safe and respectful environment. Even listening to others can be helpful. Remember, you don't have to be the most vocal person to benefit."

Psychotherapy for Psychotic Disorders

By integrating psychotherapy into treatment plans for patients with psychotic disorders, you can enhance their symptom management and improve their overall well-being. Here we review two evidence-based therapeutic approaches that are effective in various settings, including inpatient units.

Cognitive Behavioral Therapy for Psychosis (CBTp)
CBTp focuses on identifying and challenging distorted thought patterns, delusions, and hallucinations in individuals with psychotic disorders, thereby reducing distress and improving functioning.

Key steps

- Begin with a comprehensive evaluation. Assess the patient's symptoms and beliefs, focusing on identifying delusions, hallucinations, and cognitive distortions.
- Next, guide the patient in critically examining their beliefs and considering more rational interpretations. Sample dialogue:
  - *You:* "Can you share more about the belief that your thoughts are being broadcast?"
  - *Patient:* "I feel like everyone in the unit can hear my thoughts."
  - *You:* "What evidence do you have that others can hear your thoughts?"
  - *Patient:* "I see people whispering and looking at me, so they must be talking about my thoughts."
  - *You:* "Is it possible that people in the unit are engaged in conversations unrelated to you, and your perception might be influenced by your current beliefs?"
  - *Patient:* "I guess it's possible."
- Encourage the patient to maintain a daily journal to document thoughts and experiences related to their psychotic symptoms.
- During therapy sessions, jointly review these journal entries to identify cognitive distortions or delusional thought patterns.
- Regularly assess the patient's progress to tailor the therapeutic approach as necessary.

Family-Focused Therapy (FFT)
FFT involves working with patients and their families to improve family dynamics, communication, and support. Although it's typically conducted in outpatient settings, FFT can be adapted for inpatient stays.

Key steps

- Host a family meeting to evaluate family dynamics, relationships, and communication patterns.
- Educate the family about the patient's diagnosis, symptoms, and treatment.
- Help the family to improve communication:
  - Foster active listening skills by teaching techniques like nodding, eye contact, and paraphrasing to show understanding.
  - Emphasize the use of "I" statements instead of "you" statements (which can sound accusatory). For example, rather than saying, "You always make me worry when..." a family member can say, "I feel worried when..."
  - Highlight the importance of nonverbal cues, like facial expressions and tone of voice.
  - Encourage family members to validate each other's feelings with phrases like, "I see this is really hard for you."
- Teach conflict resolution techniques, like taking timeouts during heated moments or counting to 10 rather than responding impulsively.

Relaxation and Deep Breathing Exercises

Relaxation and deep breathing exercises are helpful for relieving anxiety and insomnia, and you should include them in your repertoire of therapeutic tools on the inpatient unit.

How to Introduce These Exercises to Patients

- Just about any patient can benefit from relaxation and deep breathing, but you will generally give highest priority to those with significant anxiety and insomnia—including those with depression and PTSD. Be more cautious with psychotic patients since relaxation exercises can increase focus on delusions or hallucinations.
- To introduce the concept, say something like, "Today, we're going to explore some relaxation and deep breathing exercises designed to help reduce feelings of anxiety and improve your sleep. These are simple techniques you can use anytime you're feeling stressed or unable to sleep. Let's start with something that can help you feel more at peace and grounded."
- Start with basic techniques that are universally beneficial, like diaphragmatic breathing and progressive muscle relaxation, as these form the foundation for mastering more complex exercises. Evaluate the patient's response to these initial techniques and use their feedback to guide the introduction of more specialized practices, like guided imagery or the 4-7-8 breathing technique. Your goal is to equip patients with a variety of tools so they can discover which methods provide the greatest relief from their symptoms.

Relaxation Techniques

- *Guided imagery:* Start by having patients sit or lie down in a comfortable position. Guide them through a visualization of a peaceful scene, like a beach or a forest. Encourage them to engage all their senses in this imagery to enhance the relaxation experience. Say something like, "Close your eyes and imagine you're walking down a peaceful path in a beautiful forest. With each step, you feel more at ease. The sounds of the forest, the soft rustling of leaves, and distant bird calls surround you. Breathe in the fresh air and feel the tension melting away as you become more relaxed with each breath."
- *Progressive muscle relaxation:* Teach patients to tense and then relax different muscle groups, starting from the toes and moving up toward the head. Say something like, "Let's start by focusing on your toes. Tense them as much as you can, hold for a few seconds, and then release. Notice the warmth and relaxation spreading. Now, gently move your attention up to your calves. Tense, hold, and release. We'll continue this up through each muscle group, gradually bringing relaxation to your entire body."

Deep Breathing Exercises

- *Diaphragmatic breathing:* Instruct patients to breathe deeply from the abdomen, not just the chest. This encourages full oxygen exchange and can trigger a natural relaxation response. Say something like, "Place one hand on your chest and the other on your abdomen. Take a slow, deep breath through your nose, feeling your abdomen rise more than your chest. Hold it for a moment, and then slowly exhale through your mouth. Let's repeat this a few times, each breath helping you feel more relaxed and centered."
- *4-7-8 breathing technique:* Patients breathe in for four seconds, hold their breath for seven seconds, and exhale slowly for eight seconds. This method is particularly effective in reducing anxiety and helping with sleep disturbances. Say something like, "Breathe in quietly through your nose for four seconds. Now, hold that breath for seven seconds. Next, exhale completely through your mouth, making a whoosh sound, for eight seconds. This process is a natural tranquilizer for your nervous system, reducing anxiety and aiding in sleep."

Self-Guided Practice

Encourage patients to integrate these relaxation and deep breathing exercises into their daily routine while on the inpatient unit, suggesting they set aside specific times each day to practice in their rooms or any designated quiet space available. Emphasize that these techniques are not just for moments of acute stress but are also valuable as daily practices to maintain a baseline level of calm and manageability.

When patients approach the end of their inpatient stay, have them identify specific times and places that they'll be practicing these routines after discharge, like as part of their morning routine in their home garden or during lunch breaks at a nearby park. This proactive planning will help embed these practices into their lifestyle, making the exercises more likely to become enduring habits.

Anger Management Techniques

Managing patients' anger effectively is critical for both patient well-being and the safety of the hospital environment. This fact sheet provides tips and sample dialogues to assist your patients in identifying their anger triggers, expressing their anger constructively, and reducing aggressive behaviors.

Identifying Anger Triggers

The first step in helping patients manage their anger is to help them identify what provokes it.

- "I know you sometimes have a temper, and we want to make sure you don't lose control while you're here, so let's come up with an anger management plan."
- "Tell me about triggers for your anger. Are you feeling ignored by nursing staff? Are you feeling disrespected by another patient? Is it frustrating to have to wait to speak to your doctor? Are you being annoyed by your roommate?"
- "Rate your anger on the anger meter, from 1 to 10. 1 is complete calm; 10 is losing control and doing something that causes negative consequences, like breaking something or hitting someone."
- Explore the aggression cycle, which includes three phases: escalation, explosion, and post-explosion. Discussing these phases can help patients recognize and disrupt this cycle before reaching a point of loss of control.

Anger Management Techniques

Help your patients develop a toolbox of strategies.

Timeout

Encourage patients to temporarily step away from situations that get them worked up or to ask the person with whom they are arguing if they can take a 10-minute break from the conversation.

Deep breathing

- Guide patients through deep breathing exercises to promote relaxation and reduce immediate feelings of anger.
- Example: "Get comfortable, then close your eyes or stare at the floor. Become aware of your body and scan it for any sources of tension. Let go of any tension. Now pay attention to your breathing. Take a deep breath and notice your lungs and chest expanding. Hold it for a second, then exhale through your nose. Continue to breathe this way for a couple of minutes. When you feel ready, open your eyes. You can practice this anywhere."

Progressive relaxation

- Teach patients to tense and then relax different muscle groups, helping to reduce physical tension and calm the mind.
- Example: "Start with your breathing. Now focus on your hands; clench your fists. Now relax your arms. Now raise your shoulders, neck, and face. Now relax completely."

Cognitive restructuring (ABCD method)

- Help patients understand their anger triggers and adjust their responses through the ABCD method:
  - *A:* Identify the **A**ctivating event.
  - *B:* Examine **B**eliefs about the event.
  - *C:* Consider the emotional **C**onsequences of the event.
  - *D:* **D**ispute the irrational beliefs and replace them with more rational ones.
- Example: "In the moment, you might think, 'I should be treated fairly by people,' but in reality, we can't expect to always be treated fairly by everyone."

Thought stopping

- Encourage patients to consciously interrupt and halt negative thoughts that fuel anger.
- Example: "Instead of trying to reason with yourself, just try to stop thinking the thoughts that are making you angry."

Assertiveness training

- Educate patients on expressing their needs and rights in a respectful, nonaggressive manner.
- Example: "Acting assertively is not about being aggressive—it just means standing up for your own rights in a respectful way."

Journaling

Encourage patients to journal about their anger episodes—this can help them get a better perspective on situations and develop healthier coping mechanisms.

Sample Behavior Management Plan

Behavior management plans are tools for addressing and modifying a patient's challenging behaviors. These plans typically outline specific inappropriate behaviors, set clear consequences for these behaviors, and detail rewards for appropriate behavior. Here's a sample template that you can adapt to suit each patient's unique needs and circumstances.

Patient Name: ______________________________

Expectations During Hospitalization

- Every morning: Shower, brush your teeth, get dressed, comb/brush your hair.
- Make your bed every day.
- Spend no more than ______ hours a day in bed during the daytime.
- Take your medications as prescribed by your physician.
- Attend at least one patient group in the morning and one in the afternoon.
- Take a voluntary timeout when feeling upset or angry.
- Ask staff for PRNs when necessary for anxiety, psychosis, agitation, or insomnia.
- Refrain from using profanity or insulting language.
- Other:____.

Behavioral Directives

- Maintain arm's length distance from other patients and staff.
- No self-injurious behavior.
- No damaging of personal or hospital property.
- No physical aggression toward staff or other patients.
- Limit requests at the nursing station to ______ per ______.
- Do not stand within four feet of the nursing station doors.
- Other:____.
- Other:____.

Consequences

- Restriction of the following unit privileges:______________________________.
- Emergency medications for self-injurious or aggressive/assaultive behavior.
- Seclusion room and/or restraints if your behavior puts you or others at imminent risk of harm.
- Other:____.

Rewards for Appropriate Behavior

- Access to the phone following appropriate behavior during the preceding nursing shift.
- Participation in morning outdoor activities following appropriate behavior throughout the previous day.
- Other:____.

I, ____(patient name), hereby acknowledge that I have been informed about these behavioral expectations and directives. I agree to adhere to this Behavior Management Plan as outlined.

____

Patient Name **Date**

____

Witness/Staff **Date**

Establishing a Token Economy

The token economy is a method that promotes positive behaviors in patients, such as taking medications, going to groups, or maintaining hygiene. Patients earn tokens for their desirable actions on the unit, which can later be exchanged for rewards or privileges. Token economies are sometimes used in inpatient psychiatric units, as well as in residential treatment programs.

Benefits of a Token Economy

- *Promotes positive behaviors:* Tokens are especially effective for patients who do not respond well to simple praise or encouragement.
- *Overcomes resistance:* If a patient is hesitant to engage in a certain therapeutic activity, the promise of tokens can motivate them.
- *Empowers patients:* Tokens encourage patients to assume greater control of and involvement in their treatment.

Implementation Steps

1. *Establish target behaviors*
    - Behaviors should be achievable and applicable for all patients. Examples include:
        - Going to groups.
        - Taking prescribed medication.
        - Routine hygiene tasks, such as showering and brushing teeth.
2. *Create a system of tokens*
    - Utilize a "star rewards card" for each patient.
    - Card is divided into seven days, with various categories for each day (eg, "Join group activity," "Brush teeth").
    - When a patient completes a task corresponding to one of the categories, they get a token (eg, a star-shaped stamp provided by staff) on their cards.
3. *Select rewards*
    - Choose tangible rewards that don't replace any services or privileges to which patients are already entitled (eg, meals and fresh air breaks are basic patient rights and can't be held back as rewards).
    - A mobile "store" offers a variety of reward items.
    - Rewards range from hygiene items and notebooks to cosmetics, cozy wearables like beanies, and snacks.
4. *Communicate how the system works*
    - Clearly display the rules and rewards of the token economy system, including store hours.
    - To ensure the program's smooth operation, all staff—from nurses to therapists—need to be on the same page. Everyone should understand the system's workings and objectives.
    - Maintain consistent communication to ensure every patient feels fairly treated. For instance, if one patient receives a token for a specific behavior, another patient should receive the same for exhibiting that behavior.
    - Align procedures with patients' rights policies by consulting with the local department of mental health.
5. *Monitor and adjust*
    - Collect feedback from patients and staff for continuous improvement.
    - Modify reward offerings as necessary (eg, removing beanies from the store during a lice outbreak).

Handling Undesirable Behaviors

- *Timeout mechanism:* If a patient's behavior is counter to the program's objectives, their card goes into "timeout," halting their ability to earn tokens for that day. They can start fresh the next day, keeping the focus on encouraging improved behavior.
- *Clear consequences:* Clearly outline what actions will result in a patient's card going into timeout (eg, aggressive behavior, whether verbal or physical).
- *Positive focus:* The goal isn't to punish, but to emphasize positive behavior. Therefore, even if a card is in timeout for the day, the patient has a clean slate the next day.

Medication Side Effects

Medication Side Effects

Discussing and Managing Medication Side Effects

Psychiatric medications cause plenty of side effects, yet we tend to severely underestimate the number of side effects our patients are experiencing. According to one survey, patients on antidepressants reported 20 times more side effects than were documented by their psychiatrists (Zimmerman M et al, *J Clin Psychiatry* 2010;71(4):484–490).

Sometimes we don't ask about side effects because we're not sure what to do about them—so we have created detailed fact sheets covering common side effects and suggesting management strategies. In this introductory fact sheet, we'll give you general tips on how to ask patients about side effects and how to manage them.

What to Ask About Side Effects on Admission

- Newly admitted patients probably have side effects from their current meds. In fact, some might have halted their meds due to these adverse effects, possibly contributing to their current admission. So one of the most important things you can do on admission is to ask them what side effects they are currently experiencing:
  - "Do your medications cause you any side effects?"
  - "Here are some possible side effects I often see with [medication name]. Have you had any of these since starting on your medication?"
- Give your patient a list of common side effects so they can review it at their leisure and then go over it in detail with you later in the admission. We have created such a list here: www.thecarlatreport.com/PatientSideEffectsList
- For each side effect reported, ascertain:
  - When did it begin? After medication initiation?
  - Is it a genuine side effect or a symptom of the underlying condition?
  - How bothersome is it?
    - Has the patient stopped a medication because of it?
    - Is it something they can live with if the medication is effective? (Dry mouth is a common example of this.)
    - Is it a side effect that the patient never even associated with the drug? (For example, apathy induced by a selective serotonin reuptake inhibitor may have been wrongly attributed to depression, rather than the drug.)

What to Say When Prescribing a New Medication

- Don't minimize side effects. It's tempting to talk up the benefits of a medication while glossing over its potential negatives. However, this approach can lead to long-term issues, such as unexpected severe side effects, mistrust, and avoidance of future treatment.
- Transparency is key. Before starting a medication, have an open discussion about possible side effects. Use empathy and clarity to communicate the potential risks and benefits. Highlight the importance of ongoing communication should side effects arise.
  - "Starting a new medication can cause side effects while your body adjusts to it. [List some common ones related to the medication.] Sometimes these are temporary, sometimes not. It's important for us to work together so we can adjust doses and medications to find the right balance for your treatment."

The Five R's Approach to Managing Side Effects, by Ron Pies

1. *Reduce:* Reduce the dose.
2. *Reschedule:* Adjust the timing. For example, move a sedating medication to bedtime dosing. Split dosing to BID or TID to reduce exposure at any one time.
3. *Reformulate:* Switch to a different formulation, such as from immediate release to extended release, or from a tablet to liquid or sprinkles.
4. *Rescue:* Add an antidote, like benztropine (Cogentin) for extrapyramidal symptoms.
5. *Replace:* Stop the offending medication and switch to a different one.

Metabolic Syndrome

Metabolic syndrome is a cluster of conditions that increase the risk of cardiovascular diseases, diabetes, and stroke. It includes increased abdominal fat, high blood sugar levels, high triglyceride levels, low HDL cholesterol levels, and elevated blood pressure. The Centers for Medicare & Medicaid Services (CMS) requires that inpatient psych units monitor any patient taking antipsychotics for these conditions. This fact sheet helps you make sure you know how to do this monitoring correctly—and how to mitigate these health problems in your patients.

Monitoring Requirements and Recommendations

- CMS requires monitoring for any patient on antipsychotics, even agents with a very low risk of causing problems, such as aripiprazole, ziprasidone, and lurasidone. The following four measurements must be documented within the last year (you don't have to reorder them if recent results are already in the chart):
  - BMI (this is typically calculated automatically by the electronic health record based on your patient's admission height and weight)
  - Blood pressure (this is usually obtained daily by nursing staff)
  - Glucose or HbA1c
  - Full lipid panel (cholesterol, triglyceride, LDL, HDL)
- Metabolic syndrome occurs even in the absence of weight gain, but the risk of developing metabolic syndrome and the severity of metabolic abnormalities tend to be more pronounced in patients who experience significant weight gain while on antipsychotic medications.
- Early changes in weight or metabolic parameters predict those at higher risk of developing full-blown metabolic syndrome.
- Watch for new-onset Type 2 diabetes in patients on antipsychotics, especially if they exhibit signs like increased thirst, frequent urination, or unexplained weight loss.

Recommended Actions if Patient Has Metabolic Syndrome

- *Provide education.* Educate your patient about any abnormal results and suggest things they should do.
  - Explain what metabolic syndrome is and what the health risks are.
  - Give them a fact sheet on the issue. See the patient fact sheet, "Understanding Metabolic Syndrome," here: www.thecarlatreport.com/UnderstandingMetabolicSyndrome.
  - Very important: Make sure they talk to their primary care doctor about the problem next time they see them.
- *Obtain a nutrition consultation.* A hospital dietitian or nutritionist will likely recommend things like reducing sodium and refined carbs; increasing intake of lean sources of protein like poultry, fish, and lentils; choosing healthy fats like olive oil and avocado; and boosting fiber intake.
- *Recommend exercise.* Encourage your patient to participate in any exercise program you have in your hospital.
- *Switch medications.* If possible, switch to an antipsychotic with less risk of metabolic syndrome (eg, aripiprazole, lurasidone).
- *Treat metabolic syndrome.* Start one of a range of medications that are helpful in treating aspects of metabolic syndrome:
  - Metformin XR (Glucophage XR, Glumetza) 500–2000 mg; split into two doses if needed based on GI side effects.
  - Topiramate (Topamax): Begin with 25 mg daily, then titrate up if needed, but be cautious due to potential cognitive side effects; the dose is usually capped at 200 mg daily.
  - Aripiprazole (Abilify) 15 mg/day; helps counteract weight gain and metabolic disturbances when used adjunctively.
  - Meds that are usually managed by PCPs, but that some psychiatrists will feel comfortable starting:
    - Semaglutide (Ozempic): Initiate at 0.25 mg once weekly; can titrate based on response and tolerance. Highly effective for weight loss.
    - Atorvastatin (Lipitor) 10–80 mg daily or simvastatin (Zocor) 5–40 mg at bedtime for dyslipidemia.
    - Angiotensin-converting enzyme (ACE) inhibitors like lisinopril or angiotensin II receptor blockers like losartan for hypertension.
- *Collaborate with outpatient providers.* Work with your social workers to ensure your patient has a follow-up appointment with a PCP. Make sure that you have highlighted concerning labs in your discharge summary, as this will often be the only hospital document that outpatient providers will read. If you have time, consider personally calling the PCP at the time of discharge to discuss your concerns.

Akathisia

Characteristics

A sense of restlessness, causing the patient to appear fidgety, to have difficulty sitting still, and to rock from one leg to the other while standing. It can present as an inner sense of restlessness without obvious movement. Can lead to agitation and even suicidal ideation.

Meds that Cause It

Antipsychotics, especially high-potency first-generation antipsychotics (such as haloperidol), but second-generation agents may also cause it (especially aripiprazole, brexpiprazole, paliperidone, and risperidone). Occasionally caused by selective serotonin reuptake inhibitors and buspirone.

Mechanism

D2 blockade, possibly serotonin stimulation.

General Management

- Reduce dose.
- Switch to lower-potency first-generation or second-generation agent with lower potential for akathisia.

First-Line Medications

- Propranolol (Inderal). Start 10 mg BID; increase by 10–20 mg/day increments; can go up to 30–90 mg daily in two or three divided doses. Side effects: Dizziness, fatigue, syncope, low blood pressure.
- Inderal LA (long-acting version of propranolol that can be dosed once a day). 60–80 mg daily.
- Benzodiazepines. Any of them will work (eg, lorazepam [Ativan] 0.5–1 mg BID). Dosed at the equivalent of diazepam (Valium) 10 mg BID or more frequently as needed.

Second-Line Medications

- Benztropine (Cogentin) 1 mg BID.
- Cyproheptadine (Periactin) 8–16 mg/day.
- Amantadine (Symmetrel) 100–200 mg BID.
- Clonidine 0.2–0.8 mg/day.
- Gabapentin (Neurontin) 1200 mg/day.
- Trazodone (Desyrel) 100 mg/day.
- Mirtazapine (Remeron) 15 mg/day.

Clinical Pearls

- May manifest in several ways, such as pacing, inability to sit still, crossing and uncrossing one's legs, rocking back and forth, or other purposeless repetitive motions; patients may complain of crawling feeling under skin or "shocks."
- Don't confuse akathisia with agitation due to the underlying psychiatric disorder—you might make the mistake of increasing the antipsychotic, thus worsening the akathisia.
- Risk factors include high-dose, high-potency antipsychotics, and rapid dose escalation; use of caffeine, other stimulants, or illicit drugs may also exacerbate akathisia.
- May appear within first few hours of antipsychotic exposure, but usually takes days to weeks to appear.
- Can occur in a tardive form, with symptoms lasting for greater than six months after discontinuation of the offending agent.
- Clozapine and quetiapine cause no more akathisia than placebo.

Bruxism

Characteristics

Involuntary grinding of teeth, which especially occurs during sleep but can also occur in the daytime. In 5% of cases this can cause severe health problems, such as destruction of tooth structure, temporomandibular joint dysfunction, myofascial pain, and sleep disturbances.

Meds that Cause It

A variety of medications, including antidepressants (especially selective serotonin reuptake inhibitors and the serotonin/norepinephrine reuptake inhibitor venlafaxine), psychostimulants, and antipsychotics; drugs of abuse such as methamphetamine, cocaine, and ecstasy.

Mechanism

Unclear, but likely involves central dopaminergic and serotonergic systems.

General Management

- Reduce dose or switch medication.
- Wear dental guards at night.
- Treat anxiety, which worsens bruxism.
- Decrease or stop using tobacco, caffeine, and alcohol.

First-Line Medications

Buspirone (BuSpar) 10 mg BID or TID.

Second-Line Medications

- Benzodiazepines, such as clonazepam (Klonopin) 0.5–1 mg at bedtime.
- Gabapentin (Neurontin) 300 mg at bedtime.

Clinical Pearls

- Frequency of bruxism varies from day to day, but symptoms are usually induced or worsened by anxiety and stress.
- Watching and waiting may be indicated as spontaneous remission can occur after one month.
- Botulinum toxin (Botox) injections into the masseter muscle are effective for persistent bruxism.
- Risk factors include obstructive sleep apnea and parasomnias, anxiety, heavy alcohol use, loud snoring, caffeine intake, smoking, and other psychiatric and neurologic disorders.

Constipation

Characteristics

Straining to have bowel movements, often with hard stools, and a sensation of incomplete evacuation. Not necessarily infrequent stools—patients may have a bowel movement every day, but if they strain, they are constipated.

Meds that Cause It

Antipsychotics (especially clozapine and olanzapine, but all can cause it); antidepressants, including selective serotonin reuptake inhibitors (particularly paroxetine); serotonin/norepinephrine reuptake inhibitors; mirtazapine; tricyclics; benztropine; antihistamines (eg, diphenhydramine, hydroxyzine); opioids.

Mechanism

Usually due to anticholinergic effects, which lead to decrease in bowel motility.

General Management

- Decrease dose or switch agents.
- Increase fluid intake.
- Increase dietary fiber (cereals, fruits, bran) and eat prunes.
- Increase physical activity.

First-Line Medications

- Bulk-forming laxatives (Side effects: Gas, bloating):
  - Psyllium (Metamucil) or methylcellulose (Citrucel) one tablespoon three times daily, taken with a full glass of water.
  - Avoid in patients taking clozapine as it may increase risk of perforation in slow-transit constipation.
- Stool softener (Side effects: Diarrhea):
  - Docusate sodium (Colace) 100–250 mg twice daily. Must be taken with a full glass of water.

Second-Line Medications

- Osmotic laxatives (Side effects: Bloating, gas, watery stools):
  - Lactulose (Kristalose) 15–30 mL daily or every other day.
  - Polyethylene glycol solution (MiraLax) 8–34 g in eight ounces of fluid.
  - Magnesium citrate 150–300 mL daily.
- Stimulant laxatives (Side effects: Diarrhea, cramps):
  - Sennosides (Ex-Lax, Senokot), available in different formulations (usual dose is one to two 8.6 mg tablets QD to BID as needed).
  - Bisacodyl (Dulcolax), available as suppository (usual dose is 5–15 mg daily, max 30 mg/day).
  - Magnesium hydroxide (milk of magnesia) 30–60 mL QD as needed (available also in chewable tablet form).

Clinical Pearl

Constipation can be caused by various illnesses, including irritable bowel syndrome (usually diarrhea interspersed with constipation), hypothyroidism, and colon cancer (red flags include blood in stool and weight loss).

Diarrhea

Characteristics

Passing of loose or watery stools, at least three times in a 24-hour period. Often due to infectious etiology (eg, rotovirus, norovirus, adenoviruses, *E. coli*) but can occur as a side effect to medications. Most cases resolve with routine over-the-counter treatment.

Meds that Cause It

Antibiotics, proton pump inhibitors, donepezil, galantamine, memantine, rivastigmine, sertraline, acamprosate, lithium, metformin, stool softeners and other laxatives, rapid discontinuation of anticholinergic agents (cholinergic rebound) or opioid withdrawal.

Mechanism

Increased water content of stool, usually due to impaired water absorption and/or active water secretion by the bowel.

General Management

- Push fluids and suggest dietary adjustments like the BRAT diet (bananas, rice, applesauce, and toast). Avoid high-fat foods.
- Get a travel and food history.
- Ask about recent antibiotic use.
- Assess for serotonin syndrome (presence of mental status changes, hyperthermia, hyperreflexia, autonomic instability).
- If on lithium, check serum lithium level for toxicity.

First-Line Medications

- Antimotility agents: Loperamide (Imodium) two tablets (4 mg) initially, then 2 mg after each loose stool for no more than two days with a max dose of 16 mg/day. Avoid if fever or blood in stool.
- Bismuth salicylate (Pepto-Bismol) 30 mL or two tablets every 30 minutes, up to eight doses.

Second-Line Medications

- Diphenoxylate/atropine (Lomotil) is an alternative antimotility agent that binds to opioid receptors in the gut. Start two tablets QID for no more than two days.

Clinical Pearls

- Loperamide is also an agonist at opioid receptors in the gut; misuse and abuse of this over-the-counter drug has increased in recent years. Those using opioids know it can help with withdrawal-related diarrhea. Some have discovered that in high doses (100–200 mg/day), it can produce euphoria. In rare cases, high dose use has resulted in hospitalization for arrhythmias and death.
- If persistent, bloody, or accompanied by severe pain or volume depletion (dry mucous membranes, low blood pressure), refer for further evaluation, including stool testing.

Dry Mouth (Xerostomia)

Characteristics

An uncomfortable sensation of dryness due to diminished saliva; can lead to dental caries, because saliva has an antibacterial effect. Can also cause decreased taste and inflammation of gums.

Meds that Cause It

Most psychotropic meds, especially antipsychotics, antidepressants (including selective serotonin reuptake inhibitors), lithium, psychostimulants, and medications used to treat or prevent extrapyramidal symptoms (benztropine, diphenhydramine, trihexyphenidyl).

Mechanism

Anticholinergic and other effects.

General Management

- Encourage aggressive oral hygiene, including more frequent dental cleanings.
- Chew sugarless gum to stimulate saliva production (especially gum containing xylitol, which can also reduce dental caries).
- Sip water frequently.
- Suck on ice chips.

First-Line Medications

- Biotene line of products, over the counter (most contain lubricants and humectants to "seal in" moisture):
  - Biotene gum: Use as needed.
  - Biotene toothpaste: Use as with any toothpaste.
  - Biotene oral rinse (mouthwash): Rinse up to five times per day.
  - Biotene Oralbalance Gel: Use one inch on tongue as needed (comes out of a tube).
  - Biotene moisturizing mouth spray: Spray on tongue as needed.
- Many saliva substitutes are available, such as Oralube saliva substitute, Oasis mouth spray, and others. No studies have demonstrated superiority of any single brand.

Second-Line Medications

- Procholinergic drugs:
  - Pilocarpine (Salagen) 5–10 mg two or three times daily (Side effects: Sweating, congestion, diarrhea; start with 2.5 mg test dose to ensure tolerability).
  - Cevimeline (Evoxac) 30 mg up to three times daily.

Clinical Pearls

- Caffeine can worsen dry mouth, so recommend decreasing caffeine use.
- Cigarette smoking can also worsen dry mouth, so recommend cessation.
- Don't shy away from trying procholinergic drugs—some patients prefer them over having to constantly use saliva substitute products.

Fun Fact:

Medications are often blamed, particularly in older patients, but aging itself is a common cause of dry mouth.

Dystonia

Characteristics

Involuntary contractions of muscles due to some antipsychotics. Can include torticollis (twisting neck), opisthotonos (arching spine or neck), oculogyric crisis (eyes rolling back), and trismus (jaw clenching). Rare but serious is tongue swelling, which can block the airway or cause choking when eating.

Meds that Cause It

Antipsychotics, especially high-potency first-generation antipsychotics. May rarely occur with second-generation antipsychotics.

Mechanism

D2 blockade.

First-Line Medications

Give these meds IM or IV if dystonia is severe.

- Benztropine (Cogentin) 1–2 mg once or twice per day (Side effects: Dry mouth, blurred vision, constipation, urinary retention, and cognitive changes).
- Diphenhydramine (Benadryl) 50 mg/day.
- If dystonia is severe, stop the offending drug and give either of the above agents IM or IV once or twice to stop the dystonia. Then prescribe two to three days of the oral version to prevent another episode.

Second-Line Medications

- Benzodiazepines (especially diazepam [Valium] 5–10 mg).
- Amantadine (Symmetrel) 100–200 mg BID (no injectable available).
- Trihexyphenidyl (Artane) 1–2 mg TID (no injectable available).

Clinical Pearls

- Earliest of the extrapyramidal symptoms, with an onset of hours to days after antipsychotic is started or dose is increased; 90% of reactions occur within first five days.
- Risk factors include young male patients, high-potency first-generation antipsychotics, or high dose.
- Prophylaxis with anticholinergic agent for first month of treatment in those with high risk or previous history.
- May be very frightening and painful for the patient.
- Can occur in a tardive form, with symptoms lasting for greater than six months after discontinuation of the offending agent.

Excessive Sweating (Hyperhidrosis)

Characteristics

Excessive sweating, which tends to be more prominent in the face, neck, and chest, and less prominent in the armpits and palms.

Meds that Cause It

Antidepressants, especially serotonin/norepinephrine reuptake inhibitors (venlafaxine, duloxetine, levomilnacipran) and bupropion.

Mechanism

Dysregulation of cholinergically innervated sweat glands.

General Management

Reduce dose or switch agents.

First-Line Medications

- Terazosin (Hytrin) alpha-1 blocker; start 1 mg at bedtime, then gradually increase by 1 mg/day increments up to 4–6 mg (Side effects: Dizziness, dry mouth, hypotension, rebound hypertension if stopped abruptly).
- Clonidine (Catapres) 0.1 mg daily.
- Benztropine (Cogentin) 1 mg BID.
- Glycopyrrolate (Robinul); start 1 mg twice daily and increase gradually by 1 mg/day increments up to 2 mg three times a day. Can be used PRN.

Second-Line Medications

- Oxybutynin (Ditropan) 5–10 mg daily or twice daily.
- Mirtazapine (Remeron) up to 60 mg daily as adjunct.
- Cyproheptadine (Periactin) 4 mg daily or twice daily.
- Aripiprazole (Abilify) 10 mg daily (one trial showed it alleviated hyperhidrosis due to fluoxetine or duloxetine).

Clinical Pearls

- Patients may not need to take medication for sweating in the winter.
- Often occurs in people who tended to sweat a lot before taking the medication.

Fatigue

Characteristics

Sleepiness as a result of medications. Typically, patients say they sleep more than enough at night, yet they feel like they could fall asleep at any point throughout the day.

Meds that Cause It

Antidepressants (especially paroxetine, mirtazapine, and tricyclics; bupropion is *least* likely to cause fatigue); antipsychotics (especially clozapine, quetiapine, olanzapine, but all can cause it); mood stabilizers; benztropine; benzodiazepines; antihistamines (eg, diphenhydramine, hydroxyzine); opioids.

Mechanism

Various mechanisms, often due to antihistamine or anticholinergic effects.

General Management

- Watchful waiting for spontaneous resolution (not usually effective).
- Change dosing to bedtime.
- Reduce dose.

Medications

- If not clinically contraindicated, psychostimulants such as methylphenidate or dextroamphetamine. Depending on the response, you may switch to a long-acting stimulant eventually.
- Modafinil (Provigil) 100–300 mg daily in divided doses.
- Armodafinil (Nuvigil) 150–250 mg daily in divided doses.
- If a serotonergic antidepressant is causing fatigue, consider switching to bupropion.

Clinical Pearls

- Rule out common nonmedication causes of fatigue, such as obstructive sleep apnea, hypothyroidism, and anemia.
- Fatigue can be a residual symptom of partially treated depression.
- If patients are taking a benzodiazepine for anxiety or insomnia, this could be causing daytime fatigue. Consider decreasing the dose or switching to a different agent.

Hyperprolactinemia

Characteristics

Elevated prolactin levels (>29 ng/mL in nonpregnant, nonlactating women, >18 ng/mL in men) that can cause the following symptoms:

- Women: Menstrual irregularity or amenorrhea, infertility, lowered libido, galactorrhea, decreased bone density, increase or thickening of hair in unexpected areas such as face.
- Men: Breast enlargement (gynecomastia), erectile dysfunction, low libido, infertility, galactorrhea.

Meds that Cause It

Antipsychotics, especially risperidone, paliperidone, and haloperidol. Other potential medications that cause it include estrogen, metoclopramide, and verapamil. Other causes: Hypothyroidism, pregnancy, kidney disease, polycystic ovarian syndrome, pituitary adenoma.

Mechanism

D2 blockade.

General Management

- Reduce dose or discontinue offending medication. Prolactin levels normalize within two to four days after discontinuation.
- Switch to a different agent (eg, aripiprazole, quetiapine).

First-Line Medications

(If stopping the causative drug is not feasible)

Add aripiprazole 5–20 mg daily. Aripiprazole lowers prolactin levels by partially activating dopamine receptors in the pituitary gland, thereby inhibiting prolactin release.

Second-Line Medications

- Add a dopamine agonist, such as cabergoline (Dostinex) 0.25 mg twice a week (*not* twice a day) or bromocriptine (Parlodel) 1.25–2.5 mg daily.
- Add an oral contraceptive agent to prevent bone loss in women and treat testosterone deficiency in men (it does not treat hyperprolactinemia).

Clinical Pearls

- Risperidone is the drug that causes the highest elevation, up to 300–400 mg/mL, whereas other drugs rarely cause elevations higher than 100 ng/mL.
- If your patient has a mild elevation (such as up to 40 ng/mL), get another level, but this time make sure it's a fasting level. Mild elevation can be caused by stress.
- While galactorrhea is often mentioned in discussions of high prolactin, this is a rare symptom, much less common than amenorrhea, low libido, and infertility.
- Patients with levels >100 ng/mL are generally referred for an MRI to rule out a pituitary adenoma, even if they are taking a drug known to increase prolactin.
- Use the lowest effective dose of dopaminergic agent as higher doses may worsen psychosis.

Nausea

Characteristics

Nausea or sensation of upset stomach beginning soon after first dose of a new medication.

Meds that Cause It

Serotonergic antidepressants (especially vilazodone and vortioxetine), lithium, valproic acid, naltrexone.

Mechanism

Various; may be related to stimulation of 5-HT3 receptors.

General Management

- Reduce dose.
- Wait one or two weeks since nausea is often transient.
- Switch to a nonserotonergic antidepressant.
- Start drug at half the usual dose and go up gradually.
- Take medication just after meals.
- Split the dose into BID or TID dosing.
- Switch to a delayed-release, extended-release, or enteric-coated formulation, if available (eg, valproic acid, lithium).
- Take a spoonful of peanut butter before taking the medication.

Medications

Most of these meds are well tolerated especially when used PRN. Sedation is common with many.

- Ginger root capsules two to three times per day, two capsules per dose.
- Trimethobenzamide (Tigan) 300 mg TID PRN.
- Promethazine (Phenergan) 12.5–25 mg BID PRN.
- Ondansetron (Zofran) 4–8 mg Q8 hours PRN (5-HT3 blocker).
- Mirtazapine (Remeron) 15 mg daily (5-HT3 blocker).
- Metoclopramide (Reglan) 10 mg three times a day as needed.
- Prochlorperazine (Compazine) 5–10 mg Q8 hours PRN.

Clinical Pearls

- Both metoclopramide and prochlorperazine are phenothiazines and, like others in that class, may cause extrapyramidal symptoms if continued for too long.
- Patients with preexisting GERD may be more susceptible to medication-induced nausea. Try prescribing a proton pump inhibitor, such as omeprazole (Prilosec), along with the offending agent.

Fun Fact:

Antipsychotics rarely cause nausea—in fact, several are FDA-approved antiemetics.

Neuroleptic Malignant Syndrome

Characteristics

Neuroleptic malignant syndrome (NMS) is a rare but potentially life-threatening drug reaction presenting with muscle rigidity ("lead pipe"), hyperthermia, and altered mental status. It may present similarly to serotonin syndrome although may be less acute in onset (within days vs hours).

Meds that Cause It

Antipsychotics. Occasionally other antidopaminergic medications (eg, metoclopramide).

Mechanism

D2 blockade.

General Management

- Discontinue antidopaminergic agents.
- Monitor vital signs and creatinine kinase levels to assess severity and to guide supportive care, including stabilizing vital signs and IV fluids if necessary.

First-Line Medications

Benzodiazepines. Any of them will work (eg, lorazepam [Ativan] 0.5–1 mg BID or diazepam [Valium] 10 mg BID).

Second-Line Medications

- Bromocriptine (Parlodel) 2.5–5 mg Q6–8 hours.
- For severe rigidity, dantrolene (Dantrium) 3–5 mg/kg IV divided TID or 100–400 mg/day oral divided QID. Monitor liver function.
- Bromocriptine or dantrolene should be continued for 10 days beyond symptom resolution.

Clinical Pearls

- Most cases, especially if caught early, will resolve quickly after antipsychotic discontinuation.
- Avoid bromocriptine if serotonin syndrome is not ruled out (eg, patient taking both antipsychotics and serotonergic agents). Bromocriptine has some proserotonergic activity and could worsen serotonin syndrome.
- Up to 50% of patients who have experienced NMS may have another episode. To minimize risk of recurrence in patients who require ongoing antipsychotic therapy, wait until symptoms have completely resolved (at least two weeks). Choose a different agent, ideally a second-generation antipsychotic as they are less likely to cause NMS. Never use a long-acting antipsychotic injection in patients with a history of NMS.

Orthostatic Hypotension

Characteristics

Orthostatic hypotension (OH) is caused by blood pooling in the lower extremities when people stand up, causing less blood flow to the brain and consequent dizziness. Usually caused by medications that block the alpha-1 receptors, which are responsible for telling the body to constrict blood vessels (and maintain blood pressure) after standing up. Patients will report feeling faint when they get up, and occasionally a sense of the room spinning (vertigo).

Meds that Cause It

Antipsychotics, especially clozapine, risperidone, quetiapine, and lower-potency first-generation agents. Antidepressants, especially tricyclics, monoamine oxidase inhibitors, trazodone, and sometimes mirtazapine.

Mechanism

Alpha-1 receptor blockade, also anticholinergic effects.

General Management

- Review all meds, including nonpsychiatric, since many blood pressure and cardiac meds, as well as alpha-blockers like prazosin (Minipress) and tamsulosin (Flomax) used for benign prostatic hyperplasia, can cause OH.
- Start at lower dose and titrate more slowly, especially when using higher-risk agents in higher-risk patients.
- Change dosing to minimize peak blood levels (eg, split dosing or switch to an extended-release version).
- Instruct patient to stand up slowly.
- Prevent dehydration by drinking enough fluids.
- Use compression stockings, also known as TED stockings.
- Increase salt intake. You can give salt tablets: 500–1000 mg BID or TID (use with caution in patients with hypertension or heart or kidney disease).
- Limit alcohol use.

Medications

- Fludrocortisone (Florinef) 0.1 mg daily; can increase by 0.1 mg/day increments weekly to 0.3 mg daily. Side effects: Hypokalemia. Use only in severe cases where other measures have not worked.
- Midodrine 10 mg three times daily. Side effects: Goose bumps, paresthesias. Use only in severe cases where other measures have not worked.

Clinical Pearls

- OH is defined as a 20 mm drop in systolic pressure or a 10 mm drop in diastolic pressure within three minutes of a patient moving from lying to standing position.
- Ask patients when the symptom is worse; if it is worse an hour or two after taking the medication, it is most likely medication induced.
- More common and problematic in the elderly; may contribute to fall risk.

Parkinsonism

Characteristics

Also known as pseudoparkinsonism, these drug-induced symptoms mimic those of Parkinson's disease:

- Tremor (especially apparent in the hands as a resting, "pill rolling" tremor).
- Rigidity (cog-wheel rigidity).
- Bradykinesia (slow movement), decreased arm swing.
- Shuffling gait.
- Slurred speech.
- Mask-like facies, stooped posture, drooling.
- Psychological side effects, such as cognitive dulling (bradyphrenia), worse negative symptoms (neuroleptic-induced deficit syndrome), worse depression (neuroleptic dysphoria).

Meds that Cause It

Antipsychotics, especially first-generation agents, but second-generation antipsychotics may also cause it. Least likely to cause it are clozapine, olanzapine, quetiapine, and ziprasidone.

Mechanism

D2 blockade, disruption of the balance between dopaminergic and cholinergic neurons.

General Management

Decrease dose or switch to a different antipsychotic.

First-Line Medications

- Benztropine (Cogentin) 1–2 mg once or twice per day.
- Trihexyphenidyl (Artane) 2–5 mg once or twice per day.
- Diphenhydramine (Benadryl) 50 mg/day.

Second-Line Medications

Amantadine (Symmetrel) 100–200 mg twice per day (enhances dopamine release).

Clinical Pearls

- May occur at any time, but typically seen within one to two months after antipsychotic is initiated.
- Highest-risk patients: Female, older, those taking higher-potency agents or higher doses.
- In patients at high risk of parkinsonism, start benztropine (or one of the other first-line agents) at the same time as the antipsychotic.
- Try discontinuing the anticholinergic agent after several weeks; many patients will not need to remain on it long term.

QT Interval Prolongation

What Is QT Prolongation?

The QT interval on an electrocardiogram (ECG) represents the time it takes for the heart's ventricles to depolarize (contract) and repolarize (relax). These interval times are corrected to account for variations in heart rate and are specified as "QTc." QT prolongation can lead to serious arrhythmias, including torsades de pointes (TdP), and sudden death. While the link between QT prolongation and TdP is not clear, QTc above 500 msec is a significant risk factor for TdP.

Table 4: **QTc Interval Classification for Adults**

Classification	QTc for Adult Women (msec)	QTc for Adult Men (msec)
Normal	<450	<430
Borderline	451–470	431–450
Prolonged	>480	>470

Source: Funk MC et al. *Resource Document on QTc Prolongation and Psychotropic Medications*. American Psychiatric Association. www.tinyurl.com/2p8xsf7y

How to Assess if a New Patient May Have QT Prolongation

While some units have a policy of ordering baseline ECGs on all patients, this is rare and probably an inefficient use of health care dollars. Here are some reasonable criteria for ordering an ECG to screen for QT prolongation:

- Taking a medication with a high risk of QT prolongation (see tables below and on the next page).
- Recent overdose on any medication, even if considered "low risk." Usually, such patients will have already had an ECG in the emergency room or on a medical unit.
- Taking other common medications that are not related to psychiatry, including antiarrhythmics such as sotalol, amiodarone, and quinidine; macrolide antibiotics such as azithromycin; quinolone antibiotics such as levofloxacin; some antifungals; antimalarials; and other medications such as tamoxifen.
- Significant cardiac history, such as history of myocardial infarction, arrhythmia, syncope, or prolonged QT interval.
- General risk factors for QT prolongation, such as being older, having electrolyte abnormalities (especially potassium, calcium, or magnesium), having conditions predisposing to electrolyte abnormalities (such as anorexia or bulimia), or having hepatic or renal dysfunction.

What to Do if Your Patient Has QT Prolongation

- *If borderline prolongation:* Review medications, and if necessary, switch to a less risky agent.
  - Lower-risk antipsychotics: Aripiprazole has minimal risk; asenapine, lurasidone, olanzapine, and quetiapine are also good options.
  - Lower-risk antidepressants: All antidepressants at usual therapeutic doses are relatively safe (avoid citalopram >40 mg/day). However, sertraline may be the best choice because it is the most studied in cardiac patients and has few drug interactions.
- *If marked prolongation (>500 msec):* Obtain a cardiologist consult.
- *In all cases:*
  - Periodically monitor electrolytes and ECG.
  - Manage reversible factors such as repleting electrolytes and hydration.

Table 5: **Top QT-Prolonging Non-Psychotropic Meds**

- Certain antibiotics (eg, azithromycin, levofloxacin, erythromycin)
- Antihistamines (eg, diphenhydramine, hydroxyzine)
- Antiemetics (ondansetron)
- Antiarrhythmics (eg, quinidine, amiodarone)
- Antifungals (eg, fluconazole)
- Antivirals (eg, anti-HIV meds)
- Certain anticancer medications (eg, tamoxifen)
- Certain diuretics (eg, furosemide due to its resultant hypokalemia)

Adapted from: Fazio G et al, *World J Cardiol* 2013;5(4):87–93.

Table 6: **Risk of QT Prolongation with Psychiatric Medications**

	Risk of QT Prolongation
Antidepressants	
Amitriptyline	+++
Bupropion	+
Citalopram	+++ (especially for doses >40 mg and for patients >60 years)
Clomipramine	++
Desvenlafaxine	+
Duloxetine	+
Escitalopram	+
Fluoxetine	+
Levomilnacipram	Inconclusive
Maprotiline	+++
Mirtazapine	+/++ (use cautiously for patients at risk of QT prolongation)
Paroxetine	+
Sertraline	+
Trazodone	+
Venlafaxine	++
Vilazodone	Inconclusive
Vortioxetine	Inconclusive
Antipsychotics	
Aripiprazole	--
Asenapine	+
Brexpiprazole	+
Chlorpromazine	+++
Clozapine	++
Fluphenazine	++
Haloperidol (IV)	+++
Haloperidol (oral/IM)	++
Iloperidone	++
Loxapine	++
Lurasidone	+
Risperidone	+/++
Olanzapine	+
Paliperidone	+/++
Perphenazine	++
Pimozide	+++
Quetiapine	++
Thioridazine	+++
Ziprasidone	++/+++
Mood stabilizers	
Carbamazepine	+
Lithium	++/+++ (elevated risk if level >1.2 mEq)
Valproic acid	+
Anxiolytics	
Benzodiazepines	--
Buspirone	--
Stimulants	
Amphetamines	+
Atomoxetine	+
Methylphenidate	+
Others	
Buprenorphine	--
Methadone	+++

Adapted from Funk et al 2019 and Beach SR et al, *Psychosomatics* 2013;54(1):1–13.

Serotonin Syndrome

Serotonin syndrome is a rare but potentially life-threatening emergency caused by medications that affect serotonin levels. Be vigilant when patients are on high doses or multiple serotonergic agents.

Causes

Various substances can trigger serotonin syndrome, including over-the-counter (OTC) meds and supplements:

- *Selective serotonin reuptake inhibitors (SSRIs):* The most common offenders, often in overdose or when used in combination with other serotonergic agents.
- *Monoamine oxidase inhibitors (MAOIs):* Can cause severe or fatal serotonin syndrome when combined with SSRIs or foods high in tyramine.
- *Serotonin/norepinephrine reuptake inhibitors (SNRIs):* Another class to be cautious of, particularly when used in combination with other serotonergic medications.
- *Recreational drugs:* Substances like MDMA (ecstasy) can lead to acute serotonin syndrome.
- *OTC medications and herbal supplements:* Eg, dextromethorphan and St. John's wort, respectively.
- *Other medications:* Some antipsychotics (eg, risperidone), antiemetics (eg, ondansetron), and even antibiotics (eg, linezolid) can contribute.

Diagnosis

Suspect serotonin syndrome if a patient on a serotonergic medication exhibits any of the following:

- Spontaneous clonus (rhythmic muscle contractions and relaxations occurring without provocation). This is a strong clue. It's most easily observed at the ankle but can be present in other muscle groups.
- Inducible clonus (like spontaneous clonus but occurs upon stimulation, like suddenly dorsiflexing the foot).
- Ocular clonus (rhythmic, involuntary oscillations of the eyes).
- Elevated body temperature.
- Autonomic nervous system overactivity: Tachycardia, hypertension, diaphoresis, tachypnea.
- Hyperreflexia.
- Agitation.

Differential Diagnosis

- *Neuroleptic malignant syndrome (NMS):* Often mistaken for serotonin syndrome, NMS typically features "lead pipe" rigidity rather than hyperreflexia.
- *Anticholinergic toxicity:* Presents like serotonin syndrome but generally lacks neuromuscular symptoms.
- *Sepsis and other systemic infections:* Fever and altered mental status in these conditions can be misleading, but lab findings and clinical presentation help distinguish these scenarios.

Laboratory Workup

Although there is no definitive laboratory test to diagnose serotonin syndrome, certain evaluations help in ruling out other conditions and assessing the severity of symptoms. These include:

- *Complete blood count:* To explore infectious etiologies.
- *Serum electrolytes:* To evaluate for electrolyte imbalances, like hyperkalemia, that can happen secondary to rhabdomyolysis (the breakdown of muscle tissue).
- *Renal and liver function tests:* To assess for serotonin syndrome–induced organ damage.
- *Creatine kinase levels:* To evaluate for rhabdomyolysis.
- *Blood cultures and lumbar puncture:* To exclude infectious etiologies.

Pathophysiology

Elevated levels of serotonin in the central and peripheral nervous system precipitate the syndrome.

Treatment

- Discontinue all serotonergic medications immediately.
- Provide supportive care (IV fluids, oxygen, benzodiazepines to control agitation).
- Reduce body temperature. Hyperthermia can lead to multiorgan failure and death. Use physical cooling methods (cooling blankets, cold-water immersion). Antipyretics are ineffective for serotonin syndrome.
- Prescribe cyproheptadine, an H1 antagonist with antiserotonergic properties (though with limited evidence). Give 8–12 mg PO initially, followed by 2 mg Q2 hours or 8 mg Q6 hours as needed.
- Admit to ICU in severe cases.

Sexual Dysfunction

Characteristics

Impairment of some aspect of sexual functioning, including low libido, anorgasmia, decreased sensation, erectile dysfunction, or delayed or retrograde ejaculation (in men).

Meds that Cause It

Antidepressants (paroxetine most likely, but all selective serotonin reuptake inhibitors and serotonin/norepinephrine reuptake inhibitors can cause it); antipsychotics (primarily risperidone and paliperidone); some mood stabilizers (valproic acid and carbamazepine).

Mechanism

Various, including activation of 5-HT2 receptors by antidepressants; hyperprolactinemia by antipsychotics such as risperidone; and anticholinergic and antiadrenergic effects in other antipsychotics, especially first-generation.

General Management

- Watchful waiting—works in 10%–20% of patients.
- Drug holiday—no dose Friday or Saturday, resume Sunday or Monday. (Not a good idea with paroxetine or venlafaxine due to discontinuation syndrome, nor with fluoxetine due to long half-life.)
- Decrease dose.
- Switch to a medication with low sexual side effects (eg, bupropion, mirtazapine, or an antipsychotic that does not affect prolactin).

First-Line Medications

- Add a PDE-5 inhibitor, such as sildenafil (Viagra) or tadalafil (Cialis). Works best for erectile dysfunction but may help with low libido as well. Less effective in women.
- Add bupropion (possibly more effective in women than men).

Second-Line Medications

- Buspirone (BuSpar) 30–60 mg daily.
- Cyproheptadine (Periactin) 8 mg 30 minutes before sex.
- Amantadine (Symmetrel) 100 mg daily.

Clinical Pearl

It can be hard to know if sexual dysfunction is caused by a medication, the underlying psychiatric condition, or a separate problem predating the medication. For this reason, you should try to obtain a sexual history in your patients before starting medications that can cause it.

Sialorrhea (Hypersalivation)

Characteristics

Excessive drooling, usually more severe at night.

Meds that Cause It

Clozapine is the most common cause (30%–80% incidence). Can be caused by olanzapine, risperidone, or quetiapine.

Mechanism

Procholinergic effect.

General Management

- Chew sugarless gum, which encourages more frequent swallowing of saliva.
- Place towel over pillow if main bothersome symptom is nocturnal sialorrhea.

First-Line Medications

Glycopyrrolate (Robinul): Start 1 mg at bedtime, then increase to 1–2 mg twice daily if symptoms are prominent during the day. Unlike other anticholinergics, glycopyrrolate does not cross the blood-brain barrier, so there are fewer central anticholinergic side effects. Side effects: Constipation, dry mouth, blurred vision, urinary retention.

Second-Line Medications

- Ipratropium (Atrovent) 0.03% nasal spray; use one to two sprays sublingually (rather than intranasally).
- Oxybutinin (Ditropan) 5 mg twice daily.
- Alpha agonists such as clonidine (Catapres) 0.05–0.1 mg daily or weekly transdermal patch 0.1–0.2 mg or guanfacine (Tenex).
- Benztropine (Cogentin) 1 mg twice daily.
- Trihexyphenidyl (Artane) 5 mg twice daily.
- Atropine 1% ophthalmic drops; use one drop TID PRN sublingually.

Clinical Pearls

- Dose reduction of clozapine usually is not helpful in diminishing symptoms.
- Clozapine has strong anticholinergic properties, so its procholinergic effect of excessive drooling is puzzling. Theories explaining this include specific stimulation of cholinergic salivary receptors and impairment in the autonomically mediated swallowing mechanism (which may also contribute to clozapine-related dysphagia and pneumonia).
- Sialorrhea may increase the risk of developing aspiration pneumonia in patients taking clozapine, particularly if accompanied by sedation. Monitor closely and manage accordingly.

Tardive Dyskinesia

Characteristics

Tardive dyskinesia (TD) is involuntary movements, usually occurring after months or years of antipsychotic treatment. The most common symptoms are oro-buccal-lingual, such as chewing, lip smacking, and tongue protrusion. Occasionally causes movements of fingers or toes and rarely, in severe cases, may affect torso and gait.

Meds that Cause It

Antipsychotics, especially first-generation antipsychotics (3%–5% per year); the risk is smaller with second-generation antipsychotics. Among second-generation antipsychotics, risperidone confers the highest risk.

Mechanism

D2 blockade leading to dopamine receptor supersensitivity.

Diagnosis

- Ask patients if they've ever been told they have TD or other movement disorders.
- Assess all patients who are on antipsychotics for TD by administering the Abnormal Involuntary Movement Scale (AIMS). The AIMS has 12 items to be rated and can be completed in about 10 minutes. The patient should not have anything in their mouth (dentures, gum) and should be seated in a firm, armless chair. For the full sheet and instructions, visit: www.thecarlatreport.com/AdministeringAIMS.

General Management

- Gradually discontinue the offending antipsychotic, if possible. If you abruptly discontinue a long-term antipsychotic, the TD symptoms can paradoxically worsen, because you are "uncovering" the hypersensitive dopamine receptors.
- If the patient's psychotic illness is too severe to discontinue the antipsychotic, you should gradually transition to a second-generation antipsychotic with low dopamine occupancy, such as quetiapine, clozapine, or lurasidone.

First-Line Medications

Vesicular monoamine transporter type 2 (VMAT2) inhibitors are clearly the most effective medications for reducing TD symptoms and should be the first-line agents—and they take about six weeks to yield measurable improvement. All three VMAT2 inhibitors are likely equally effective, but valbenazine is generally the first choice simply because it can be dosed once daily. Tetrabenazine has the advantage of being generic but lacks FDA approval for TD (though data show it is effective) and must be dosed three times daily.

- Valbenazine (Ingrezza): 40 mg/day; increase to 80 mg/day after a week. FDA approved for TD.
- Deutetrabenazine (Austedo): Start 6 mg BID; increase weekly by 6 mg/day increments to maximum dose of 48 mg/day (divide doses >12 mg/day BID); use QD dosing with extended-release formulation. FDA approved for TD.
- Tetrabenazine (Xenazine): Start 12.5 mg QD for one week, increase by 12.5 mg/day increments weekly to usual dose of 75–150 mg QD (divided doses >37.5 mg TID). FDA approved for Huntington's disease. Not FDA approved for TD but likely effective.

Side effects of VMAT2 inhibitors

- Most common side effect: Sedation, which generally improves over time.
- Less common: Akathisia, tremor, depression, anxiety.
- Both deutetrabenazine and tetrabenazine are contraindicated in patients with suicidal ideation or untreated/inadequately treated depression.

Second-Line Medications

- Benzodiazepines (eg, clonazepam [Klonopin] or lorazepam [Ativan] 0.5–1 mg daily or BID). Can help with both dyskinesia and anxiety associated with TD.
- Amantadine (Symmetrel) 100–300 mg/day.
- Gingko biloba extract 240 mg/day.

Clinical Pearls

- Risk factors for TD include first-generation antipsychotics more so than second-generation antipsychotics, higher-potency agents, duration of exposure, higher dose, elderly age, and Black ethnicity.
- Increasing the dose of the antipsychotic will improve symptoms temporarily but probably make them worse in the long run.

Tremor

Characteristics

Rapid regular movements of body parts, especially hands. Classified as fine vs coarse, and as resting vs postural vs intention.

Meds that Cause It

Lithium (fine intention tremor); valproic acid (fine); lamotrigine; bupropion; antipsychotics (parkinsonian, resting coarse tremor), especially high-potency first-generation agents and risperidone. Occasionally selective serotonin reuptake inhibitors and buspirone.

Mechanism

Multiple mechanisms depending on cause. Medication-induced tremor may be induced by excitability in muscle receptors and neuronal reflexes.

General Management

- Rule out unrelated causes, such as essential tremor or hyperthyroidism.
- Most drug tremors are fine postural tremor (seen best when patient is holding a fixed posture, such as holding hands up with arms extended).
- Reduce use of caffeine, which can worsen all tremors.
- Change dosing to minimize peak blood levels (eg, split dosing, switch to an extended-release version, or give full dose before sleep).
- Reduce dose or switch agents.

First-Line Medications

- Propranolol (Inderal) 10 mg BID as needed; increase by 10–20 mg/day increments weekly; can go up to 30–120 mg daily in two or three divided doses. Side effects: Dizziness, fatigue, syncope, low blood pressure.
- Inderal LA. Long-acting propranolol that can be dosed 60–80 mg once a day.
- Benztropine (Cogentin) 1 mg BID for parkinsonian tremor (due to antipsychotics).

Second-Line Medications

- Primidone (Mysoline) 100 mg three times a day.
- Vitamin B6 for lithium tremor 900–1200 mg daily.
- Amantadine (Symmetrel) 100–200 mg BID for parkinsonian tremor (due to antipsychotics).
- Various anticonvulsants such as topiramate (Topamax), gabapentin (Neurontin), oxcarbazepine (Trileptal).

Clinical Pearls

- Try to systematically track the severity of the tremor over time. Options include taking a quick video at each appointment, having patients copy a design or write their name and address, or having them drink a cup of water. Take notes or include samples during visits.
- Don't forget that tremor can signal alcohol or benzodiazepine withdrawal—something you might want to ask patients about.

Weight Gain

Characteristics

Typically, patients will report food craving and binging. Medication-induced weight gain is rapid in the first three months, more gradual over the following year, then often plateaus. Rapid initial weight gain is correlated with greater eventual cumulative weight gain. FDA definition of weight gain is an increase of 7% or more in weight from baseline.

Meds that Cause It

Antipsychotics, especially clozapine, olanzapine, and quetiapine. Somewhat less weight gain with risperidone and paliperidone. Least weight gain with aripiprazole, haloperidol, ziprasidone, and lurasidone. Antidepressants: Mirtazapine, tricyclics, paroxetine. Mood stabilizers: Lithium, valproic acid.

Mechanism

Blockade of histamine and serotonin-2A receptors, leading to increased hunger.

General Management

- Monitoring: Weight, BMI, waist circumference every four weeks for three months, then every three months.
- Lifestyle modification, including exercise and dietary changes, is helpful for patients who are motivated; several studies have shown some benefit, but in actual clinical settings it may be difficult to match their results.
- Switch to a medication that is more weight neutral.

First-Line Medications

These meds have some evidence specifically for reducing psychotropic-induced weight gain.

- Topiramate (Topamax) 100–300 mg/day. Side effects: Cognitive dulling.
- Metformin XR (Glucophage XR, Glumetza) 500–2000 mg; take with largest meal, split into two doses if needed (based on GI side effects).
- Olanzapine/samidorphan (Lybalvi) as an alternative to olanzapine alone to reduce weight gain.
- Orlistat (Xenical) 120 mg three times daily after meals. Interferes with fat absorption. Side effects: Diarrhea.
- Aripiprazole (Abilify) 15 mg/day. Antipsychotic. May be useful for olanzapine-induced weight gain as adjunct.
- Glucagon-like peptide-1 agonists (GLP1 agonists), such as liraglutide (Saxenda) or semaglutide (Ozempic).

Second-Line Medications

These meds are effective for weight loss but have little or no evidence specifically for psychotropic-induced weight gain.

- Bupropion SR (Wellbutrin SR) 300–400 mg daily.
- Any psychostimulant of the methylphenidate or amphetamine class.
- Naltrexone/bupropion (Contrave) 8 mg/90 mg up to two tabs twice daily. Antiobesity drug.
- Phentermine (Adipex-P, Lomaira) 15–37.5 mg daily. Antiobesity drug.
- Phentermine/topiramate (Qsymia) 7.5 mg/46 mg up to two tablets daily. Antiobesity drug.
- Nizatidine (Axid) 150–300 mg daily. Antacid, H2 blocker, available over the counter.
- Amantadine (Symmetrel) 100–300 mg/day.

Clinical Pearls

- Weight gain is most likely in the first six weeks of taking an antipsychotic, and it's difficult for patients to ever lose this weight. As such, you should monitor weekly initially and switch to a more weight-neutral agent at the first sign of weight gain.
- If patient gains 5% or more of body weight, switch to a different drug.
- Ziprasidone and aripiprazole are probably the most weight-neutral antipsychotics and may even cause weight loss, especially if switching from another agent.
- Weight gain tends to be most severe in patients who are taking an antipsychotic for the first time.
- Ask weight-gaining patients about dry mouth; many psychotropics cause this, and such patients may gain weight from drinking sugary beverages to deal with this side effect.

Diagnostic and Monitoring Tools

Which Diagnostic Labs Should You Order?

In this fact sheet, we present our approach to ordering lab tests for psychiatric patients, focusing on those most relevant to patients newly admitted to psychiatric units. In this section's other fact sheets, we'll drill down into more detail on specific labs (eg, thyroid tests) to help you interpret abnormalities.

Reasons to Order Labs in Psychiatry

- To rule out medical conditions that might present with psychiatric symptoms.
- To monitor potential side effects of psychiatric medications that could alter lab values.

Guidelines for Ordering Lab Tests

- *Avoid routine screenings for all patients:* Consider the patient's history and current presentation to select the most appropriate tests.
- *But adhere to guidelines from your state or your hospital:* Many regulatory agencies require that you order specific tests for all patients on certain medications. Examples include ordering lipid panels and hemoglobin A1c (HbA1c)/fasting glucose for all patients on antipsychotics, or lithium levels and renal function tests for those on lithium therapy.
- *Refrain from repeating recent tests:* The exception is if there's a significant change in the patient's condition that warrants reevaluation.
- *Be prepared to act on abnormal results:* Ordering tests without the readiness to interpret and respond to the findings does not contribute to effective patient care. While this may seem obvious, in practice we have seen many abnormal results languishing in patients' charts without proper follow-up.

Commonly Ordered Labs in Inpatient Psychiatry

- Complete blood count (white blood cell [WBC] with differential, red blood cell, hematocrit, hemoglobin, platelets).
  - Low hematocrit (anemia) can cause fatigue and depression.
  - Elevated WBC may reflect infection or dehydration.
  - Low WBC leukopenia is common in drug detox or as a side effect of some psych meds like clozapine and carbamazepine.
  - Low platelet count can occur from valproate exposure and can cause abnormal bruising and bleeding.
- Basic metabolic panel, also called a chem 7 panel (sodium, potassium, blood urea nitrogen [BUN], creatinine [Cr], chloride, carbon dioxide, glucose).
  - Hyponatremia in dehydration, psychogenic polydipsia, side effect of some psych meds like selective serotonin reuptake inhibitors, carbamazepine, oxcarbazepine.
  - Low bicarbonate (acidosis) side effect of topiramate.
  - Hypokalemia in dehydration and bulimia nervosa.
  - Low BUN/Cr in renal impairment.
  - High BUN/Cr in dehydration.
  - High glucose in diabetes.
- Urine pregnancy test.
- HbA1c.
  - Screen for diabetes; can be elevated by several antipsychotics.
- Magnesium, calcium, phosphate.
  - Rule out elevations or deficiencies.
- Thyroid-stimulating hormone (TSH).
  - Rule out hypo- or hyperthyroidism, which can contribute to mood disorders.
- Liver function tests (LFTs; alanine transaminase [ALT], aspartate transaminase [AST], alkaline phosphatase [ALP], bilirubin).
  - Detect liver impairment, which can affect choice of medications.
- Lipid panel.
  - Can be elevated by a variety of medications, especially certain antipsychotics.
- Vitamin B12/folate.
  - Deficiencies can contribute to depression/fatigue/cognitive impairment.
- Vitamin D.
  - Deficiency is common in patients with chronic mental illness and can exacerbate mood and anxiety disorders.
- Rapid plasma reagin (RPR).
  - Used to screen for syphilis, as neurosyphilis can present with psychiatric symptoms.

- If positive, follow up with confirmatory treponemal testing, such as fluorescent treponemal antibody absorption (FTA-ABS) or *T. pallidum* particle agglutination (TP-PA).

- HIV.
  - To detect HIV-associated neurocognitive disorders.
- Urine drug screen (UDS).
  - To identify substance use that may affect mental status or interact with medications.
- Troponins.
  - To rule out myocarditis in patients on clozapine, especially in the first four weeks of treatment.
- Medication blood levels.
  - Therapeutic levels:
    - Lithium: 0.6–1.2 mEq/L.
    - Valproate (valproic acid): 50–125 mcg/mL.
    - Carbamazepine: 4–12 mcg/mL.
    - Clozapine: 350–600 ng/mL.
- Urinalysis.
  - Useful for detecting urinary tract infections or kidney issues that can present with altered mental status.
- Neuroimaging.
  - To identify structural brain abnormalities that might contribute to psychiatric symptoms, such as tumors, strokes, or traumatic brain injuries.
- TB screening (Tuberculin Skin Test [TST] or QuantiFERON-TB Gold).
  - If indicated, screen for latent TB infection, especially in high-risk populations. QuantiFERON-TB Gold (a lab-based blood test) is preferred over TST in certain cases, such as in individuals who have received the BCG vaccine (a vaccine used to protect against TB).

Labs and Tests that May Be Altered by Certain Psychiatric Medications

This section provides a guide on which lab and other tests to consider based on the psychiatric medications your patient might be taking. Obtain pregnancy tests in reproductive-age patients prior to initiating any psychiatric medications.

Table 7: **Recommended Diagnostic Tests**

Medications	Recommended Diagnostic Tests
Antipsychotics—second generation, primarily clozapine, olanzapine, quetiapine, paliperidone, risperidone	Fasting glucose or HbA1c and lipids
Atomoxetine	LFTs
Carbamazepine	Carbamazepine level, CBC, sodium, LFTs, HLA-B*1502 in Asians[1]
Citalopram	ECG if cardiac disease or age >60 or dose >40 mg daily
Clozapine	Fasting glucose and lipids, CBC, troponins
Desvenlafaxine	Periodic blood pressure (BP)
Haloperidol	Prolactin level
Levomilnacipran	Periodic BP/pulse rate
Lithium	Lithium level, TSH, BUN/Cr[2], ECG if cardiac disease
Mirtazapine	Lipids
Naltrexone	LFTs if suspect liver disease
Oxcarbazepine	Sodium, HLA-B*1502 in Asians[2]
Paliperidone	Prolactin, fasting glucose and lipids

[1] HLA-B*1502 is a gene that increases the risk of developing toxic epidermal necrolysis and Stevens-Johnson syndrome in response to taking carbamazepine. Asians, especially the Han Chinese, are much more likely to have the gene than other populations.

[2] The serum Cr is used to compute the estimated glomerular filtration rate (eGFR), a more precise measure of kidney functioning. Increasingly, laboratory test results include the eGFR. You can calculate it yourself using an online calculator at www.tinyurl.com/mrywv5dh.

Complete Blood Count

The complete blood count (CBC) is one of the most commonly ordered lab tests—it is fundamental because it offers insights into many medical conditions that can have psychiatric implications. As psychiatrists, we often order and review CBCs, but we may not remember how to interpret the various abnormalities. This fact sheet will guide you through the essentials of the CBC, including when to order it, how to interpret its elements, and its relevance in psychiatry.

Elements of the CBC: A Basic Review

White blood cells (WBC)

- *Function:* WBCs are crucial for the immune response. Normal range: 4,000–10,000 WBCs per microliter (μL) of blood.
- *Differential:* Lists types of WBCs both as percentages of the total count and absolute numbers.
  - *Neutrophils (~60% of WBC):* Elevated in bacterial infections. Neutrophils are typically the first WBCs that the bone marrow produces when battling an infection. You'll often hear terms like "bands," "segs," and "shift to the left." A band means an immature neutrophil, in which the nucleus looks like a simple band or U shape. A segmented neutrophil (a seg) is a regular mature cell, with a nucleus that is segmented into several lobes. A shift to the left means that there are more bands than normal—in other words, lots of new neutrophils are being produced to fight infection.
  - *Lymphocytes (~20%):* Elevated in viral infections or tuberculosis (TB).
  - *Monocytes (~5%):* Also higher in viral infections and TB.
  - *Eosinophils:* Elevated in allergic reactions and parasitic infections. Significant increases might suggest a drug reaction in psychiatric patients, especially if accompanied by symptoms like rash or itching.

Red blood cells (RBC)

- *Function:* RBCs transport oxygen. The CBC offers several indices for evaluating RBCs:
  - *Hematocrit (Hct):* This measures the proportion of blood volume that is made up of RBCs. Normal ranges vary by sex, typically 38%–48% for males and 35%–45% for females.
  - *Hemoglobin (Hgb):* Hemoglobin is the protein in RBCs that carries oxygen. Normal values are usually 14–17 g/dL for males and 12–15 g/dL for females.
  - *Mean corpuscular volume (MCV):* Average volume of individual red blood cells. Useful in classifying anemias as microcytic, normocytic, or macrocytic.
  - *Mean corpuscular hemoglobin (MCH) and mean corpuscular hemoglobin concentration (MCHC):* Average hemoglobin amount and concentration in RBCs, aiding in anemia diagnosis.
  - *Red cell distribution width (RDW):* Variability in RBC size, differentiating anemia causes.

Platelets

- *Function:* Critical for blood clotting. Normal range: 150,000–450,000 platelets/μL.
- *Thrombocytopenia:* Low platelet count.
- *Thrombocytosis:* High platelet count.

Terminology Related to CBC Elements

- *Leukopenia:* Overarching term meaning a low WBC count, generally below 4 (4000 cells/μL). This doesn't specify which type of WBC is low—for that, you have to look at the differential.
- *Neutropenia:* Lower than normal neutrophil count (below 1500). In drug-induced neutropenia, the total WBC count may be normal even in the presence of neutropenia.
- *Agranulocytosis:* Severe version of neutropenia in which there are essentially no neutrophils in the blood.
- *Pancytopenia:* Reduction in *all* types of blood cells, including WBCs, RBCs, and platelets. It is usually caused by bone marrow suppression.
- *Bone marrow suppression:* Can be caused by various psychiatric medications and can lead to various hematological problems.

Reasons to Order CBC in Psychiatry

- Rule out hidden medical issues that may be masquerading as or contributing to psychiatric symptoms.
- Investigate physical symptoms and general health status in newly admitted psychiatric patients, especially those who have had poor outpatient medical follow-up.
- Detect hematological side effects of psychiatric medications (eg, neutropenia due to clozapine or carbamazepine).

How to Interpret the CBC in Inpatient Psychiatry

Elevated WBC (leukocytosis)

- *Infection:* A WBC count over 10,000/μL could indicate an infection. Assess the differential for a shift to the left.

- Common signs of infection include fever, urinary symptoms, upper respiratory symptoms, and skin changes indicative of cellulitis.
- Common infections that you may see in your psychiatric inpatients include:
  - Urinary tract infections: A frequent cause of delirium, especially in patients with dementia.
  - Upper respiratory infections: Such as bronchitis, potentially progressing to pneumonia.
  - Cellulitis: Often resulting from IV drug use or self-injury.
  - Sinusitis.

- *Lithium*: Lithium therapy can cause benign leukocytosis.
- *Steroid use:* Steroid use (such as for COPD exacerbations) can cause leukocytosis.
- *Dehydration:* Apparent leukocytosis due to hemoconcentration. Factors like homelessness or reduced food and fluid intake from depression might lead to dehydration in newly admitted patients. This usually resolves with adequate hydration.
- *Psychological stress:* The stress associated with psychiatric illness can induce leukocytosis through cortisol and catecholamine release, prompting the release of WBCs from the bone marrow.

Low WBC (leukopenia)

- *Medication side effect:*
  - In about 3% of patients, clozapine can cause a low neutrophil count. If your patient's absolute neutrophil count (ANC) is at least 1500, you can start clozapine and then follow standard monitoring guidelines (see the "Clozapine: Guidelines for Use and Monitoring" fact sheet in the Common Psychiatric Conditions section, Schizophrenia and Other Psychotic Disorders subsection). Neutropenia is defined as an ANC below 1500. Agranulocytosis is a very severe form of neutropenia implying near-absence of neutrophils. (Granulocytes are named for their visible granules in the cytoplasm—granules that contain substances crucial for fighting bacteria. While two other types of WBCs, eosinophils and basophils, are also called granulocytes, neutrophils are the most abundant and important ones.)
  - Carbamazepine can rarely cause neutropenia, anemia, and pancytopenia.
  - Valproic acid can cause general bone marrow suppression, often initially indicated by thrombocytopenia (low platelet count).
- *Drug or alcohol use disorder:* Chronic drug or alcohol use can lead to various hematological changes, including the potential for bone marrow suppression. The mechanisms involve direct toxicity to the bone marrow, nutritional deficiencies (such as folate or vitamin B12 deficiency), and the harmful effects of substances or their metabolites on the production of WBCs.

Elevated RBC (polycythemia)

- *Primary polycythemia (polycythemia vera):* A rare condition that results in increased RBC production due to abnormalities in the bone marrow. This condition requires specialist management.
- *Secondary polycythemia:* More common in the psychiatric setting; can be caused by chronic hypoxia or smoking. It may also be induced by testosterone replacement therapy. Symptoms include headaches, dizziness, and an increased risk of blood clots.
- *Dehydration:* Similar to leukocytosis, high RBC count can be due to hemoconcentration. It's reversible with proper hydration.

Low RBC (anemia)

- *Iron deficiency anemia (microcytic anemia):*
  - Iron deficiency anemia is classified as microcytic, meaning the RBCs are smaller than normal. It is diagnosed with low Hct and Hgb levels. Key laboratory findings include a low MCV (typically below 80 fL) and an MCH and MCHC within or below the lower limits of normal (MCH: 27–32 pg; MCHC: 31–36 g/dL).
  - The most common causes include chronic blood loss (eg, from gastrointestinal bleeding or heavy menstrual periods), dietary iron deficiency, or malabsorption syndromes (eg, celiac disease).
  - To confirm iron deficiency and its severity, standard follow-up labs include serum ferritin, serum iron, total iron binding capacity (TIBC), and transferrin saturation. A low serum ferritin is the hallmark of iron deficiency. Additional tests may include stool occult blood test to rule out GI bleeding as a cause.
- *Vitamin B12 or folate deficiency anemia (megaloblastic anemia):*
  - This type of anemia is known as megaloblastic due to the presence of unusually large RBCs, with an elevated MCV (>100 fL), indicating a macrocytic anemia. The Hct and Hgb are usually low, and the MCH and MCHC can be elevated or within the upper limits of normal.
  - B12 deficiency can result from poor dietary intake, malabsorption (as seen in pernicious anemia or after gastric surgery), or certain medications. Folate deficiency is often due to dietary deficiency, malabsorption, or increased need (as in pregnancy).

- To distinguish between B12 and folate deficiencies, the following labs are recommended: serum B12 level, red cell folate level, and homocysteine and methylmalonic acid levels (elevated in B12 deficiency).

Elevated platelets (thrombocytosis)

- *Causes:* Often a reactive process due to inflammation or infection, or as an acute phase reactant. Less commonly, it can be due to a primary hematological disorder.
- *Psychiatric relevance:* Elevated platelet counts may indicate an underlying inflammatory or infectious process that could be affecting the patient's psychiatric status or response to treatment.

Low platelets (thrombocytopenia)

- *Causes:* Can result from bone marrow suppression due to medication effects (eg, valproic acid, some antipsychotics), viral infections, or autoimmune diseases, or as a part of pancytopenia.
- *Psychiatric relevance:* Patients with low platelet counts may present with easy bruising or bleeding, which can be concerning and require medical evaluation. Monitoring platelet counts is essential when initiating or managing treatment with medications known to impact bone marrow.

Basic Metabolic Panel

The basic metabolic panel (BMP) is a commonly ordered test on admission to most psychiatric units. This fact sheet focuses on five components relevant to psychiatric care: sodium (Na), potassium (K), chloride (Cl), bicarbonate (HCO3), and glucose. Mostly excluded from this discussion are blood urea nitrogen (BUN) and creatinine (Cr), which are covered in the "Kidney Function Testing" fact sheet in this section.

Reasons to Order BMP in Psychiatry

- Monitor potential side effects of psychiatric medications that may impact liver, kidney, or metabolic functions.
- Evaluate unexplained symptoms such as fatigue, confusion, or abdominal pain that could be related to metabolic disturbances.
- Assess overall health status in patients with psychiatric conditions, especially those with suspected or known substance use disorders.

BMP Abnormalities Commonly Seen in Psychiatric Inpatient Units

Sodium

Essential for nerve and muscle function. Normal range: 135–145 mmol/L.

- *Hyponatremia (low sodium):* Typical causes in psychiatric patients include:
  - Dehydration due to decreased food and fluid intake (eg, depression, homelessness, or substance use disorders with poor self-care). A clue to dehydration is an elevated BUN/Cr ratio.
  - Bulimia nervosa due to self-induced vomiting and/or diuretic abuse.
  - Psychogenic polydipsia, which involves compulsive water drinking that dilutes sodium levels.
  - Drug side effects: Selective serotonin reuptake inhibitors, carbamazepine, oxcarbazepine, thiazide diuretics.
- *Symptoms of hyponatremia:*
  - Mild (130–135 mmol/L): May be asymptomatic but can cause unsteadiness and falls.
  - Moderate (125–130 mmol/L): Headache, lethargy, restlessness, disorientation, muscle twitching.
  - Severe (<125 mmol/L): Confusion, seizures, and potential coma.
- *Initial management of hyponatremia:* Water restriction and addressing underlying cause.

Potassium

Key for heart function. Normal range: 3.5–5.0 mmol/L.

- *Hypokalemia (low potassium):* Can result from dehydration due to diarrhea and vomiting, or from laxative abuse (often in patients with eating disorders). Hypokalemia is a concern in alcohol withdrawal due to the potential for cardiac arrhythmias.
- *Hyperkalemia (high potassium):* Often elevated in kidney failure. If elevated, use kayexalate 15 mg daily. Can repeat dose as needed, up to four times daily, to normalize potassium.

Chloride

Helps maintain fluid balance. Normal range: 98–106 mmol/L. It's not usually abnormal in isolation from other electrolytes.

Bicarbonate

Regulates blood pH. Normal range: 22–29 mmol/L.

- *Decreased bicarbonate (leading to metabolic acidosis):*
  - Conditions and causes include topiramate use (due to inhibition of carbonic anhydrase), diabetic ketoacidosis, anorexia (starvation leading to fat breakdown and ketosis), and alcohol use disorder (poor liver function leading to a buildup of lactic acid and ketones).
  - Management generally involves stopping the offending agent (like topiramate), insulin and fluid replacement for diabetic ketoacidosis, nutritional support for anorexia, and abstinence plus liver support for alcohol use disorder.
- *Increased bicarbonate (metabolic alkalosis):*
  - Rare in psychiatry but can occur in conditions such as bulimia nervosa due to vomiting up stomach acid.

Glucose

The primary energy source for the body's cells. Normal range: 70–100 mg/dL fasting.

- *Elevated glucose (hyperglycemia):*
  - May indicate diabetes mellitus, prediabetes, or stress hyperglycemia. Psychiatric medications, especially some antipsychotics, can increase the risk of developing diabetes or exacerbate preexisting diabetes.
  - Diagnosis of diabetes is confirmed by a fasting blood glucose >125 mg/dL on two separate occasions or a random blood glucose >199 mg/dL accompanied by diabetes symptoms like frequent urination, increased thirst, unexplained weight loss, intense hunger, visual changes, fatigue, and slow wound healing. An HbA1c level

above 6.5%, which reflects average blood glucose levels over the past two to three months, further supports the diagnosis.
  - Prediabetes is a condition characterized by blood glucose levels that are higher than normal but not yet high enough to be classified as diabetes. It's a critical stage where intervention can significantly delay or prevent the development of Type 2 diabetes. Diagnosis is based on certain criteria, including HbA1c of 5.7%–6.4% or a fasting glucose level of 100–125 mg/dL.
  - Elevated glucose levels may affect cognitive function, mood, and overall mental health. Check glucose levels regularly in patients on antipsychotic medications.
- *Decreased glucose (hypoglycemia):*
  - Insufficient glucose level in the blood, which can cause symptoms such as dizziness, sweating, confusion, irritability, and even seizures or loss of consciousness.
  - Causes include insufficient glucose intake or excessive insulin in patients with diabetes, prolonged fasting, and excessive alcohol consumption.

Kidney Function Testing

The kidneys filter the blood, eliminating unwanted chemicals (such as metabolic byproducts of medications) from the body. The three most common kidney function labs that we order in psychiatry are blood urea nitrogen (BUN), creatinine (Cr), and glomerular filtration rate (GFR).

The Basics

Blood urea nitrogen

Tests kidney function and hydration status. Normal range: 7–20 mg/dL.

- When amino acids (proteins) are metabolized, one of the breakdown products is ammonia—which is toxic and can cause sedation and coma in high concentrations. The liver detoxifies ammonia by combining it with carbon dioxide to create urea.
- When labs report "blood urea nitrogen," they are actually reporting the urea concentration. The reason for using the confusing term "BUN" is that it's cheaper and easier for labs to measure just the nitrogen portion of urea.
- The body can live with a certain concentration of urea, but when it gets too high, it can cause sedation and other problems. The kidney keeps the concentration of urea down by clearing it into the urine, but kidney impairment leads to abnormally high BUN.
- BUN is not specific to kidney failure. In dehydration, the kidney tubules reabsorb more water, and urea often follows that water into the bloodstream—resulting in a high BUN that has nothing to do with kidney failure.

Creatinine

Tests kidney function. Normal range: 0.5–1.1 mg/dL.

- Creatinine is a waste product produced by the muscles from the breakdown of a compound called creatine. Creatine (as phosphocreatine) is needed for the production of adenosine triphosphate, which is used for muscle contraction. When phosphocreatine gives up its phosphate group, it becomes creatinine, which must be cleared by the kidneys.
- The kidneys filter creatinine from the blood into the urine. Because muscle mass in individuals tends to be stable, creatinine production and its filtration rate by the kidneys are relatively constant.
- High levels of creatinine in the blood are specific to kidney impairment because they indicate the kidneys are not effectively filtering this waste. This makes creatinine a more reliable marker of kidney function than BUN.

Glomerular filtration rate

Best test of kidney function. Normal range: 90 mL/min or above.

- GFR is the best overall index of kidney function. It measures how well the kidneys filter a specific volume of blood over a set period, typically expressed in milliliters per minute.
- Direct measurement of GFR is complex and time-consuming, involving the injection of a specific substance and measuring its clearance from the blood. Because of this, it's rarely done in clinical practice.
- The estimated GFR (eGFR) is commonly reported and is calculated using formulas that take into account the patient's age, gender, body size, and serum creatinine levels.

Interpreting and Acting on Abnormalities

Dehydration

BUN/Cr ratio is elevated, typically exceeding 20:1. In psychiatry units, this often reflects poor self-care due to homelessness, psychiatric illness, or substance use. Push oral fluids and food intake, monitor vital signs, and reorder BUN/Cr within 24–48 hours. If this conservative approach isn't working to normalize kidney function tests, obtain a medical consult for assistance.

Lithium use

About 20% of patients on long-term lithium will develop some degree of kidney impairment, usually signaled by a "creeping creatinine." When creatinine reaches 1.5, this is the standard cutoff for renal impairment. While not a medical emergency, you should refer such patients to their primary care physician after discharge from inpatient psychiatry.

Patients on dialysis

Patients on dialysis will be followed closely by nephrology. Most psychiatric meds can be continued during dialysis and can typically be administered on the same schedule as for patients who aren't receiving dialysis, as they are primarily metabolized and cleared by the liver. However, lithium is usually given after a dialysis session because it is almost entirely removed by the procedure.

Liver Function Tests

Liver function tests (LFTs) are important in psychiatry for various reasons. The liver metabolizes most of the medications we prescribe, so we need to ensure that liver functioning is adequate. In addition, excessive substance use can seriously damage the liver. This fact sheet provides an overview of the most relevant LFTs, including their normal ranges, interpretation, and clinical relevance in psychiatry.

Standard LFT Panel

- *Alanine transaminase (ALT) and aspartate transaminase (AST):* Elevated levels indicate liver inflammation from various causes. Normal ranges vary but are generally <50 units per liter for ALT and <40 units per liter for AST.
  - Mild elevation = Up to five times the upper limit of normal (eg, ALT and AST no higher than about 200). Don't freak out when AST and ALT are double or triple normal levels—this means mild inflammation but not liver impairment. Such patients can usually take regular doses of all psychiatric drugs.
  - Moderate elevation = Five to 10 times the upper limit of normal.
  - Marked elevation = More than 10 times the upper limit of normal.
  - An AST:ALT ratio equal to or greater than 2:1 suggests alcoholic liver disease (Mnemonic: S is higher than L in the alphabet).
  - Nonalcoholic fatty liver disease is the most common cause of mild liver enzyme elevation in absence of alcohol use. It's often related to obesity, diabetes, hypertension, and hyperlipidemia, all of which are frequently seen in patients with psychiatric disorders. In other words, elevated liver enzymes don't necessarily mean your patient has a drinking problem.
  - In alcoholic cirrhosis, AST and ALT may be abnormally low due to extensive scarring of hepatic cells.
- *Gamma-glutamyltransferase (GGT):* Normal range: 7–48 units per liter; range varies by sex.
  - GGT levels can rise due to excessive alcohol consumption, even when other liver enzymes like ALT and AST remain normal. This increase is because chronic alcohol use prompts the liver to produce more enzymes, including GGT, to metabolize and detoxify alcohol.
  - Elevated GGT serves as an early indicator of heavy alcohol intake, often before any liver damage is visible. Thus, high GGT levels with normal ALT and AST suggest significant alcohol use, making GGT a critical marker for assessing alcohol use disorder in patients without overt liver damage.
- *Alkaline phosphatase (ALP):* Another enzyme related to liver and bone health. Normal range: 20–140 units per liter.
  - Elevations may mean cholestasis (any blockage in ducts), pregnancy, or various bone diseases (including cancers).
- *Bilirubin:* Bilirubin is a breakdown product of red blood cells, which have a lifespan of about 120 days. The liver creates bilirubin via enzymes, then adds it to bile for eventual excretion via the GI tract. Thus, the bilirubin level is a measure of the liver's ability to process waste.
  - Total bilirubin range: 0.1–1.2 mg/dL. It is composed of both direct and indirect bilirubin.
  - Direct bilirubin is bilirubin that has been conjugated to other molecules, rendering it water soluble and able to be excreted.
  - Indirect bilirubin is the form released from the breakdown of red blood cells not yet processed by the liver.
  - Excessive bilirubin leads to jaundice (yellow skin and eyes) and can be caused by liver dysfunction, bile duct obstruction ("cholestatic jaundice"), or excessive breakdown of red blood cells, as in hemolysis. The levels of indirect vs direct bilirubin will help specialists determine the pathology, but it's not something psychiatrists need to learn.
- *Albumin:* Main protein made by the liver; a measure of nutrition and liver function. Normal range: 3.5–5.0 g/dL.
  - Albumin is an important transporter of various substances in the bloodstream (such as many medications). Since albumin has a long half-life of about 20 days, low levels indicate chronic liver disease and malnutrition rather than acute liver injury.
- *Total protein:* Includes albumin and all other blood proteins. Normal range: 6.3–7.9 g/dL.

Other Labs Relevant to Liver Function

- *Prothrombin time (PT):* Measures the time it takes for blood to clot (range 11–13.5 seconds).
- *International normalized ratio (INR):* The INR is a standardized way of expressing PT and is used primarily to monitor patients on the anticoagulant warfarin. Normal INR range is 0.8–1.1; target INR for those on warfarin is 2.0–3.0. Both PT and INR assess the liver's ability to produce clotting factors.
- *Ammonia:* Normal range: 15–45 µmol/L. The liver metabolizes ammonia, which is a toxic byproduct of protein metabolism. Elevated levels cause lethargy and confusion. Poor liver function may lead to high ammonia levels, though a more common cause of hyperammonemia in psychiatric patients is valproic acid (Depakote). Management includes stopping the offending agent and administering lactulose.
- *Viral hepatitis titers:* See the "Viral Hepatitis" fact sheet in the Managing Comorbid Medical Conditions section for details.

Urinalysis

In this fact sheet, we discuss when to order and how to interpret a urinalysis in psychiatric inpatients. We won't cover the urine tox screen (or drug screen) here, as it is already covered in the "Urine Drug Screening" fact sheet in this section.

Table 8: **Elements of a Urinalysis: Quick Reference Chart**

Element	Normal Range	Significance
Color and appearance	Pale to dark yellow, clear	Dark urine may indicate dehydration; cloudy urine suggests infections
Specific gravity (SG)	1.005–1.030	High SG points to dehydration; low SG may signal kidney issues or overhydration
pH	4.6–8.0	Affected by diet, diseases, and medications; abnormal levels may indicate metabolic or renal disorders
Protein	Little to none	Presence indicates potential kidney disease; transient increases can occur with stress or exercise
Glucose	Absent	Presence suggests diabetes
Ketones	Absent	May indicate diabetes mellitus, starvation, or a low-carbohydrate diet
Blood (hematuria)	Absent	Sign of infection, injury, stones, cancer, or kidney disease
Leukocyte esterase and nitrite	Absent	Indicate urinary tract infection (UTI)—leukocyte esterase for white blood cells; nitrites suggest bacterial conversion from nitrate
Microscopic examination	—	Identifies cells, crystals, casts, bacteria, or yeast; crucial for diagnosing infections, stones, or kidney diseases

When to Order a Urinalysis in Psychiatry

Order a urinalysis as part of initial screening for symptoms like dysuria (painful or burning urination), hematuria, or flank pain. In addition, order a urinalysis in geriatric patients who are agitated or delirious for no clear reason. Sometimes such patients—especially those with dementia—may have a UTI without a fever and may not be able to communicate clear urinary symptoms.

- *Typical UTI findings:* Cloudy or odorous urine, positive leukocyte esterase, positive nitrites, increased white blood cells, hematuria, and presence of bacteria on microscopic exam.
- *Contamination signs:* Large numbers of squamous cells and common skin flora (eg, *Staphylococcus epidermidis* or *Staphylococcus aureus*) suggest contamination. Order a "clean catch" repeat test if necessary.
- *Should you order a culture?* If your patient is otherwise healthy and has UTI symptoms, empiric treatment with nitrofurantoin (Macrobid) or trimethoprim/sulfamethoxazole (Bactrim) is usually recommended. Order a medicine consult if a clinical decision hinges upon culturing the sample to identify a specific pathogen.
- *Assessment for dehydration:* While often signaled by orthostatic vital signs and a high blood urea nitrogen/creatinine ratio, the urinalysis may also show findings of a dark color and elevated SG.
- *Psychogenic polydipsia:* Patients with psychogenic polydipsia may have urinalysis findings like low specific gravity and low osmolality.

Additional Urine-Based Testing

While not part of a routine urinalysis, you can use urine tests for these purposes:

- STD screening (for chlamydia, gonorrhea, or trichomoniasis).
- Substance use screening.
- Pregnancy testing (critical before starting medications that might be teratogenic).
- Urine osmolality (to measure the concentration of particles in urine; relevant for patients with psychogenic polydipsia or those at risk of dehydration due to neglect of basic needs).

Therapeutic Drug Monitoring

Therapeutic drug monitoring (TDM) means measuring blood levels of medications to guide dosing and detect toxicity or nonadherence. Its usefulness is the subject of continuing debate. For many psychiatric drugs, blood levels are useful only to see if the patient is adherent or if they have a genetic variation affecting their ability to metabolize the drug normally.

Reasons to Order Drug Levels

- *Fine-tune the dose:* For a very few drugs in psychiatry, we have some evidence that certain serum levels are correlated with efficacy—these are lithium, valproic acid, carbamazepine, clozapine, and nortriptyline.
- *Understand poor tolerability:* Some patients seem to have significant side effects on low doses of medications, and for such patients you might consider ordering serum levels just to see if the serum level is very high. If this is true, your patient may be a genetically poor metabolizer (which you can investigate with genetic testing) or there may be a drug-drug interaction.
- *Understand poor response:* If your patient is consistently not responding to medications at robust doses, it's possible that they are not adherent, that they are genetically ultrarapid metabolizers, or that there is a drug interaction causing rapid metabolism of the medication. Ordering TDM and finding atypically low blood levels can help you decide what to do next.

Practical Issues

The best time to draw a drug level is during steady state, which is five half-lives after initiating the medication or after making a dosage change; for most medications below, this means about five days. You should measure the trough level (the lowest level), which is best done right before a dose is taken (eg, if the drug is taken in the morning, draw the blood before the morning dose; if it is given twice a day, draw it at least 12 hours after the last dose).

TDM to Fine-Tune Dosing

For the following medications, there is reasonably good evidence correlating specific ranges of blood levels with therapeutic efficacy. The usual procedure is to titrate the medication up to the standard recommended dosage, then order blood levels to guide any further titration.

Lithium

- *Clinical efficacy:* Widely accepted evidence of the following:
  - 0.6–0.8: Correlated with prevention of depression.
  - 0.9–1.2: Correlated with treatment and prevention of mania.
- *Toxicity:* Levels above 1.2 are correlated with side effects and toxicity, though select patients may require higher blood levels for a clinical response without becoming toxic.

Valproic acid

- *Clinical efficacy:* 50–100 mcg/mL for bipolar disorder, though correlation is weak.
- *Toxicity:* Levels above 100 mcg/mL increase risk of side effects.

Carbamazepine

- *Clinical efficacy:* 4–12 mcg/mL for bipolar disorder.
- *Toxicity:* Levels above 12 mcg/mL increase risk of side effects.

Clozapine

- *Clinical efficacy:* 350 ng/mL is generally considered the minimal blood level for a response. There is some limited evidence that efficacy falls off above 600 ng/mL, but many individual patients require higher doses. Note that some labs also report norclozapine levels, but this is not useful for making dosing decisions, so just ignore that value if you see it.
- *Toxicity:* Levels above 1000 ng/mL increase risk of side effects, especially seizures.

Nortriptyline

- *Clinical efficacy:* 50–150 ng/mL for depression.
- *Toxicity:* Levels above 150 ng/mL increase risk of side effects.

Clomipramine

- *Clinical efficacy:* Clomipramine 50–250 mcg/L; desmethylclomipramine 150–350 mcg/L; total 200–500 mcg/L.
- *Toxicity:* Levels above 500 mcg/L (total) increase risk of side effects.

TDM to Assess Nonresponse or Toxicity

The following medications and classes of medications have no conclusive evidence of a correlation between blood levels and efficacy. The only reason to draw their levels is in cases of nonresponse, suspected overdose, or specific side effects.

- Antipsychotics other than clozapine.
- Antidepressants other than tricyclics.
- Lamotrigine.

Urine Drug Screening

Urine drug screening (UDS) is used to determine whether a patient has used a drug in the recent past.

What Is the Basic UDS?

- Based on immunoassay technology, which uses enzymes, fluorescent particles, or radioisotopes to enhance visual detection of the binding between the antibody and the antigen.
- Most commonly used due to low cost (<$30) and quick results.
- Very sensitive (only misses a few cases) but not very specific (prone to false positives).
- Procedure:
  - A typical multipanel test card has 10 test strips attached to the bottom, one for each drug of interest.
  - Strips are dipped into the urine sample for a few seconds, then allowed to incubate for about five minutes.
  - Each strip has a specific antibody on it that will bind to a specific drug compound, or antigen.
  - As the urine is absorbed by the paper and moves up the strip, the antibody will react with the drug (if present).
  - Based on presence or absence of control lines and test lines, results are interpreted as positive or negative for the drug corresponding to its strip.

How Does Confirmatory ("Reflex") Testing Work?

- Based on gas chromatography–mass spectrometry, which identifies the precise substances present.
- Used to verify questionable UDS results.
- Expensive ($200+) and slow (three days or more).
- Highly sensitive and specific; won't give false results.

What Is Included in a UDS?

In most facilities across the US, a UDS detects a standard "bundle" of substances. However, the specific substances can vary by region or institution. For example, in some areas, buprenorphine may be included in the standard panel, while in others, it might not. Typically, a UDS screens for the following nine substances:

- Nonopioids: Amphetamines, barbiturates, benzodiazepines, cannabinoids, cocaine.
- Opioids: Fentanyl, methadone, oxycodone, opiate screen.

These are self-explanatory—except for the "opiate screen," which is a catch-all for a group of opioids that are not included in the four specific screens. Typically, the opiate screen is positive in the presence of heroin, morphine, codeine, hydrocodone (Vicodin, Norco, Lortab), or hydromorphone (Dilaudid). A patient might report using street drugs and have a UDS that is negative for everything except the opiate screen. If you want to know exactly which opioids the patient has been using, ask your lab to do confirmatory testing for specific substances.

Which Patients Should Get a UDS?

Most patients who present to an ED get a UDS as part of the standard medical workup. In addition, the following groups of patients should get one:

- Patients with a current or recent substance use disorder (SUD).
- Patients with a remote SUD to whom you are considering prescribing a medication with potential for abuse.
- Patients with psychiatric disorders who are not responding to evidence-based treatment—this may be a sign of undisclosed drug use.
- Patients who are prescribed controlled substances and have been requesting early refills.

Potential false positives

- Opioids: Poppy seeds, fluoroquinolones, dextromethorphan.
- Amphetamines: Selegiline, cold medications containing pseudoephedrine.
- Barbiturates: Certain migraine medications.
- Cocaine: Topical anesthetics.

False negatives

- Uncommon if the UDS includes a catch-all opiate screen.
- May reflect use of a substance outside of the detection window.

Table 9: **Urine Drug Screening**

Drug	Detection Period	Agents Potentially Causing Positive Result
Alcohol	7–12 hours (80 hours for alcohol metabolites EtG and EtS)	Short-chain alcohols (eg, isopropyl alcohol)
Amphetamine/methamphetamine	1–2 days	ADHD medications (atomoxetine, stimulants) Amantadine (Symmetrel) Antipsychotics (aripiprazole, chlorpromazine, thioridazine) Bupropion (Wellbutrin) Ephedrine (Primatene, Bronkaid) Isometheptene (Midrin) MDMA (ecstasy) Phentermine (Adipex-P, Qsymia) Phenylephrine (Sudafed PE) Promethazine (Phenergan) Pseudoephedrine (Sudafed) Ranitidine (Zantac) Selegiline (Eldepryl, Emsam) TCAs (desipramine, trimipramine) Trazodone (Desyrel) Trimethobenzamide (Tigan)
Barbiturates	2–4 days (2–3 weeks for long-acting phenobarbital)	Ibuprofen (Advil, Motrin) Naproxen (Naprosyn)
Benzodiazepines (alprazolam, clonazepam, lorazepam, triazolam may not be detected on some assays)	24 hours (short-acting); 2–4 days (long-acting); >7 days for chlordiazepoxide, diazepam	Oxaprozin (Daypro) Sertraline (Zoloft)
Cocaine	6–8 hours (2–4 days for benzoylecgonine metabolite)	Coca leaf tea Topical anesthetics containing cocaine
LSD	2–4 days	Trazodone (Desyrel)
Marijuana	3 days for single use; 5–7 days for moderate use (4x/week); 10–15 days for daily use; >30 days for long-term heavy use	Dronabinol (Marinol) Efavirenz (Sustiva) Hemp-containing foods NSAIDs Proton pump inhibitors
MDMA	1–2 days	
Nicotine	12 hours	
Opioids: Buprenorphine Codeine Heroin, hydromorphone, morphine, oxycodone Methadone	 2–3 days (5–7 days for metabolites) 1–2 days 2–4 days 2–3 days; 7–9 days for chronic use	Dextromethorphan (Robitussin DM) Diphenhydramine (Benadryl) Doxylamine (Unisom) Poppy seeds Quinolones Rifampin (Rifadin) Verapamil (Calan)
PCP	2–8 days; up to 30 days for chronic use	Dextromethorphan (Robitussin DM) Diphenhydramine (Benadryl) Doxylamine (Unisom) Ibuprofen (Motrin) Imipramine (Tofranil) Ketamine (Ketalar, Spravato) Lamotrigine (Lamictal) MDPV (bath salts) Meperidine (Demerol) Tramadol (Ultram) Venlafaxine (Effexor), desvenlafaxine (Pristiq)

Adapted from: Moeller KE et al, *Mayo Clin Proc* 2008;83(1):66–76; Moeller KE et al, *Mayo Clin Proc* 2017;92:774–796; Verebey KG, Meenan G. Diagnostic laboratory: Screening for drug abuse. In: Ruiz P, Strain E, eds. *Lowinson and Ruiz's Substance Abuse: A Comprehensive Textbook.* 5th ed. Philadelphia: Wolters Kluwer, Lippincott Williams & Wilkins, 2011:123–137; Warner EA, Sharma N. Laboratory diagnosis. In: Ries RK, Miller SC, Fiellen DA, Saitz R, eds. *Principles of Addiction Medicine.* 4th ed. Philadelphia: Lippincott Williams & Wilkins; 2009:295–304.

Neuroimaging in Psychiatry

Ordering neuroimaging for psychiatric inpatients can be a complex decision. In the past, many inpatient units ordered these tests as a routine measure. However, unnecessary tests can drive up costs and lead to benign but distracting findings. This fact sheet serves as a quick guide to help you decide which neuroimaging tests might be appropriate for your psychiatric inpatients.

Common Types of Neuroimaging in Psychiatry

Computed tomography (CT) scan

A CT scan uses x-rays to create cross-sectional images of the brain. Denser structures like bones block the x-rays, appearing white on the scan, while less dense areas like cerebrospinal fluid appear dark. Fresh blood (eg, from a hemorrhagic stroke) appears whiter than surrounding cerebral tissue, making CT scan a great modality to diagnose an acute cerebral bleed. Rarely used in psychiatry because MRIs provide better spatial resolution.

Magnetic resonance imaging (MRI)

MRI uses strong magnetic fields and radio waves to create detailed images of the brain's internal structure. Unlike a CT scan, MRI doesn't use x-rays, making it safer for repeated use. MRI with contrast is generally preferred for better visualization.

Positron emission tomography (PET)

PET uses a radioactive compound to trace metabolic activity in the brain. It's ideal for tracking changes in active brain regions.

Single photon emission computed tomography (SPECT)

SPECT is similar to PET but uses different radioactive tracers and gamma rays to create 3D images of blood flow and metabolic activity in the brain.

When to Consider Neuroimaging

The primary reason to use neuroimaging is to exclude brain pathology that might be causing psychiatric symptoms. MRI with contrast is usually preferred, but a CT scan can be used if MRI is not available. Order neuroimaging selectively to avoid unnecessary costs and patient anxiety. Here are some cases where it may be useful:

- Neurological signs or symptoms (eg, weakness, numbness, cranial nerve abnormalities).
- Preexisting comorbid neurological condition or brain pathology (eg, a history of stroke or multiple sclerosis).
- Significant head injury history.
- Late-onset psychiatric symptoms (eg, first-onset psychosis after age 50).
- Unexplained worsening of symptoms.
- Lack of response to effective medications.

The most common brain pathologies detected on an MRI or CT scan include brain tumors, stroke, multiple sclerosis, temporal lobe epilepsy, neurodegenerative disorders (eg, Alzheimer's, Parkinson's), traumatic brain injury, and inflammatory or infectious conditions.

Dementia diagnosis

- MRI:
  - Rules out conditions like normal pressure hydrocephalus, vascular disease, or trauma.
  - Can reveal typical patterns of Alzheimer's dementia, such as hippocampal atrophy.
  - Detects white matter hyperintensities (WMH), which are a marker of impairment in the integrity of the white matter. There's an association between WMH and the development of some late-life conditions, such as major depression and vascular dementia.
- PET or SPECT scan:
  - Helpful for distinguishing Alzheimer's from frontotemporal dementia (FTD). In FTD, you will see lower metabolism in the frontal lobe area; in Alzheimer's, you will see lower metabolism in the medial temporal lobe.
  - Ligands for amyloid and tau can help assess a patient's risk of progressing from mild cognitive impairment to Alzheimer's disease.

Pharmacogenetic Testing

Pharmacogenetic testing looks at genetic variations that can impact an individual's response to psychiatric medications. Some genes influence how quickly the body metabolizes medications (pharmacokinetics), while other genes impact how medications act in the body, including their effects in the brain (pharmacodynamics).

Genetic Variations in Metabolizer Status

- *Poor metabolizer:* Having inactive copies of certain genes can lead to slower metabolism of medications, higher blood levels, and increased side effects. For example, 7%–10% of people have inactive CYP2D6 genes and metabolize CYP2D6 substrates like antidepressants and antipsychotics poorly.
- *Extensive metabolizer:* Having normal copies of metabolic genes leads to expected rates of medication metabolism and typical blood levels. Most people (90%–93%) are extensive metabolizers for enzymes like CYP2D6.
- *Ultrarapid metabolizer:* Having extra copies of metabolic genes leads to faster than normal metabolism and lower medication blood levels. For CYP2D6, 2%–5% of people are ultrarapid metabolizers.

Commercially Available Tests

Most commercial pharmacogenetic tests bundle together analyses of many genes. The most heavily marketed tests include GeneSight, Genomind, and Genecept. However, these tests combine some clinically useful genetic tests with many others that are not evidence based. Reliability between different labs is also a concern. Professional guidelines do not recommend using any of these tests.

Individual Genetic Testing

Ordering specific pharmacokinetic genes like CYP2D6 or CYP2C19 may be warranted in certain situations. However, pharmacodynamic gene testing is not currently supported by strong evidence.

Clinical Situations When Testing May Help

- Your patient has unusual sensitivity to medication side effects, which could indicate poor metabolizer status.
- Your patient has had multiple ineffective medication trials, in which case testing may identify if drugs are being metabolized too quickly.

FDA Recommendations

The FDA suggests genetic testing in specific situations with certain psychiatric medications, outlined in the following table.

Table 10: **Pharmacogenetic Recommendations from the FDA**

	Medication	Gene	Risk	Action
Testing required	Carbamazepine (and possibly oxcarbazepine)	HLA-B*1502	Stevens-Johnson syndrome (SJS)	In patients of Asian descent, test is required before starting carbamazepine and recommended (but not required) before oxcarbazepine; a positive result in this population means they are 80 times more likely to develop SJS on carbamazepine and 30 times more likely on oxcarbazepine
	Pimozide	2D6	Arrhythmias	Test is required before dosing pimozide above 4 mg/day (or 0.05 mg/kg/day in children) because of risk of arrhythmias; in poor metabolizers, wait 14 days between dose adjustments
Testing recommended[1]	Thioridazine	2D6	Arrhythmias	Contraindicated in poor metabolizers
	Citalopram	2C19	Arrhythmias	Max dose of 20 mg/day in poor metabolizers
	Deutetrabenazine	2D6	Arrhythmias	Max dose 18 mg BID in poor metabolizers (must be divided BID)
	Valbenazine	2D6	Arrhythmias	Lower the dose by 50% and divide it twice a day in poor metabolizers
Adjust dose if testing results are known	Atomoxetine, clozapine, perphenazine, venlafaxine, vortioxetine, and various tricyclics (amitriptyline, clomipramine, desipramine, doxepin, imipramine, nortriptyline, protroptyline, trimipramine)	2D6	Various	Lower the dose by 50% in poor metabolizers; for clozapine and tricyclics, adjust based on serum levels; for venlafaxine, keep in mind that the active metabolite (desvenlafaxine) will be low in poor metabolizers and high in rapid metabolizers
	Aripiprazole, brexpiprazole, iloperidone	2D6, 3A4	Various	Lower the dose by 50% in poor metabolizers at either enzyme, or by 75% if both enzymes are poor
	Flibanserin	3A4	Syncope	Lower the dose in poor metabolizers

[1] In these cases, the FDA does not require the test but does require dose adjustment if the test was done and an abnormality found (a slightly inconsistent recommendation). Sources: www.cpicpgx.org/genes-drugs, www.tinyurl.com/mshes7dd

ECG in Inpatient Psychiatry

This fact sheet aims to provide an evidence-based guide on when and why to order an ECG, medications that may necessitate an ECG, and basic ECG interpretation tips.

Indications for Ordering an ECG

- *Routine screening for patients with preexisting cardiac issues:* Most patients with a history of arrhythmias, coronary artery disease, or other cardiac disorders should have a routine ECG on admission to assess whether their psychiatric symptoms may be related to cardiac issues, and in preparation for possible prescriptions of meds that may affect cardiac function.
- *Cardiac symptoms:* Any patient with chest pain, palpitations, shortness of breath, dizziness, or other symptoms should get an ECG.
- *Prior to starting or increasing the dose of certain medications:* Note that there is no requirement to check an ECG before starting any of these medications; rather, there are various recommendations, depending on risks such as age, underlying diseases that might affect cardiac functioning, and presence of other medications that affect the heart.

Antipsychotics

- *Clozapine:* Sinus tachycardia, QT prolongation, myocarditis, cardiomyopathy.
- *Ziprasidone:* QT prolongation.
- *First-generation antipsychotics:* QT prolongation with IV haloperidol, high-dose chlorpromazine, thioridazine.

Antidepressants

- *Tricyclic antidepressants:* QRS widening (also known as heart block), prolonged QT interval. ECG is strongly recommended in patients older than 40.
- *Citalopram:* Can cause prolonged QT interval at doses >40 mg daily; however, the clinical significance of this is debatable.

Mood stabilizers

- *Lithium:* Can cause T wave flattening or inversion. ECG is recommended in patients with preexisting heart disease.
- *Lamotrigine:* Can cause arrhythmias. ECG is recommended if there is cardiac disease or in patients older than 60.

Methadone

QT prolongation.

Stimulants

Can cause tachycardia and arrhythmia. ECG is recommended only if there is a history of heart disease.

Basic ECG Interpretation Primer

- *P wave:* Atrial contraction.
- *QRS complex:* Ventricular contraction.
- *T wave:* Ventricular relaxation.
- *PR interval:* Time from atrial to ventricular contraction.
- *QT interval:* Total time of ventricular activity.

Evaluate the rhythm

- *Normal sinus rhythm:* Regular P waves before each QRS complex.
- *Atrial fibrillation:* Irregular P waves.

Look at the rate

- *Normal:* 60–100 beats per minute (BPM).
- *Tachycardia:* >100 BPM.
- *Bradycardia:* <60 BPM.

Inspect the intervals

- *QT interval:* Varies by rate; use QTc to correct for rate (should be <450 msec for males, <470 msec for females).
- *PR interval:* 0.12–0.20 seconds.

Look for abnormal patterns

- *ST elevation:* May indicate myocardial infarction.
- *T wave flattening or inversion:* May indicate ischemia.

ECG of Normal Sinus Rhythm

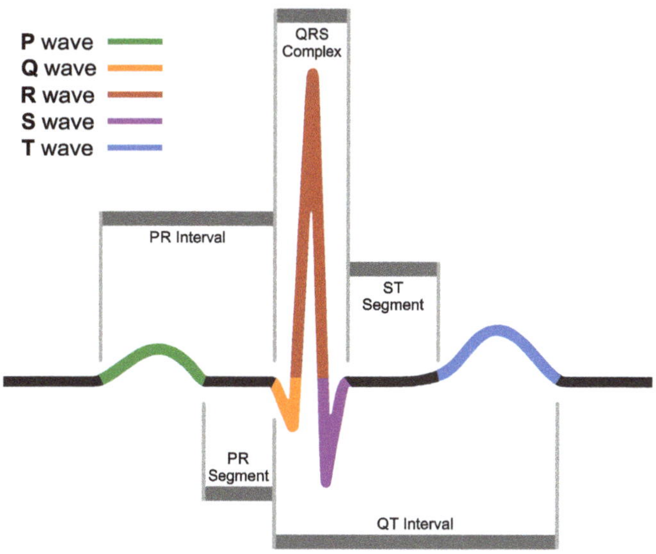

Prescribing and Medication Management

Clinically Significant Drug Interactions

Drug Interactions in Psychiatry

Generally, when pressed for time, most clinicians will use one of the following online drug interaction checkers:

Free

- Medscape (https://reference.medscape.com/drug-interactionchecker)
- www.epocrates.com (you'll need to register first)
- www.drugs.com/drug_interactions.html

Paid

- Lexicomp (www.wolterskluwer.com/en/solutions/lexicomp/lexicomp)

Most interactions in psychiatry will not result in a serious outcome. Many interactions, however, may result in decreased efficacy or increased adverse effects, and these can be easily avoided. To understand drug-drug interactions, you'll need to refamiliarize yourself with some basic terms. Drugs are substrates of specific enzymes, meaning that drugs rely on specific enzymatic pathways for metabolism. An inhibitor is a drug that binds more tightly to an enzyme than the usual substrate and prevents the enzyme from doing its job; as a result, the substrate for that enzyme gets stuck in a game of musical chairs as it scurries around looking for a free enzyme system to break it down. Since this drug is not getting metabolized as quickly as it otherwise would (the inhibitor is preventing it from doing so), its serum levels become higher than expected. On the other hand, inducers stimulate the production of extra enzymes. With more enzymes around, the substrate for that enzyme is broken down more rapidly, leading to lower serum drug levels.

Another important concern with drug interactions is timing. Inhibition happens quickly. It can occur with the first dose of a medication and can subside quickly when an inhibitor is discontinued. How long it takes to subside depends on the inhibitor's half-life. Generally, the inhibition will stop after five half-lives of the inhibitor drug. On the other hand, for induction to occur, the body has to synthesize more CYP450 enzymes, and this can take up to four weeks. This accounts for the delayed "auto-induction" of carbamazepine. Likewise, for induction to subside, these extra enzymes need to be broken down, a process that could also take several weeks. As a general rule of thumb, any drug prescribed with its inhibitor should be started at half the usual dose and titrated more slowly. Conversely, a drug prescribed with its inducer may need to be dosed higher after the few weeks it takes for induction to occur. One exception to the rule of inhibitors increasing substrate levels is when the substrate is a prodrug. Tamoxifen, hydrocodone, and tramadol are prodrugs that rely on CYP2D6 to be converted into an active metabolite. In the presence of a potent inhibitor like fluoxetine or paroxetine, patients may see a drop in therapeutic effects rather than increased effects.

Practical Tips for Quickly Identifying Significant Drug Interactions

- Identify the 10 drugs that you most commonly prescribe and memorize their major drug interactions.
- Antidepressants, antipsychotics, antibiotics, antiretrovirals, and older anticonvulsants have a high likelihood of significant drug interactions—so be particularly vigilant if your patient is taking any of these.
- Recognize the drugs with a narrow therapeutic window, ie, drugs for which the toxic dose is not much higher than the therapeutic dose. Commonly used drugs with narrow therapeutic windows include lithium, carbamazepine (Tegretol), warfarin (Coumadin), digoxin (Lanoxin), phenytoin (Dilantin), and phenobarbital.
- Recognize drugs that cause serious side effects and outcomes if blood levels are significantly increased or decreased (eg, oral contraceptives, lamotrigine, clozapine, tricyclic antidepressants, warfarin).
- Drugs with long half-lives, such as diazepam (Valium) or aripiprazole (Abilify), can be particularly troublesome when involved in drug interactions, because metabolic inhibitors—or hepatic dysfunction—can make them ultra-long lasting. Be cautious with any new or rarely prescribed drugs: Neither you nor anybody else has had much experience with them, and unreported drug interactions can appear.
- The risk of drug interactions can increase exponentially as the number of drugs increases. Setting a threshold to check for interactions is helpful (eg, any patient on three or more drugs).

Table 11: **Most Common Clinically Significant Drug Interactions in Psychiatry**

Clinical Consequence	Medications Most Commonly Contributing	Comments
Decreased efficacy of psychiatric medications	Carbamazepine, St. John's wort, cigarette smoking strongly induce metabolism and decrease serum levels of many psychotropics	Smoking may reduce olanzapine, clozapine levels; carbamazepine can reduce levels of many medications
Decreased efficacy of opioids	Potent 2D6 inhibitors (paroxetine, fluoxetine, duloxetine, bupropion) prevent conversion of certain opioids (codeine, hydrocodone, oxycodone) to active metabolites, thereby decreasing pain relief	Use alternative antidepressants (eg, sertraline, citalopram, escitalopram)
Decreased efficacy of oral contraceptive pills (OCPs)	Carbamazepine, St. John's wort, cigarette smoking strongly induce metabolism and decrease serum levels of OCPs	Avoid these meds in women taking OCPs
Increased side effects or toxicity of psychiatric medications	The most common and potent CYP450 inhibitors are paroxetine, fluoxetine, duloxetine, bupropion, valproic acid, asenapine, and grapefruit juice—all may lead to increased substrate levels and increased side effects or toxicity	Adjust dose of substrate or use alternative medications
Serotonin syndrome	High doses or combinations of the following: SSRIs, SNRIs, TCAs, MAOIs, buspirone, dextromethorphan, lithium, tramadol, trazodone	Caution patients to report new sudden onset of fever, agitation, tremor, sweating, diarrhea; discontinue offending agents and provide supportive care
QT prolongation	Monotherapy or combined therapy with the following: ziprasidone, thioridazine, TCAs, methadone, and certain cardiac meds and antibiotics (amiodarone, ciprofloxacin, clarithromycin, erythromycin, ketoconazole, quinidine)	May lead to potentially fatal arrhythmias; monitor ECG and electrolytes and use alternative medications in patients with borderline or increased QT interval
Increased risk for bleeding	Serotonergic antidepressants (SSRIs, SNRIs) especially when combined with anticoagulants (warfarin), antiplatelets (aspirin), or NSAIDs	May lead to bruising or minor bleeding (nosebleed, gum bleed); GI bleeds and more severe bleeding also rarely reported; use alternative in patients at highest risk, such as the elderly
Lowered seizure threshold	Bupropion, clozapine	Use with caution in patients with a history of seizures, electrolyte disturbances, or head trauma; consider concomitant antiepileptic for seizure prophylaxis
Lithium toxicity	Lithium used in combination with NSAIDs, ACE inhibitors, angiotensin II receptor blockers, diuretics (especially thiazides)	Use alternative agents or monitor lithium levels closely and adjust dosing
Anticholinergic delirium	Anticholinergics (benztropine, trihexyphenidyl), antihistamines (diphenhydramine, doxylamine), low-potency first-generation antipsychotics (chlorpromazine), olanzapine, clozapine, TCAs, others (oxybutynin)	High anticholinergic burden may lead to confusion and delirium, particularly in older patients; minimize use or use alternative medications

Recommended Labs for Psychiatric Medications

This is a short and sweet table listing the medications that most psychiatrists would agree require lab monitoring. Our recommendations are quite abbreviated, and we haven't spelled out whether you should order labs before or after starting the medications, nor how you should do follow-up monitoring. There's just too much variation in practice for us to give authoritative detailed guidelines. These medications are mainly here to jog your memory so you don't forget to at least consider what type of monitoring to do.

Table 12: **Recommended Laboratory Tests for Psychiatric Medications**

Medications	Recommended Laboratory Tests
Acamprosate	BUN/creatinine if renal impairment is suspected
Amantadine	BUN/creatinine if renal impairment is suspected
Antipsychotics—second generation, primarily clozapine, olanzapine, quetiapine, paliperidone, risperidone[1,2]	Fasting glucose and lipids
Atomoxetine	LFTs
Carbamazepine	Complete blood count (CBC), sodium, LFTs, pregnancy test, HLA-B*1502 in Asians[3] Carbamazepine level (at least 3 days on stable dose, trough level, 12 hours after last dose); target: 4–12 mcg/mL
Chlorpromazine	ECG if cardiac disease
Citalopram	ECG if cardiac disease, dose ≥40 mg/day
Clomipramine	Clomipramine/norclomipramine levels (at least 5 days on stable dose, trough level, 12 hours after last dose); target: 220–500 ng/mL
Clozapine	Fasting glucose and lipids, CBC Clozapine/norclozapine level (at least 3 days on stable dose, trough level, 12 hours after last dose); target: >350 ng/mL; toxicity: >700 ng/mL
Desvenlafaxine	Periodic BP
Deutetrabenazine	ECG if cardiac disease
Disulfiram	LFTs if liver disease is suspected
Duloxetine	LFTs if liver disease is suspected[4]
Gabapentin	BUN/creatinine if renal impairment is suspected
Levomilnacipran	Periodic BP/pulse rate
Lithium	TSH, BUN/creatinine[5], pregnancy test, ECG if cardiac disease Lithium level (at least 5 days on stable dose, trough level, 12 hours after last dose); target: 0.8–1.2 mEq/L (acute mania) and 0.6–1.0 mEq/L (maintenance)
Methadone	ECG if cardiac disease
Mirtazapine	Lipids
Naltrexone	LFTs if liver disease is suspected
Nortriptyline	Nortriptyline level (at least 5 days on stable dose, trough level, 12 hours after last dose); target: 50–150 ng/mL
Oxcarbazepine	Sodium, HLA-B*1502 in Asians[3]
Paliperidone	Prolactin if symptoms, fasting glucose and lipids
Pregabalin	BUN/creatinine if renal impairment is suspected

[1] Some guidelines recommend monitoring glucose and lipids with all second-generation antipsychotics.

[2] Utility of routine therapeutic monitoring is unclear for antipsychotic medications other than clozapine; reference ranges are available for many agents, and blood levels may help in establishing whether a patient is taking the medication.

[3] HLA-B*1502 is a gene that increases the risk of developing toxic epidermal necrolysis (TEN) and Stevens-Johnson syndrome (SJS) in response to taking carbamazepine. Asians, especially Han Chinese, are much more likely to have the gene than other populations.

[4] Duloxetine should not be prescribed in patients with significant alcohol use of evidence of chronic liver disease as it can lead to hepatic failure in rare cases (Cymbalta prescribing information). While the manufacturer does not recommend baseline LFTs for all patients, some clinicians do so anyway to be extra cautious.

[5] The serum creatinine is used to compute the estimated glomerular filtration rate (eGFR), a more precise measure of kidney functioning. Increasingly, laboratory test results include the eGFR. You can calculate it yourself using an online calculator at www.kidney.org/professionals/kdoqi/gfr_calculator.

(table continues)

Table 12 (continued): **Recommended Laboratory Tests for Psychiatric Medications**

Medications	Recommended Laboratory Tests
Risperidone	Prolactin if symptoms, fasting glucose and lipids
SSRIs	Sodium in elderly if fatigue, dizziness, confusion
Stimulants	ECG if cardiac disease
Thioridazine	ECG if cardiac disease
Topiramate	Bicarbonate
Tricyclic antidepressants	ECG if cardiac disease
Valbenazine	ECG if cardiac disease
Valproic acid	LFTs, CBC for platelets, pregnancy test, ammonia if confusion Valproic acid level (at least 3 days on stable dose, trough level, 12 hours after last dose with IR or 21–24 hours with ER); target: 50–125 mcg/mL
Venlafaxine	Periodic BP
Ziprasidone	ECG if cardiac disease

[1] Some guidelines recommend monitoring glucose and lipids with all second-generation antipsychotics.

[2] Utility of routine therapeutic monitoring is unclear for antipsychotic medications other than clozapine; reference ranges are available for many agents, and blood levels may help in establishing whether a patient is taking the medication.

[3] HLA-B*1502 is a gene that increases the risk of developing toxic epidermal necrolysis (TEN) and Stevens-Johnson syndrome (SJS) in response to taking carbamazepine. Asians, especially Han Chinese, are much more likely to have the gene than other populations.

[4] Duloxetine should not be prescribed in patients with significant alcohol use of evidence of chronic liver disease as it can lead to hepatic failure in rare cases (Cymbalta prescribing information). While the manufacturer does not recommend baseline LFTs for all patients, some clinicians do so anyway to be extra cautious.

[5] The serum creatinine is used to compute the estimated glomerular filtration rate (eGFR), a more precise measure of kidney functioning. Increasingly, laboratory test results include the eGFR. You can calculate it yourself using an online calculator at www.kidney.org/professionals/kdoqi/gfr_calculator.

Prescribing Psychiatric Medications in Kidney Impairment

Most psychotropic medications can be used safely in patients with kidney disease, although you will need to adjust doses in some cases. This fact sheet tells you what you need to know.

Stages of Chronic Kidney Disease

These stages are based on glomerular filtration rate (GFR) (in mL/min/1.73m^2):

- *Mild:* GFR 60–89.
- *Moderate:* GFR 30–59.
- *Severe:* GFR 15–29.
- *End-stage renal disease (ESRD), need for dialysis:* GFR <15.

Key Factors Influencing Medication Adjustments in Kidney Disease

- *Route of elimination:* Drugs that are mostly metabolized by the liver and then excreted by the bowel into the feces don't need to be adjusted as significantly as drugs that are primarily eliminated by the kidneys. Gabapentin is an example of a drug primarily eliminated by the kidneys that might need significant adjustment in renal disease.
- *Metabolites:* Some medications are metabolized into active metabolites that require renal excretion. For example, desvenlafaxine, venlafaxine's metabolite, requires renal excretion.
- *Therapeutic index:* Drugs with a narrow therapeutic index, like lithium, require more precise dosing adjustments to avoid toxicity.
- *Protein binding:* Kidney disease can reduce protein levels in the blood. For drugs that are highly protein bound, like valproate, lower protein levels lead to a greater proportion of the free (active) form.

Best Medication Options for Patients with Kidney Impairment

- *Antidepressants:* Mirtazapine, sertraline, trazodone.
- *Mood stabilizers:* Carbamazepine, valproate (but start at lower doses).
- *Anxiolytics:* Lorazepam, oxazepam, temazepam.
- *Antipsychotics:* Aripiprazole, olanzapine, quetiapine.
- *Sleeping medications:* Eszopiclone, temazepam, zolpidem.
- *Medications for side effects (eg, anticholinergics for EPS):* Diphenhydramine.

Medications to Be Most Careful with in Kidney Impairment

Antidepressants

- Bupropion: Use with caution; consider dose adjustment as elevated serum levels will increase the seizure risk.
- Duloxetine: Requires dose adjustment; avoid in severe renal impairment due to risk of accumulation.
- Phenelzine: Can accumulate in renal impairment, leading to increased side effects.
- Venlafaxine: Risk of accumulation and increased side effects.

Mood stabilizers/anticonvulsants

- Gabapentin: Requires significant dose adjustment in kidney impairment; risk of accumulation and side effects.
- Lamotrigine: Requires dose adjustment in severe kidney impairment; use with caution.
- Lithium: Primarily excreted by the kidneys; requires significant dose adjustment and close monitoring in kidney impairment.
- Topiramate: Requires dose adjustment in kidney impairment; risk of metabolic acidosis and kidney stones.

Anxiolytics

- Alprazolam: Metabolized by the liver but may accumulate in kidney impairment; use with caution.
- Buspirone (BuSpar): Avoid using in severe kidney impairment due to the risk of accumulation and increased side effects.
- Clonazepam: Use with caution; may require dose adjustment in severe kidney impairment.

Antipsychotics

- Lurasidone: Requires dose adjustment in kidney impairment; avoid in severe cases.
- Paliperidone: Requires dose adjustment in moderate to severe kidney impairment; avoid in severe cases.
- Risperidone: Requires dose adjustment in severe kidney impairment due to the risk of accumulation.

Medications for side effects

- Metformin: Contraindicated in severe renal impairment due to the risk of lactic acidosis.

Important Considerations

- Consult with a nephrologist for complex cases.
- Educate patients on how to recognize signs of potential kidney impairment (eg, dark urine, reduced urine output, swelling in the legs or ankles, fatigue, confusion) or worsening medication side effects and to report them immediately.

Prescribing Psychiatric Medications in Liver Impairment

Prescribing psychiatric medications for patients with liver impairment is a complex task, given the liver's critical role in drug metabolism. A good rule of thumb is to start at lower doses than you would for healthy patients, monitor closely for side effects, and avoid some medications in certain cases. Here we provide tips for the safe use of psychotropic medications in patients with liver disease.

Key Factors Influencing Medication Adjustments in Hepatic Dysfunction

- *Metabolism and clearance:* Liver impairment can lead to elevated serum levels of drugs that require extensive hepatic metabolism.
- *Protein binding:* Liver disease can impair production of proteins like albumin, increasing the bioavailability of highly protein-bound drugs, thereby upping the risk of drug side effects or toxicity.
- *Active metabolites:* May accumulate in liver disease and increase the risk of side effects.

Understanding Liver Disease Severity

The most common liver function test abnormality we see in psychiatric inpatients is a mild to moderate elevation of liver enzymes (defined as alanine transaminase [ALT] and aspartate transaminase [AST] less than five times the upper limit of normal). This degree of elevation is common in inflammation due to alcohol use, nonalcoholic fatty liver disease, and viral hepatitis. In the absence of other liver abnormalities (see below), these patients are generally able to metabolize psychiatric medications normally and don't require major dosage adjustments.

Patients with more severe or advanced liver disease may not be able to metabolize drugs normally. The Child-Pugh classification for degree of liver disease is useful because it focuses on actual hepatic dysfunction as opposed to inflammation. Here are the definitions of mild, moderate, and severe dysfunction:

- *Child-Pugh Class A (mild):* Well-compensated disease with no ascites, mild encephalopathy, and relatively preserved hepatic function. No dosing modifications needed. Criteria include:
  - Total bilirubin <2 mg/dL.
  - Albumin >3.5 g/dL.
  - International normalized ratio (INR; prothrombin time measure) <1.7 seconds.
- *Child-Pugh Class B (moderate):* Significant functional compromise with obvious symptoms like ascites and encephalopathy, requiring substantial modification in medication dosing. Criteria include:
  - Total bilirubin 2–3 mg/dL.
  - Albumin 2.8–3.5 g/dL.
  - INR 1.7–2.3 seconds.
- *Child-Pugh Class C (severe):* Advanced liver disease with poor hepatic function, marked ascites, and encephalopathy, often contraindicating many medications due to high risk of toxicity. Criteria include:
  - Total bilirubin >3 mg/dL.
  - Albumin <2.8 g/dL.
  - INR >2.3 seconds.

Best Medication Options for Patients with Liver Impairment

Antidepressants

- Mirtazapine: Generally safe in mild/moderate liver impairment.
- Sertraline: Has a relatively favorable hepatic metabolism profile and is less likely to cause liver enzyme elevations compared to other antidepressants.
- Trazodone: Generally safe, but start at a lower dose.

Mood stabilizers

- Lithium, topiramate: Primarily excreted by the kidneys; no liver metabolism is needed.
- Gabapentin: Primarily excreted unchanged by the kidneys.

Anxiolytics

- Lorazepam, oxazepam, temazepam: Undergo minimal hepatic metabolism.

Antipsychotics

- Haloperidol: Long history of safe use in liver impairment, though dosages may need reduction.
- Quetiapine: Safe in mild to moderate liver impairment; in severe impairment, start at a lower dose (eg, 25 mg/day) and titrate slowly.
- Ziprasidone: Primarily metabolized by aldehyde oxidase so does not require dosage adjustments in mild to moderate hepatic impairment.

Sleeping medications

- Eszopiclone (Lunesta): Safe in mild to moderate impairment.
- Zolpidem: Generally safe but start at 5 mg/day.

Medications for side effects

- Diphenhydramine (Benadryl): Generally safe but monitor for potential side effects.

Medications to Be Most Careful with in Liver Impairment

Antidepressants

- Bupropion: Metabolized by the liver, risk of hepatotoxicity; use with caution.
- Duloxetine: Avoid in severe liver impairment due to the risk of hepatotoxicity.
- Isocarboxazid: Risk of hepatotoxicity; use with caution in liver impairment, particularly in moderate to severe cases.
- Paroxetine: Requires dose reduction in severe liver impairment; potential for increased side effects.
- Phenelzine: High potential for hepatotoxicity; use with extreme caution or avoid in moderate to severe liver impairment.

Mood stabilizers/anticonvulsants

- Carbamazepine: Metabolized by the liver, risk of hepatotoxicity; requires dose reduction and close monitoring.
- Lamotrigine: Requires dose adjustment in moderate to severe liver impairment due to reduced clearance.
- Valproate (valproic acid): High risk of hepatotoxicity, particularly in patients with preexisting liver impairment; avoid in severe cases.

Anxiolytics

- Buspirone (BuSpar): Avoid using in severe liver impairment due to the risk of accumulation and increased side effects.
- Clonazepam: Metabolized by the liver; risk of accumulation and prolonged sedation.
- Diazepam: Extensively metabolized by the liver; prolonged effects in liver impairment; use with caution.

Antipsychotics

- Clozapine: Metabolized by the liver; risk of hepatotoxicity; requires close monitoring and dose adjustment.
- Risperidone: Metabolized by the liver, especially in severe liver impairment; use with caution.

Sleeping medications

- Flurazepam: Metabolized by the liver; long half-life, increased risk of accumulation and sedation in liver impairment.
- Zolpidem: Requires dose reduction in severe liver impairment due to prolonged sedation.

Medications for side effects

- Metoclopramide: Risk of hepatotoxicity; use with caution in liver impairment.
- Valbenazine: Metabolized by the liver; requires dose adjustment in moderate to severe liver impairment.

Important Considerations

- Consult with a gastroenterologist or hepatologist for complex cases.
- Educate patients on how to recognize signs of potential liver impairment (jaundice, severe nausea, or unusual fatigue) or worsening medication side effects and to report them immediately.

Routine Medications for Common Patient Needs

When patients are admitted to psychiatric units, they often present with miscellaneous medical needs alongside their psychiatric conditions. The simple interventions listed below help address these needs and promote patients' overall comfort and well-being.

Allergies and Sleep Aids

For allergies

- Diphenhydramine (Benadryl): 25–50 mg every four to six hours as needed.
- Loratadine (Claritin): 10 mg once daily.
- Cetirizine (Zyrtec): 10 mg once daily.

For sleep

- Melatonin: 1–5 mg at bedtime.
- Diphenhydramine (Benadryl): 25–50 mg at bedtime.

Digestive Issues

For constipation

- Docusate (Colace): 100 mg twice daily.
- Senna: One to two tablets at bedtime.
- Milk of magnesia: 30–60 mL once daily.
- Polyethylene glycol 3350 (MiraLAX): 17 grams in four to eight ounces of liquid, once daily.

For loose stool/diarrhea

- Loperamide (Imodium): 4 mg initially, then 2 mg after each loose stool; max 16 mg/day.
- Bismuth subsalicylate (Pepto-Bismol): 525 mg (two tablets or 30 mL) every 30–60 minutes as needed; not to exceed eight doses in 24 hours.

For indigestion and acid reflux

- Famotidine (Pepcid): 20–40 mg once or twice daily.
- Omeprazole (Prilosec): 20 mg once daily for up to 14 days.
- Aluminum hydroxide/magnesium hydroxide (Mylanta, Maalox): Two to four teaspoons (10–20 mL) up to four times a day.

For nausea and vomiting

Ondansetron (Zofran): 4–8 mg every six hours as needed.

Pain, Fever, and Muscle Soreness

For pain and fever

- Acetaminophen (Tylenol): 500–1000 mg every four to six hours as needed.
- Ibuprofen (Advil, Motrin): 400–800 mg every six to eight hours as needed.
- Naproxen (Aleve): 220–550 mg every 12 hours; max 1100 mg/day.

For muscle soreness

Cyclobenzaprine (Flexeril): 5–10 mg three times a day.

For muscle, joint, and neuropathic pain

- Capsaicin 0.1% cream (Capzasin): Apply a thin layer to the affected area three to four times daily.
- Topical analgesic patch (containing menthol and methyl salicylate, eg, Salonpas): Apply one patch to the affected area; max three patches per day. Each patch can be worn for up to eight hours.
- Topical NSAIDs (eg, diclofenac gel, Voltaren): Apply to the affected area as directed.
- Lidocaine 5% patch: Apply to the affected area for up to 12 hours in a 24-hour period.

Respiratory Symptoms

For wheezing or shortness of breath

Albuterol: One to two puffs every four to six hours as needed.

For nasal congestion

- Oxymetazoline (Afrin): Two to three sprays in each nostril every 10–12 hours; not to exceed two doses in 24 hours. Use for a maximum of three days.
- Fluticasone propionate (Flonase): Two sprays in each nostril once a day.
- Nasal saline spray: Two to three sprays.

For cough

- Dextromethorphan (eg, Robitussin): 10–20 mg every four hours or 30 mg every six to eight hours as needed.
- Guaifenesin (an expectorant): 200 mg every four hours as needed.

For sore throat

Throat lozenges (eg, with menthol or benzocaine): One lozenge every two hours as needed.

Skin and Eye Care

For skin irritations and rashes

- Hydrocortisone cream 1%: Apply to the affected area two to three times daily.
- Triamcinolone cream 0.1%: Use for three weeks, then take a one-week break.
- Clotrimazole 1% or Nystatin: Apply to fungal rash areas one to two times per day.

For fungal infections (athlete's foot, jock itch, ringworm, etc)

- Lotrimin cream 1%: Apply twice daily.
- Lamisil cream/tablet: Apply cream or take 250 mg tablet once daily as directed.
- Fungal nail infections (onychomycosis): Apply cream to the affected nail or take 250 mg tablet once daily for six weeks (fingernails) or 12 weeks (toenails).

For eye care

Artificial tears: One to two drops in each eye every six hours as needed.

For dry lips

Lip balm with moisturizers (eg, petrolatum, lanolin, or beeswax): Apply as needed.

Smoking Cessation

Nicotine gum (Nicorette)

- Light smokers: 2 mg gum; take one piece every one to two hours as needed for cravings; max 24 pieces/day.
- Heavy smokers: 4 mg gum; same frequency and maximum as light smokers.

Nicotine patch (Nicoderm CQ)

- Light to moderate smokers: 7–14 mg patch daily.
- Heavy smokers: 21 mg patch daily.

Managing Comorbid Medical Conditions

Abnormal Lipid Levels

You'll frequently encounter cases of dyslipidemia among your patients on the psychiatric unit. Individuals with chronic mental illnesses are at a higher risk due to poor dietary habits, inadequate health care follow-up, smoking, and lack of physical exercise. Their use of antipsychotic medications further exacerbates the risk. Like most psychiatric hospitals, yours probably has a policy requiring that you order a lipid panel on any patients taking an antipsychotic. Here we review evaluation and management approaches.

What Is a Lipid Panel?

The lipid panel measures cholesterol and triglycerides. Cholesterol is a fat-like substance found in every cell of the body and is essential for creating cell membranes, for producing hormones like testosterone and estrogen, for creating bile, and for synthesizing vitamin D when we are exposed to sunlight. The liver produces most of the cholesterol we need, and we also consume it from animal-based foods. The bad side of cholesterol is that high levels are correlated with a higher risk of heart disease and stroke.

Elements of a Lipid Panel

- *Total cholesterol (Optimal: <200 mg/dL):* Reflects all cholesterol in the blood, including HDL and LDL. The commonly used calculation formula is: Total cholesterol = HDL + LDL + (triglycerides/5).
- *High-density lipoprotein (HDL) cholesterol (Optimal: >60 mg/dL):* The "good" cholesterol; helps remove other cholesterol forms from the bloodstream. Higher levels are protective against heart disease.
- *Low-density lipoprotein (LDL) cholesterol (Optimal: <100 mg/dL):* The "bad" cholesterol; high levels can lead to atherosclerosis. Of particular concern for patients on antipsychotics that can elevate LDL levels.
- *Triglycerides (Optimal: <150 mg/dL):* Triglycerides are a type of fat created by the liver from excess calories, to be used for energy between meals. High levels are correlated with obesity, heart disease, and diabetes.

Reasons to Order a Lipid Panel

- Evaluate heart disease and stroke risk, especially for patients with contributing risk factors.
- Monitor medication side effects, particularly for antipsychotics known to cause dyslipidemia.
- Select medications with minimal impact on lipid levels for patients with preexisting dyslipidemia.

What to Do When There Is Hyperlipidemia

- *Ensure your patient was fasting:* Accurate results require nine to 12 hours of fasting.
- *Consult with medicine:* Addressing hyperlipidemia during hospitalization is critical, especially given that many psychiatric inpatients have poor outpatient follow-up. Initiating treatment while hospitalized can help demonstrate to patients that the therapy is manageable and encourage adherence after discharge.
- *ASCVD (atherosclerotic cardiovascular disease) risk calculator:* Estimates a person's 10-year risk of having a cardiovascular event, such as a heart attack or stroke. The calculator considers factors like age, cholesterol levels, blood pressure, smoking status, and diabetes. The decision to initiate statins is based on the patient's risk level. It can be found online at the American College of Cardiology (ACC) website: https://tools.acc.org/ASCVD-Risk-Estimator-Plus/
- *Review metabolic profile of psychiatric medications and make changes when possible:*
  - The antipsychotics most likely to cause dyslipidemia include olanzapine, clozapine, and quetiapine.
  - Antipsychotics less likely to alter lipid levels include aripiprazole, asenapine, cariprazine, haloperidol, lurasidone, and ziprasidone.
  - Other psychiatric medications that may worsen lipid levels include certain mood stabilizers (like valproate and lithium), and some antidepressants (particularly older tricyclics and the selective serotonin reuptake inhibitor paroxetine).
- *Reinforce long-term interventions:* These include dietary changes, exercise, and taking lipid-lowering medications like statins if prescribed by a medical consultant.
- *Monitor periodically:* It's recommended to monitor lipid levels every two months until goals are reached, then monitor them every six to 12 months.

Lifestyle Modifications

- *Heart-healthy diet:* Encourage a diet rich in fruits, vegetables, whole grains, and nuts while minimizing saturated fats. Your hospital will provide dietary options (eg, cardiac, low-fat, or Mediterranean) that can be tailored to meet these needs.
- *Regular exercise:* Encourage participation in the unit's daily exercise groups.
- *Nicotine cessation:* Help patients quit smoking with the use of nicotine replacement therapies, like nicotine gum, lozenges, or patches.
- *Healthy weight:* Assist patients in achieving and maintaining a weight that keeps them within their ideal BMI range. Minimize the use of medications that cause weight gain and consider adding medications like topiramate or semaglutide to promote weight loss.

Medication Options

When lifestyle modifications are insufficient, you may need to initiate medication.

- *Statins:* First-line treatment; include atorvastatin (10–80 mg daily) and simvastatin (20–40 mg nightly).
  - Common side effects: Muscle aches (myalgia), which are the most common reason for medication discontinuation; headache; and gastrointestinal disturbances.
  - Monitoring: Baseline liver function tests (LFTs) and creatinine kinase (CK), and LFTs 12 weeks later.
  - If severe muscle symptoms develop, check CK levels to assess for muscle injury. Myalgia typically resolves within two months of discontinuing the statin, and you can restart the same or a different statin once symptoms resolve. Be cautious of interactions with grapefruit and drugs (eg, verapamil) that can increase the risk of statin-induced muscle damage (rhabdomyolysis).
- *Fibrates:* Primarily for high triglycerides—but these can interfere with other medications' absorption.
  - Fenofibrate 54–160 mg daily.
  - Gemfibrozil 600 mg twice daily, 30 minutes before the morning and evening meals.
- *Bile acid sequestrants:* These can also interfere with other medications' absorption.
  - Cholestyramine 4–16 g daily, divided into two doses.
- *Niacin (vitamin B3):* 500 mg daily at bedtime, gradually increasing to 1–2 g daily, but its use is limited by side effects like flushing, itching, headaches, and dose-dependent hepatoxicity.
- *Ezetimibe (a cholesterol absorption inhibitor):* 10 mg daily, often used in conjunction with statins when further reduction of LDL cholesterol is needed.

Referral Guidelines

Initiating lifestyle modifications and statin therapy on the psychiatric unit is reasonable for uncomplicated cases of dyslipidemia, but consult with an internist or cardiologist if lipid levels remain significantly abnormal despite initial treatment, or if the patient has multiple cardiovascular risk factors (particularly a history of heart disease or stroke).

Abdominal Pain

Abdominal pain, whether acute or chronic, can signal serious medical conditions. Intervene promptly, especially as patients with psychiatric conditions may underreport or misinterpret their symptoms. Below is a guide for understanding and managing abdominal pain on a psychiatric unit.

Possible Etiologies and Distinguishing Features

- *Appendicitis:* Dull periumbilical pain shifting to the right lower quadrant, becoming intense within 12–24 hours, often with nausea, vomiting, and fever.
- *Cholecystitis and gallstones:* Right upper quadrant pain radiating to the shoulder.
- *Constipation:* Generalized abdominal pain, bloating, and discomfort.
- *Diverticulitis:* Left lower quadrant pain with fever, nausea, and bowel habit changes.
- *Gastritis and GERD:* Chronic or recurring epigastric (upper abdominal) pain related to meals.
- *Hepatitis:* Right upper quadrant pain with jaundice and liver enlargement.
- *Hernias:* Painful bulges that worsen with straining. Can cause severe pain if strangulated.
- *Inflammatory bowel disease (IBD):* Recurrent episodes of abdominal pain, often with diarrhea (which may be bloody), weight loss, and fatigue. Includes Crohn's disease and ulcerative colitis.
- *Irritable bowel syndrome (IBS):* Chronic abdominal pain with changes in bowel habits (diarrhea, constipation, or both), often related to stress or certain foods.
- *Ischemic bowel:* Severe pain with systemic symptoms like tachycardia and hypotension.
- *Myocardial infarction (MI):* Epigastric pain with shortness of breath or sweating.
- *Pancreatitis:* Sudden, severe epigastric pain radiating to the back.
- *Peptic ulcer disease (PUD):* Epigastric pain related to meals.
- *Peritonitis:* Generalized abdominal pain with severe tenderness.
- *Somatic:* Diffuse abdominal pain linked to anxiety or depression, without a clear physical cause. Stress and emotional distress may exacerbate symptoms.
- *Urinary tract infection (UTI):* Lower abdominal pain with urinary symptoms. May progress to pyelonephritis (ie, UTI that reaches the kidneys), leading to flank pain, fever, and chills.

When to Refer

- *Immediate referral to IM or GI:*
  - Signs of acute abdomen (severe pain, rigidity).
  - Suspected appendicitis, cholecystitis, strangulated hernias, ischemic bowel, kidney stones, myocardial infarction, pancreatitis, or peritonitis.
- *Routine referral to IM or GI:*
  - Persistent or recurrent symptoms without clear etiology.
  - Symptoms suggestive of diverticulitis, hepatitis, IBD, or PUD.

Manage on the Psych Unit

- *Constipation:* Increase fiber intake, encourage physical activity, use stool softeners or laxatives, and adjust or switch any contributing medications if possible.
- *Gastritis and GERD:* Dietary modifications (avoid spicy, acidic, and fatty foods); provide medications like antacids, H2 blockers (eg, ranitidine [Zantac], famotidine [Pepcid]), or proton pump inhibitors (eg, omeprazole [Prilosec], lansoprazole [Prevacid]), and encourage smaller, frequent meals. Elevate the head of the bed for GERD.
- *Hernias:* Instruct patients to avoid activities that cause straining (eg, heavy lifting), maintain a healthy weight, and consume a fiber-rich diet. Hernia belts can help, but their use is typically restricted in psych units due to safety concerns.
- *IBS:* Dietary management, stress reduction techniques, and fiber supplements (eg, Metamucil, Fibercon). Refer to IM or GI if symptoms are severe or unresponsive to initial management.
- *UTIs:* Administer antibiotics based on culture results and ensure adequate hydration.

Acute Stroke Symptoms

Identifying a potential acute stroke in the psychiatric unit is crucial because immediate treatment can usually prevent permanent neurologic damage. As a psychiatric clinician, you won't have primary responsibility for stroke assessment and management, but you should understand current standards in stroke care so that you can coordinate treatment when such an emergency occurs.

Stroke Symptoms

- Sudden onset of neurological deficits, such as weakness or numbness of the face, arm, or leg, especially on one side of the body.
- Confusion, trouble speaking, or difficulty understanding speech.
- Visual disturbances in one or both eyes.
- Trouble walking, dizziness, loss of balance, or lack of coordination.
- Severe headache with no known cause.

Diagnostic Approach

- Call medical staff urgently if you suspect a stroke. Hospitals usually have specific protocols for stroke diagnosis and management (often called "code stroke"), and these should be implemented by trained staff in order to prevent further neurologic damage.
- Here is the typical diagnostic sequence that medical consultants will use; if no consultant is available promptly, you should initiate the exam.
  - *Immediate assessment:* Perform the **BE-FAST** test as a quick screening tool. Any positive sign warrants urgent further evaluation.
    - **B**alance: Check for loss of balance or dizziness.
    - **E**yes: Ask about any sudden vision problems, like blurred vision or loss of vision in one or both eyes.
    - **F**ace: Ask the patient to smile to see if one side of the face droops.
    - **A**rms: Have the patient raise both arms. Observe if one arm drifts downward or cannot be raised.
    - **S**peech: Ask the person to repeat a simple sentence (eg, "The sky is blue"). Check for slurred or unusual speech.
    - **T**ime: If you observe any of these signs, activate the hospital's rapid response team. Time is critical in stroke treatment.
  - *Expedited neurological examination:* Conduct a brief but comprehensive neurological exam to evaluate the extent of the stroke and pinpoint neurologic deficits.
  - *Urgent imaging:* Obtain a CT scan as soon as possible. CT scans are effective at distinguishing between hemorrhagic and ischemic strokes and guiding initial treatment.
  - *Laboratory tests:* Order stat labs, including a complete blood count, coagulation profile (prothrombin time [PT]/activated partial thromboplastin time [aPTT], international normalized ratio [INR]), and a basic metabolic panel. These tests help rule out other conditions that might mimic stroke symptoms, such as metabolic disturbances.

Management Strategies

- Acute care: Your patient should be immediately transferred to a stroke unit or ICU. In preparation for transfer:
  - *Monitor vital signs:* Blood pressure, heart rate, respiratory rate, and oxygen saturation.
  - *Restrict oral intake:* Avoid administering anything by mouth, including medications, to reduce the risk of aspiration, since stroke patients may have swallowing difficulties.
- Post-transfer management will depend on the type of stroke:
  - *Ischemic stroke:* Involves reperfusion therapy to dissolve the clot obstructing blood flow to the brain, ideally administered within 4.5 hours from the onset of symptoms.
  - *Hemorrhagic stroke:* Focuses on stabilizing vital signs, controlling high blood pressure to minimize the risk of further bleeding, and in some cases surgical interventions to alleviate pressure caused by bleeding in the brain.

Anti-NMDA Receptor Encephalitis

Anti-NMDA receptor encephalitis is a serious autoimmune condition where the body produces antibodies against N-methyl-D-aspartate (NMDA) receptors in the brain, leading to psychiatric and neurological symptoms. While uncommon, consider it in your psychosis differential, especially for young women with new-onset psychosis, prodromal symptoms like fever or fatigue, and subtle neurological abnormalities.

Who's Most at Risk?

This condition primarily affects young women and is often linked to ovarian teratomas. However, it can occur in individuals of any age and gender.

Symptoms

- *General:* Fever, headache, fatigue.
- *Psychiatric:* Acute psychosis, hallucinations, behavioral changes.
- *Neurological:* Seizures, memory deficits, abnormal movements, speech dysfunction, altered level of consciousness.
- *Autonomic instability:* Blood pressure fluctuations, heart rate changes.

Diagnostic Approach

- *Cerebrospinal fluid (CSF) analysis:* Testing for NMDA receptor antibodies in CSF is the most reliable diagnostic method.
- *Serum antibodies:* Blood tests for NMDA receptor antibodies can support the diagnosis but are less reliable than CSF analysis.
- *Neuroimaging:* MRI may show subtle abnormalities but is often unremarkable.
- *EEG:* Often reveals generalized slowing or seizure activity.

Treatment Protocols

- Prompt consultation with neurology is essential.
- Patients will need immunosuppressive therapy:
  - *Corticosteroids:* High-dose steroids to reduce inflammation.
  - *Plasmapheresis:* To remove antibodies from the bloodstream.
  - *Intravenous immunoglobulin (IVIG):* Neutralizes harmful antibodies.
  - *Rituximab:* A monoclonal antibody targeting B cells.
  - *Cyclophosphamide:* Used in severe or refractory cases.
- Supportive care in an intensive care setting may be necessary for severe cases.

Prognosis

With early and aggressive treatment, many patients experience significant and even full recovery within weeks to months. Delayed treatment can result in substantial residual disability and increased mortality.

Chest Pain in Psychiatric Settings

The sudden onset of chest pain in a patient is always a cause for concern. Your immediate goal is to distinguish between non-life-threatening conditions, like panic attacks or heartburn, and medical emergencies like myocardial infarction. Here we provide a systematic approach to diagnosing and managing chest pain on the psychiatric unit.

Initial Evaluation of Chest Pain: Quick Assessment

- *Onset:* Determine if the pain began suddenly or gradually. A sudden onset can indicate a myocardial infarction or pulmonary embolism, while a gradual onset may suggest GERD or an anxiety disorder.
- *Location:* Identify if the pain is localized or widespread. Central chest pain often relates to cardiac issues, whereas side-located pain might indicate musculoskeletal or pulmonary problems.
- *Associated symptoms:* Note accompanying symptoms such as shortness of breath, palpitations, nausea, or sweating. These may suggest serious conditions like myocardial infarction or pulmonary embolism.
- *Intensity:* Have the patient rate the pain on a scale of 1–10 to help determine urgency.
- *Aggravating factors:* Determine if pain worsens with movement or exertion, which could indicate costochondritis or a cardiovascular origin, respectively. Pain after eating might suggest a GI issue.
- *Radiation:* Ask if the pain extends to the shoulders, arms, neck, jaw, or back. Radiation particularly to the left arm and jaw is often related to cardiac problems.
- *Quality:* Ask the patient to describe the pain (sharp, dull, crushing, burning), noting that a crushing sensation typically indicates cardiac pain.
- *Duration:* Establish how long the pain lasts and whether it is constant or intermittent. Persistent pain may be due to musculoskeletal issues, while intermittent pain could be angina or related to panic attacks.
- *Previous episodes:* Gather information on any past episodes and their management, including response to medications like antacids or nitroglycerin.
- *Psychosocial factors:* Consider stress, anxiety, and depression, which can also present with chest pain.
- *Cardiac risk factors:* Assess for hypertension, diabetes, smoking, and family history of heart disease to evaluate the likelihood of a cardiac event.

Physical Examination

- Vital signs: Check temperature (fever may indicate infections), heart rate, blood pressure, and respiratory rate to identify any immediate abnormalities.
- Check respiratory systems for signs of distress like labored breathing, or cyanosis (bluish coloration of the skin due to lack of oxygen).
- Palpate the chest area for tenderness (which might indicate musculoskeletal issues).
- Assess for signs of heart failure (eg, jugular venous distension, peripheral edema).
- Auscultate the lungs for wheezing or crackles that could suggest respiratory issues.

Psychiatric Evaluation

- Assess for:
  - Panic attacks and other anxiety disorders.
  - Depression presenting with somatic symptoms.
  - Somatic symptom disorder.

Differential Diagnosis

- *Cardiovascular:* Acute coronary syndrome, including ST-segment elevation myocardial infarction (STEMI) and non-ST-segment elevation MI (NSTEMI); angina; arrythmias; and pericarditis.
- *Respiratory:* Pulmonary embolism, pneumothorax, pneumonia.
- *Gastrointestinal:* GERD, esophageal spasm, peptic ulcer.
- *Musculoskeletal:* Costochondritis, myofascial pain, rib fractures.
- *Psychiatric:* Panic attacks, anxiety disorders, depression with somatic complaints, somatic symptom disorder.

Diagnostic Approach

- *ECG:* Obtain a stat ECG (see "ECG in Inpatient Psychiatry" fact sheet in the Diagnostic and Monitoring Tools section).
- Laboratory tests:
  - *Troponins:* Cardiac biomarkers that are highly specific for cardiac muscle injury. Levels typically rise three to 12 hours from the onset of myocardial injury.
  - *Complete blood count:* To identify signs of infection (eg, elevated white blood cells) or other hematologic conditions (eg, leukemia) that can cause chest pain.
  - *Electrolytes:* Electrolyte imbalances can cause or exacerbate cardiac arrhythmias, which might present as or contribute to chest pain. For example, hypokalemia and hypomagnesemia can increase the risk of ventricular arrhythmias.

- *D-dimer:* if pulmonary embolism is a concern, like if the patient has a sudden onset of shortness of breath, chest pain with a deep breath, or unexplained cough.

- *Imaging:* Chest x-ray to rule out pneumothorax, pneumonia, or rib fractures.
- *Oxygen saturation:* Measure oxygen saturation levels using pulse oximetry.
- *Medication review:* Check for psychiatric and cardiovascular medications that might prolong the QT interval.

Management Strategies

- *Medical emergencies:* Immediate transfer to the medical unit for patients with suspected myocardial infarction, pulmonary embolism, or other life-threatening conditions.
- *Gastrointestinal causes:* Manage GERD or esophageal spasm with antacids (eg, calcium carbonate [Tums]), proton pump inhibitors (PPIs, eg, omeprazole [Prilosec]), or H2 antagonists (eg, famotidine [Pepcid]). Treat peptic ulcers with PPIs; patients with ulcers caused by *H. pylori* may also need antibiotics. Advise patients to eat smaller and more frequent meals, stop smoking, and practice stress management techniques like deep breathing exercises.
- *Musculoskeletal pain:* Acetaminophen or NSAIDs; referral to physical therapy.
- *Psychiatric causes:* Psychotherapy and pharmacotherapy (eg, selective serotonin reuptake inhibitors, benzodiazepines).

Chronic Obstructive Pulmonary Disease (COPD)

COPD is progressive lung disease usually caused by cigarette smoking. It's a common comorbidity of psychiatric illness that can complicate your treatment of patients. In this fact sheet, we give you a brief refresher on the pathophysiology and treatment of this illness, and then focus on how a psychiatrist can be helpful.

Capsule Summary

- *Pathophysiology:* COPD is an umbrella term that includes various lung conditions that diminish airflow. Emphysema refers to the destruction of the alveoli (lung air sacs), reducing the surface area for gas exchange, making it hard to exchange oxygen for carbon dioxide—causing both hypoxia and hypercapnia (high carbon dioxide). Chronic bronchitis refers to inflammation and narrowing of the bronchial tubes, leading to mucus buildup and difficulty clearing the airways.
- *Symptoms:* Chronic cough sometimes with sputum, wheezing, shortness of breath (dyspnea on exertion), frequent colds. Can lead to heart disease as it progresses. Hypoxia and hypercapnia.
- *Diagnosis:* Spirometry will show low forced vital capacity (FVC, meaning the total amount of air the patient can exhale after a taking a deep breath), and low forced expiratory volume 1 second (FEV1, meaning the percentage of FVC exhaled in the first second). Chest x-ray or CT scan is used to rule out other lung problems. Arterial blood gas analysis measures levels of oxygen and carbon dioxide in the blood.
- *Differential diagnosis:* Distinguish from asthma by history and lack of complete reversal of symptoms after puffs of bronchodilator (known as the bronchodilator reversibility test).

Treatment

Lifestyle changes

- *Smoking cessation:* The most crucial step; slows progression.
- *Avoidance of lung irritants:* Like pollution, dust, and fumes.
- *Pulmonary rehabilitation:* Exercise training, nutritional advice, and education.

Medications

Although you will not be initiating these treatments, you will be continuing meds prescribed by PCPs or specialists, so it's helpful to have some familiarity with the more common examples.

- *Beta agonists, or bronchodilators:* Beta receptors relax the muscles lining the bronchioles, causing the tubes to widen, making breathing easier. These are usually prescribed as short-acting bronchodilators and are commonly used as rescue inhalers. They are prescribed for virtually all COPD patients. Most end in "ol." Examples: Short-acting albuterol (Ventolin, Proventil) and long-acting salmeterol (Serevent).
- *Muscarinic receptor blockers (also called muscarinic antagonists or anticholinergics):* Since muscarinic receptors cause smooth muscle contraction, you want to inhibit these to widen the bronchi, hence they are muscarinic antagonists (as opposed to the beta agonists above). Most end in "ium." Examples: ipratropium (Atrovent), tiotropium (Spiriva).
- *Inhaled corticosteroids:* To reduce inflammation. Usually prescribed in long-acting form. Often end in "one." Examples: Fluticasone (Flovent), budesonide (Pulmicort).
- *Combination inhalers:*
  - Advair: Fluticasone and salmeterol.
  - Breo Ellipta: Fluticasone and vilanterol.
  - Symbicort: Budesonide and formoterol.
  - Combivent: Albuterol and ipratropium.
  - Note that hospitals often do not carry inhalers, so you usually have to order them as nebulizers; for example, instead of ordering Serevent two puffs BID, you would order one nebulizer BID.
- *Oxygen therapy:* Supplemental oxygen is needed for patients with severe COPD and low blood oxygen levels.

Psychiatric Implications

- *Anxiety and depression:* Having COPD is both depressing and anxiety-provoking. Patients worry about becoming short of breath, and they often have to limit activities that might otherwise enhance their moods, like working, exercise, recreation, and being with friends. In addition, bronchodilators can lead to tachycardia and jitteriness, which can feel like panic and may worsen anxiety in those already prone to panic attacks.
- *Sleep:* COPD patients have a higher prevalence of insomnia. However, primary care doctors are often reluctant to prescribe benzodiazepines due to concerns about worsening respiratory status, despite the lack of conclusive evidence. Retrospective studies show an association between benzodiazepine use and more severe COPD, but this may simply reflect their use in response to respiratory distress rather than as a cause.
- *Smoking cessation:* This is a key part of treating COPD, and psychiatrists are generally pretty expert at helping patients kick the habit. Ask patients how much they smoke, discuss nicotine replacement therapy options (usually

they will need to be started on nicotine patch 21 mg weekly or nicotine gum 2–4 mg every one to two hours as needed for cravings), and educate them about medication options like bupropion and varenicline.

The takeaway is that you should ask your COPD patients how their illness has been affecting their lives and if it contributed to their psychiatric admission. If it is a big factor, make sure to get a medical consult to beef up their treatment regimen, and involve social work to enhance community supports like visiting nurses and home health aides.

CPR Guidelines for Inpatient Psychiatry

If you are primarily an inpatient psychiatrist, it's pretty likely you will be called upon to participate in CPR at some point in your career—especially if you work in a geriatric setting. While most hospitals require recertification in CPR (usually called Basic Life Support, or BLS) every two years, we may forget the specifics in the heat of the moment—so we have created this quick reference fact sheet for you to review periodically, and perhaps especially at the time of a medical emergency.

Vignette

You are rounding on your patients and see some commotion outside one of your patient's rooms—she is a 75-year-old woman admitted for depression and suicidality. You go into the room and find her seated but slumped over in a chair, with two nurses calling her name. She is not responding. You ask what's going on and one of the nurses says, "I passed by her room and saw her slumped over like this." You are the only MD on the unit, and you are trying to recall what you should do first—it has been at least two years since you had CPR training.

CPR Overview

When to perform CPR

CPR is necessary when a patient becomes unresponsive and is not breathing normally or at all. In inpatient psychiatric settings, this will usually be the result of cardiac arrest or drug overdose.

Purpose of CPR

The purpose is to maintain blood flow to the brain and the heart until more advanced medical help arrives—via three processes:

- *Chest compressions:* The most important aspect of CPR is administering chest compressions, which manually pump blood through the heart and circulate oxygenated blood to the brain and other organs.
- *Rescue breathing:* Rescue breathing maintains oxygenation of the blood.
- *Automated external defibrillator (AED):* When available, an AED is used to convert an irregular heart rhythm (such as ventricular fibrillation) to a normal rhythm.

How to Do CPR

1. *Assess the situation*
   - *Take charge if needed:* Usually in these situations there is an initial stage of chaos, with many staff milling around trying to figure out the situation. If you are the only MD or NP in the room, it's likely that you will be expected to take charge and lead the team. That said, every unit is different, and there may be a nurse or other staff member who is clearly more experienced with medical emergencies—in which case they should take the lead.
   - *Communicate your intentions:* Let other staff know what you plan to do every step of the way. For example, before starting chest compressions, say, "I'm going to start chest compressions." This allows staff to facilitate the process and gives them a chance to chime in if they have concerns—for example, the patient may have a do not resuscitate (DNR) advance directive, in which case you should not perform CPR.
   - *Check responsiveness:* Gently tap the person and shout, "Are you okay?"
   - *Call for help:* If there's no response, direct staff to call a code (often a "code blue," but the name may vary from hospital to hospital).
   - *Call for the AED:* If others are present, instruct someone to call and bring an AED if available. Usually, the AED is on a crash cart on the unit. Once the AED arrives, immediately stop chest compressions and use it (see below for instructions).
2. *Position the person*

   Carefully place the person on their back on a firm, flat surface, such as the floor.
3. *Check for breathing and pulse*
   - *Open airway:* Tilt the person's head back slightly to open the airway.
   - *Check for breathing:* Look for chest movement, listen for breath sounds, and feel for air on your cheek for no more than 10 seconds.
   - *Check pulse:* Quickly check the carotid pulse (located on the side of the neck) for no more than 10 seconds. If you are unsure or do not feel a pulse, start CPR.
4. *Begin chest compressions*
   - *Hand placement:* Place the heel of one hand in the center of the chest, between the nipples. Place your other hand on top, interlocking your fingers.
   - *Body position:* Position yourself directly over your hands, with straight arms.
   - *Compressions:* Push hard and fast, compressing the chest at least 2 inches deep at a rate of 100–120 compressions per minute. Allow the chest to recoil completely between compressions. Use songs to help you maintain the right rhythm—traditionally the Bee Gees song "Stayin' Alive" is used.
   - *Cycle:* Maintain a cycle of 30 chest compressions and two rescue breaths.

5. *Provide rescue breaths*
    - *Head tilt–chin lift:* Ensure the airway is open by tilting the head back.
    - *Pinch nose:* Pinch the person's nose shut.
    - *Deliver breaths:* If an Ambu bag is available, use that to give breaths. Give two breaths, each lasting about one second, watching for the chest to rise. If the chest does not rise, retilt the head and try again.
6. *Continue CPR*
    - *Cycle:* Continue the cycle of 30 chest compressions and two rescue breaths.
    - *Rotating chest compressors:* Doing chest compressions right is tiring, and to maintain the quality of the compressions, you should rotate staff every two minutes. When you are tired, ask another staff member to take over for you at the end of your current cycle.
    - *Reassessment:* Reassess every two minutes. If there are signs of life, stop CPR. Otherwise, continue until professional help arrives or an AED is ready to use.
7. *Use an AED*

    The AED should be used the moment it becomes available. Interrupt CPR to use it.
    - *Turn on AED:* Follow the voice prompts.
    - *Attach pads:* Place the adhesive pads on the person's bare chest as shown in the diagrams on the AED.
    - *Analyze rhythm:* Allow the AED to analyze the heart rhythm. Ensure no one is touching the person during analysis.
    - *Deliver shock:* If advised by the AED, ensure everyone is clear of the person and press the shock button. Immediately resume CPR after the shock.

Key points to remember

- *High-quality compressions:* Focus on depth and rate; let the chest recoil.
- *Minimize interruptions:* Keep interruptions in chest compressions to a minimum.
- *AED use:* Follow AED instructions promptly.

Diabetes

Diabetes is notably common among patients with chronic mental illness, often due to a combination of factors such as poor diet, lack of physical activity, and the metabolic effects of psychotropic medications. Here's a detailed guide on the diagnosis and management of diabetes for patients on the psychiatric unit.

Key Tasks for the Psychiatrist

- Assess glycemic control and adherence to treatment.
- Educate patients on glycemic control and long-term complication risks.
- Evaluate psychotropic medications for their impact on diabetes and weight.

Pathophysiology

Normally, the beta cells of the pancreas produce insulin and release it continuously into the bloodstream. Insulin acts as a key to unlock receptors on cells, opening them up like pores to allow the entry of glucose. Insulin levels normally rise after a meal to allow our cells to absorb more glucose.

In Type 1 diabetes (insulin-dependent diabetes mellitus) the pancreas stops producing insulin (an autoimmune process destroys the cells that manufacture it). Therefore, blood glucose can't get into the cells, and glucose blood levels rise.

In Type 2 diabetes, or adult-onset diabetes, the pancreas produces less insulin than normal and the insulin receptors are less sensitive, or more resistant, to insulin. Type 2 diabetes is more related to poor diet and obesity than Type 1, and patients can sometimes improve their condition by diet and exercise.

Diagnosis

- Fasting blood glucose >125 on at least two occasions; symptoms plus a random blood glucose >199.
- Other lab tests: Glycosylated hemoglobin (HbA1c) above 7% (measure of average glucose level over past two to three months; percentage of Hb molecules with glucose attached); urinalysis with acetone; diabetic retinopathy on eye exam.

Symptoms

- Polyuria (caused by kidney trying to filter out excessive sugar, which increases urine output), polydipsia (polyuria causes dehydration and therefore thirst), polyphagia (glucose can't enter cells effectively, causing hunger to increase energy input), weight loss (body breaks down muscle and fat to provide energy to starved cells), fatigue (glucose not optimally being processed, leading to fatigue), blurred vision, slow-healing wounds.
- Diabetic ketoacidosis: High levels of glucose cause diuresis and severe dehydration; in addition, cells start metabolizing fat for energy, converting it into fatty acids, which get converted into ketones, which in turn causes acidosis.
- Long-term complications: When the bloodstream is extremely concentrated with glucose, the blood becomes stickier and more viscous and binds to proteins in vessel walls, causing vessels to stiffen. This decreases circulation to vital organs, causing complications such as coronary artery disease, stroke, kidney damage, blindness, nerve damage, and problems with wound healing.

Treatment

- Dietary management: Follow the ADA diet: 45% carbs, 15%–20% proteins, no more than 20% fats.
- Regular exercise: Improves insulin sensitivity, helps decrease weight, reduces cardiovascular risks.

Medications

- *Metformin:* First-line therapy for Type 2 diabetes. Increases sensitivity to insulin and decreases the amount of sugar released by the liver into the bloodstream.
- *Sulfonylureas (eg, glyburide, glipizide):* Stimulate insulin production from pancreatic beta cells. Patients should avoid alcohol when on these drugs because the combination can cause hypoglycemia.
- *Meglitinides (eg, repaglinide):* Stimulate beta cells to make insulin.
- *GLP-1 receptor agonists (eg, liraglutide, semaglutide):* Enhance glucose-dependent insulin secretion, suppress glucagon release, and slow gastric emptying. They are associated with weight loss and reduced cardiovascular risk, making them an excellent option for patients with Type 2 diabetes, especially those with obesity or cardiovascular disease.
- *Insulin:* There are four types of insulin: rapid acting (eg, Humalog [Lispro] insulin), short acting (eg, insulin regular), intermediate acting (eg, insulin NPH), and long acting (eg, Lantus).

Table 13: **Illustrative Insulin Sliding Scale Protocol**

Blood Glucose	Regular Insulin Dose*
Less than 70	OJ, hypoglycemia protocol**
70–150	0 units
151–200	2 units (0 if at bedtime)
201–250	4 units (2 if at bedtime)
251–300	5–6 units (3 if at bedtime)
301–350	6–8 units (4 if at bedtime)
351–400	7–10 units (5 if at bedtime)
>400	8–12 units and call MD (6 if at bedtime)

*Doses may be higher depending on a patient's suspected insulin sensitivity.

**In case of hypoglycemia (lightheadedness, sweatiness, and clammy palms), a typical protocol is to immediately give a cup of juice, a tablespoon or two of sugar, or Life Savers candy, and to recheck blood sugar after 15 minutes. Once normalized, patients are often given a more complex carbohydrate, such as graham crackers or regular Saltine crackers, to tide them over until the next regular meal.

Psychiatric Aspects of Diabetes

- *Psychotropic medications:* Be especially vigilant about metabolic side effects of antipsychotics. Olanzapine and clozapine present the highest risk; quetiapine and risperidone are intermediate risk.
- *Psychological issues:* Patients may have difficulty accepting the diagnosis, fear of hypoglycemia, fear of complications, or difficulties with adherence to treatment and self-care.
- *Depression and anxiety:* Some psych meds can treat both psychiatric issues and diabetic neuropathy (eg, duloxetine, amitriptyline, nortriptyline, gabapentin).
- *Substance use:* Drinking impairs management of diabetes, whether via lifestyle alterations or medication compliance. Therefore, in patients who have comorbid diabetes and substance use, you can use the diabetes as a leverage point to increase motivation to stop using substances.
- *Insulin overdose:* Among diabetics with psychiatric disorders, an insulin overdose is a common type of suicide attempt. Such patients will be treated initially in the ICU. They will usually be hypoglycemic, sometimes severely so (less than 50 mg/dL) and will often receive a bag of IV "D5W," which means saline with 50% dextrose. One of the common dramatic symptoms of hypoglycemia is a seizure. They will be observed for a couple of days to make sure they are stabilized, and then may be transferred to the psychiatric unit, where you will have an endocrinologist or hospitalist see them daily and make any required adjustments in their insulin dose.

Gastroesophageal Reflux Disease (GERD)

GERD occurs when stomach acid flows back into the esophagus and causes irritation. You will likely encounter this condition among patients with psychiatric disorders because two major risk factors—smoking and obesity—are prevalent in this population. Additionally, many of the medications we prescribe tend to relax the lower esophageal sphincter, like antipsychotic medications with anticholinergic properties, and benzodiazepines due to their muscle relaxant effects. Here's a guide to help you recognize and treat GERD.

Symptoms to Look Out For

- *Typical symptoms:* Heartburn, regurgitation, dysphagia (difficulty swallowing).
- *Less common symptoms:* Chest pain, chronic cough, laryngitis, and/or asthma-like symptoms (due to acid reflux irritating the esophagus, throat, and airways).

Ask Patients

- Do you experience heartburn? If so, how often?
- Is there a pattern to your symptoms, like occurrence after meals or when lying down?
- Do you notice symptoms getting worse with certain foods or beverages, like spicy foods, caffeine, chocolate, or alcoholic beverages?
- Do you have any symptoms that might not seem related to heartburn, like persistent cough, hoarseness, wheezing, shortness of breath, or chest pain?

When to Consult Medicine

- For uncomplicated GERD, you can initiate treatment without a medical consult—though in many hospitals medicine is happy to assist you with this.
- If you are unsure about the symptoms and suspect a potential cardiac cause, consult medicine for a more thorough evaluation.

Lifestyle and Dietary Modifications

- Have patients elevate the head of their bed at night with extra pillows.
- Instruct them to avoid large meals, especially before bedtime.
- Work with the hospital dietitian to eliminate trigger foods from the patient's diet.
- Advise patients to work toward a healthy weight if they're overweight.

Medications

- Antacids (eg, calcium carbonate [Tums, Rolaids]).
- H2 receptor antagonists (eg, ranitidine [Zantac] 150 mg twice daily, famotidine [Pepcid] 20 mg twice daily).
- Proton pump inhibitors (PPIs; eg, omeprazole (Prilosec) 20 mg once daily, esomeprazole (Nexium) 20–40 mg once daily, lansoprazole (Prevacid) 30 mg once daily).
  - PPIs should be taken 30 minutes before the first meal of the day.
  - Increase the dose to twice daily (before breakfast and before dinner) if symptoms don't resolve after four to eight weeks.
  - PPIs increase the risk of osteoporosis, kidney disease, and vitamin B12 deficiency, so the goal is to eventually taper and discontinue their use once the patient's GERD improves, except for patients with erosive esophagitis or Barrett's esophagus—a condition where the esophageal lining becomes red and thickened, placing patients at a heightened risk of esophageal cancer.

Headaches

Headaches are common in inpatient psychiatry. This guide will help you to distinguish potentially life-threatening headaches from chronic headaches, provide advice on the psychiatric-headache intersection, and discuss treatment options that might address both psychiatric conditions and headaches.

How to Distinguish Types of Headaches

- *Migraine:* Typically unilateral, pulsating or throbbing pain; often accompanied by nausea and light sensitivity; worsens with physical activity; may include aura (visual disturbances, sensory changes, speech difficulties).
- *Tension headache:* Presents as a dull, constant, pressing pain on both sides of the head. Unlike migraines, these headaches don't throb and do not involve nausea.
- *Medication side effect headache:* Typically a dull headache, similar to a tension headache, that starts after a new medication or a change in dose. The most common culprits are antidepressants, especially bupropion and escitalopram.
- *Emergency/life-threatening:* A sudden, severe headache, often described as the worst headache ever felt (a "thunderclap"), warrants immediate action. This could signal something serious like a subarachnoid hemorrhage or meningitis. Obtain immediate medical consultation.

Interaction Between Headaches and Psychiatric Disorders

- *Comorbidity:* Migraine is very common in both mood disorders and anxiety disorders.
- *Psychological impact of headaches:* Migraine pain and associated symptoms like photophobia can exacerbate depression and anxiety. The unpredictability of a migraine attack can escalate anxiety, and the constant pain leads to a sense of helplessness and depression.
- *Psychiatric triggers of headaches:* Stress and anxiety can trigger or worsen headaches. Also, depression might make patients less responsive to headache treatments due to poor adherence to the medication regimen.
- *Substance use disorders:* These can complicate headache management, as substances like alcohol can induce headaches during withdrawal or contribute to chronic headache conditions.

Medications for Headaches and Their Psychiatric Implications

Navigating the medication maze is crucial in ensuring that treatment for headaches doesn't throw psychiatric treatments off balance:

Analgesics

Acetaminophen 325–650 mg PRN or ibuprofen 200–800 mg PRN are effective. Opiate agonists are sometimes used to abort severe headaches, such as hydrocodone/acetaminophen (Vicodin), but this is considered a last resort due to potential for dependency.

Triptans

Effective specifically for aborting migraines (eg, sumatriptan 25–50 mg as needed at first sign of a migraine). In the past there were warnings about serotonin syndrome with the combination of triptans and selective serotonin reuptake inhibitors (SSRIs), but several large studies have debunked this concern (Orlova Y et al, *JAMA Neurol* 2018;75(5):566–572).

Combination meds

Many patients swear by Fiorinal, one to two capsules PRN, which is a combination of butalbital (sedative), aspirin (analgesic), and caffeine (vasoconstrictor). But overuse often leads to rebound headaches.

Newer medications

Many new migraine medications and devices have been approved recently. As a psychiatrist, you won't be expected to keep up with these new treatments, but they are listed here so you can understand why some of your patients are taking these meds.

- *Calcitonin gene-related peptide (CGRP) receptor blockers:* Collectively known as "gepants" (ubrogepant, rimigepant, atogepant). Generally used as abortants, especially for patients who can't take triptans.
- *Lasmiditan:* Similar to triptans (aborts migraines) but has fewer side effects.
- *Monoclonal antibodies for migraine prevention:* These include erenumab (Aimovig), fremanezumab (Ajovy), galcanezumab (Emgality), and eptinezumab (Vyepti). Expensive, but a game-changer for people with migraines.
- *Portable neurostimulation devices:* Several portable devices stimulate various nerves to inhibit migraine attacks. They include Cefaly, Relivion, Nerivio, and SAVI Dual (a portable transcranial magnetic stimulation device).

Medications for both headaches and psychiatric disorders

- *Antidepressants:* Tricyclic antidepressants, especially amitriptyline and its metabolite nortriptyline, have the best evidence for migraine treatment among antidepressants. Serotonin/norepinephrine reuptake inhibitors, such as venlafaxine and duloxetine, are also effective in the higher dose range. SSRIs, bupropion, and mirtazapine don't help with migraines but are effective for tension headaches.

- *Valproic acid:* FDA approved for both bipolar disorder and migraine, so it can be a good "twofer" for some patients.
- *Topiramate:* Effective for migraine and better tolerated than valproic acid. In psychiatry, it's often used for alcohol use disorder and weight loss, as well as an adjunct to mood stabilizers.
- *Beta-blockers:* Effective for both migraine prevention and social anxiety (eg, propranolol starting at 40 mg BID).
- *Dopamine blockers:* Can help with acute migraine, especially if there's prominent nausea. Try promethazine (Phenergan) 25 mg PRN or prochlorperazine (Compazine) 10 mg PRN. Chlorpromazine (Thorazine) 25–50 mg is also used for severe migraine.

Headache meds that help psychiatric conditions

On the flip side, certain migraine treatments can alleviate psychiatric symptoms. For instance, onabotulinumtoxinA (Botox), while primarily for chronic migraines, has shown benefits in treating depression.

Psychiatric meds that can make headaches worse

Trazodone produces a metabolite that can cause migraine-type headaches. Also avoid the other "azodones"—nefazodone and vilazodone.

Psychological Treatments

- *Relaxation techniques:* Introduce patients to relaxation techniques, including deep breathing exercises, which can help reduce the frequency of headaches. (See the "Relaxation and Deep Breathing Exercises" fact sheet in the Psychotherapy on the Inpatient Unit section.)
- *Cognitive behavioral therapy (CBT):* CBT helps patients understand the stress-headache connection and develop coping strategies. (See the "Cognitive Behavioral Therapy Techniques" fact sheet in the Psychotherapy on the Inpatient Unit section.)
- *Mindfulness and acceptance therapies:* These therapies aid patients in accepting their pain and reducing the psychological distress associated with chronic headaches.

Lifestyle Interventions

- *Education on habits:* Inform patients about the benefits of maintaining regular sleep patterns and staying well hydrated. Help them identify their headache triggers, which may include caffeine, alcohol, and sensory stimuli like bright lights or strong smells.
- *Medication use awareness:* Educate patients on the risks associated with the regular, long-term use of headache medications, especially analgesics and triptans. Explain that overuse can paradoxically increase the frequency and severity of headaches.

HIV

Pathophysiology

Human immunodeficiency virus (HIV) targets the immune system, specifically CD4+ T-cells, leading to their gradual depletion. This impairment of the immune response makes the body more susceptible to infections and certain cancers. The virus can also cross the blood-brain barrier, affecting the central nervous system and potentially leading to neurocognitive disorders.

Key Tasks for the Psychiatrist

- *Monitor for neuropsychiatric complications:* HIV can affect the nervous system, leading to cognitive impairments, mood disorders, and psychotic disorders.
- *Assess adherence to antiretroviral therapy (ART):* Nonadherence can lead to treatment failure and the development of resistant HIV strains.
- *Address psychiatric comorbidities:* Patients with HIV are at increased risk for depression, anxiety, and substance use disorders.
- *Evaluate psychotropic medications:* Consider the potential interactions between psychotropic medications and ART.

Diagnosis

- *Screening tests:* Enzyme-linked immunosorbent assay (ELISA) followed by confirmatory Western blot or polymerase chain reaction (PCR) tests. These tests detect antibodies against HIV in the blood, allowing for early diagnosis and treatment.
- *CD4 count:* A measure of immune function; levels below 200 cells/mm^3 are indicative of progression to acquired immunodeficiency syndrome (AIDS).
- *Viral load:* This is a measure of the amount of virus in the blood, important for monitoring treatment response. An important goal of treatment is to achieve and maintain an undetectable viral load (<20 copies/mL), as it prevents disease progression and reduces transmission risk.

Symptoms

HIV vs AIDS

With the wide availability of ART, many patients with HIV will experience few symptoms. However, if left untreated, HIV can lead to AIDS.

AIDS-defining conditions

- Opportunistic infections:
  - *Pneumocystis pneumonia:* Prevalent when CD4 counts drop below 200 cells/mm^3. Symptoms include shortness of breath, dry cough, fever, and fatigue.
  - *Toxoplasmosis:* A brain infection that presents with neurological symptoms like headache, weakness, seizures, or confusion.
  - *Tuberculosis (TB):* Symptoms include cough, night sweats, fever, and weight loss. Always screen for TB in HIV-positive patients.
- Severe weight loss, also known as wasting syndrome; neurocognitive disorders due to HIV-associated neurocognitive disorders; and cancers such as Kaposi's sarcoma and non-Hodgkin's lymphoma are considered AIDS-defining conditions.

Treatment

- *Vaccinations:* Ensure vaccinations are up to date, including hepatitis A and B, HPV, COVID-19, and seasonal flu shots, to prevent infections that can be more severe in individuals with HIV.
- *ART:* A combination of medications that reduce HIV viral load, maintain or increase CD4+ T-cell counts, and prevent the progression to AIDS. Psychiatric patients with HIV often have poor adherence to ART. Educate your HIV+ patients about the risk of developing resistance to the medications unless they take them consistently.
  - ART medications are chosen based on the patient's stage of infection, coexisting conditions (eg, liver disease, mental health conditions), treatment history, drug resistance profiles, drug interactions, pill burden, and dosage frequency. Genetic testing for drug resistance is also important before choosing the right medication.
  - Classes of ART medications:
    - Nucleoside reverse transcriptase inhibitors (NRTIs): Tenofovir, emtricitabine, etc.
    - Non-nucleoside reverse transcriptase inhibitors (NNRTIs): Often used initially. Efavirenz, etc.
    - Protease inhibitors (PIs): Darunavir, etc.
    - Integrase strand transfer inhibitors (INSTIs): Often used due to fewer side effects and interactions. Dolutegravir, etc.
- *Prevention of opportunistic infections:* Prophylactic treatments based on CD4 count and exposure risks.

Psychiatric Aspects

Major depression

- Assessment
  - Some symptoms commonly associated with depression, like fatigue and poor concentration, might be side effects of medications (like efavirenz and corticosteroids) used in HIV/AIDS treatment. If the patient's mood changes began shortly after initiating a medication for HIV, work with the infectious disease service to reassess and potentially modify the patient's treatment regimen.
  - Alternatively, depressive-like symptoms might reflect HIV-associated neurocognitive impairment rather than depression.
  - If a patient's HIV infection is well controlled and their viral load is undetectable, treat any depressive symptoms as primary depression. In patients with more advanced infections or poor compliance with treatment, lethargy and cognitive impairment may be secondary to the HIV infection rather than depression.
- Medications
  - Selective serotonin reuptake inhibitors (SSRIs): First-line therapies for the treatment of depression and anxiety in patients with HIV.
  - Tricyclic antidepressants: Beneficial for patients with diarrhea and wasting, but their anticholinergic properties can produce or exacerbate cognitive impairment.
  - Mirtazapine: Stimulates appetite without producing anticholinergic side effects.
  - Bupropion: Helpful in cases where fatigue and impaired concentration are primary symptoms, but its dose-dependent seizure risk complicates treatment in patients with neurologic complications from HIV (eg, cerebral toxoplasmosis).
  - Psychostimulants: Modafinil, methylphenidate, and dextroamphetamine can be helpful adjunctive treatments for fatigue and apathy.

Cognitive impairment

- Neuropsychiatric complications can lead to AIDS-related neurocognitive disorder. Consider neuropsychiatric screening tests, such as the Montreal Cognitive Assessment (MoCA).

Anxiety

- Assessment
  - Evaluate whether a patient's symptoms of anxiety stem from an anxiety disorder or are secondary to medical conditions linked to HIV, like chronic illnesses or opportunistic infections. These health issues can cause symptoms (eg, night sweats and difficulty breathing) that mimic those of anxiety disorders. Similarly, side effects from certain antiretroviral drugs, including insomnia, restlessness, and heart palpitations, can be confused with an anxiety disorder. If symptoms appear to be directly related to medical conditions or medication side effects, address these underlying causes.
- Treatment
  - SSRIs and serotonin/norepinephrine reuptake inhibitors (SNRIs) are generally safe and effective for treating anxiety in HIV-infected patients, but monitor for potential interactions with ART.
  - While benzodiazepines can be effective for the temporary relief of acute anxiety symptoms, use them cautiously due to their risks of dependency, withdrawal, and potential interactions with some ART medications.
  - Use cognitive behavioral therapy (CBT) and other psychotherapeutic approaches as first-line treatments or adjuncts to medication, particularly for mild to moderate anxiety or when pharmacotherapy is contraindicated or limited by drug interactions.

Substance use disorders

- Assessment
  - Evaluate the presence and extent of substance use, including alcohol, illicit drugs, and nonmedical use of prescription medications. Assess how the substance use impacts the patient's HIV management, including adherence to ART.
- Treatment
  - Medication-assisted treatment (MAT): For opioid use disorder, use methadone, buprenorphine, or naltrexone, but be mindful of their interactions with ART—especially methadone. For alcohol use disorder, consider prescribing naltrexone or acamprosate.
  - Screen for kidney and liver function in patients on MAT and ART to prevent drug-induced hepatotoxicity and nephrotoxicity and to adjust treatments as necessary.
  - Behavioral therapies such as CBT, motivational interviewing, and contingency management help address substance use and promote adherence to HIV treatment.
  - At discharge, arrange for outpatient support groups and community resources, including 12-step programs.

Potential interactions between psychiatric medications and ART

- Protease inhibitors inhibit the CYP3A4 enzyme, leading to elevated serum concentrations of several psychiatric medications, while NNRTIs induce CYP3A4 activity, thereby reducing the levels.
- Carbamazepine is a potent inducer of CYP3A4, which can decrease the levels of some PIs and NNRTIs.

Huntington's Disease

Huntington's disease (HD) is a genetic neurodegenerative disorder. This disease occurs due to an abnormality in the HTT gene located on chromosome 4—specifically, the above-normal repetition of a particular sequence of DNA, known as CAG repeats. If a parent has the condition, their child's risk of inheriting the disease is 50%. There's no cure, but supportive care helps manage symptoms.

Symptoms

- *Neuromuscular:* Patients exhibit chorea, characterized by unpredictable movements of the face, limbs, and trunk, as well as rigidity and dystonia.
- *Cognitive:* Includes declines in memory, attention, and executive functions.
- *Psychiatric:* Symptoms like depression, irritability, and anxiety can precede neuromuscular symptoms by years, with psychosis developing in advanced stages.

Disease Onset and Progression

- The age when symptoms first appear and their severity correlate with the number of CAG repeats.
- A repeat count above 40 guarantees disease manifestation.
- Most patients develop symptoms between 30 and 50 years old, but juvenile-onset HD can emerge before age 20.
- Life expectancy is shortened, with the average life expectancy 15–20 years after onset of symptoms.

Diagnosis

If a patient displays a mix of movement, cognitive, and psychiatric symptoms, especially with a family history of HD, obtain genetic testing. Prior to testing, ensure your patient receives genetic counseling, given the profound implications a diagnosis can have for them and their family.

Management

A multidisciplinary approach is essential (eg, with neurologists, physical therapists, etc).

- *Medication management:*
  - VMAT-2 inhibitors: Tetrabenazine, deutetrabenazine, and valbenazine can mitigate choreic movements. Watch for side effects, including depression and suicidal thoughts.
  - Antidepressants: Selective serotonin reuptake inhibitors or serotonin/norepinephrine reuptake inhibitors help with depression and obsessive-compulsive symptoms.
  - Antipsychotics: Useful for controlling both chorea and psychosis, but monitor for worsening tremors and muscle stiffness.
  - Mood stabilizers: For mood swings.
  - Benzodiazepines: For anxiety, but use cautiously as they can worsen cognition.
- *Psychotherapy:* Cognitive behavioral therapy helps in managing anxiety, obsessive-compulsive symptoms, and depression.
- *Physical therapy:* To enhance mobility and reduce fall risk.
- *Nutritional guidance:* To assess the patient's dietary needs and make recommendations (eg, pureed food to prevent choking).
- *Speech therapy:* Helpful for patients who struggle with speech due to dysarthria.
- *Capacity evaluation:* Regularly assess the patient's ability to understand and make decisions about their care; maintain a clear line of communication with their designated decision makers.
- *Advanced care planning:* Initiate early, before the patient's decision-making capacity becomes compromised.
- *Family support:* Family therapy or support groups on the unit can be invaluable for relatives feeling stressed or overwhelmed.
- *Post-discharge planning:* Ensure patients and families are aware of community resources, such as the Huntington's Disease Society of America (www.hdsa.org).

Hypertension

Hypertension is fairly common in patients admitted to psychiatric units. Causes range from transient anxiety to substance withdrawal to cardiovascular issues. Your job as a psychiatric provider is to assess whether there is an urgent situation needing immediate treatment or an issue that can wait for your medical colleagues to do a thorough evaluation and come up with a treatment plan. Occasionally, depending on your training and comfort level, you can also initiate treatment for moderate hypertension, and we suggest an approach should you decide to do so.

Measurement and Actions if Hypertension Is Severe

Definition of hypertension

While definitions vary, the standard definition of hypertension is a sustained blood pressure above 140/90.

Was the reading accurate?

Many hospitals use automated cuffs, which are inaccurate in 10%–15% of patients, so ask nursing to confirm with a manual reading. In addition, you should obtain readings on at least two separate occasions while the patient is sitting and calm before concluding they have hypertension.

Hypertensive emergency

Your first job is to determine if this is a medical emergency. Typically if the systolic is >180 mmHg and/or the diastolic is >120 mmHg, you are going to want to consult medicine immediately—especially if there are any accompanying symptoms suggesting potential heart, kidney, or brain damage, like chest pain, shortness of breath, back pain, numbness/weakness, change in vision, difficulty speaking, or severe headache.

- While awaiting transfer to medicine, you can administer clonidine 0.1–0.2 mg orally. It should work in 20–30 minutes.
- In cases where anxiety is contributing to elevated blood pressure, administer lorazepam (Ativan) IM 1–2 mg. This should work within 30–60 minutes.

Assessment and Management of Nonurgent Hypertension

Common causes of hypertension in psychiatric units

- Stress/agitation due to underlying psychiatric illness.
- "Essential" hypertension (cause unknown) in 90% of patients.
- Obesity.
- Chronic alcohol use.
- Methamphetamine or cocaine use.
- Withdrawal from alcohol, benzodiazepines, or opiates.
- Obstructive sleep apnea.
- Medications:
  - Venlafaxine.
  - Duloxetine.
  - Bupropion at higher doses.
  - Amphetamines (especially Adderall).
  - NSAIDs.
  - Corticosteroids.
  - Anabolic steroids.
  - Oral contraceptives.

Evaluation

- Ask your patient if they have a history of any of the typical causes listed above. Also inquire about a history of cardiovascular or kidney disease.
- Assess for the following symptoms, all of which can indicate serious medical conditions requiring prompt attention:
  - Headache.
  - Chest pain.
  - Shortness of breath.
  - Dizziness or lightheadedness.
  - Nausea or vomiting.
  - Palpitations.
  - Nosebleeds.
  - Neurological symptoms such as numbness or weakness, vision changes, or difficulty speaking.
  - Swelling in the legs or feet.

Psychiatric treatment

- If your history indicates that the cause may be related to a psychiatric or substance use issue, begin standard psychiatric treatment and monitor daily vitals for improvement in blood pressure. If the hypertension is moderate and there are no concerning medical symptoms, no medical consultation is needed right away.
- If hypertension persists after psychiatric symptoms have improved, consult medicine for further evaluation, or if the patient is ready for discharge, refer to a primary care physician for follow-up.

Medical workup and treatment

If you order a medical consult for evaluation and treatment of moderate hypertension (or if you choose to do this medical workup yourself), here is a common protocol for assessment and initial treatment. In most cases, you won't find a specific treatable cause, so the treatment will involve targeting blood pressure with specific meds and recommending lifestyle changes.

- Medical workup:
  - Lipid profile to screen for dyslipidemia and risk for cardiovascular disease.
  - Electrolytes and kidney function.
  - Fasting glucose or hemoglobin A1c to screen for diabetes.
  - Urinalysis to screen for proteinuria (sign of kidney impairment).
  - Electrocardiogram to screen for left ventricular hypertrophy or prior infarction.
- Medications: The following are all reasonable options for initial treatment of uncomplicated hypertension. If these don't work, there are various protocols for escalating treatment by adding a second or third medication, but this is typically done as an outpatient, and the decision will be made by a primary care provider or a cardiologist.
  - Thiazide diuretics: Hydrochlorothiazide (start at 12.5 mg daily; maximum 25 mg daily). This is a good initial choice for most patients except those with impaired kidney function (eg, glomerular filtration rate <30).
  - ACE inhibitors: Lisinopril (start at 10 mg daily; can increase up to 40 mg daily). Good choice for patients with diabetes or heart failure.
  - Angiotensin II receptor blockers: Losartan (start at 25 mg daily; can increase to 100 mg daily). Good choice for patients who can't tolerate the common side effects from ACE inhibitors, like a persistent cough.
  - Calcium channel blockers: Amlodipine (start at 5 mg daily; can be increased to 10 mg daily). Good choice for patients with angina or peripheral artery disease.
  - Beta-blockers: Metoprolol (start at 25 mg twice daily; can be increased to 100 mg twice daily). Good choice for patients with tachycardia or a history of myocardial infarction, as it reduces heart rate and decreases the workload on the heart. Don't use for patients with asthma due to the risk of bronchoconstriction.
- Lifestyle modifications on the inpatient unit:
  - Place patients on a heart-healthy diet that is low in sodium, saturated fat, and cholesterol.
  - Encourage patients to engage in regular physical activity on the unit, such as walking or light stretching exercises, but to avoid strenuous activities.

Hyponatremia

Hyponatremia is the most common electrolyte imbalance you will encounter on the psych unit. It's easy to miss, so keep a low threshold for suspicion, especially since psychotropic medications are among the most common causes. Here are key principles to identify and manage this condition.

What Is Hyponatremia?

Hyponatremia is defined as a serum sodium level of less than 135 mEq/L. The lower the level, the more symptomatic patients will typically be. However, the speed at which a patient becomes hyponatremic also matters. A patient whose serum sodium acutely (ie, within 48 hours) drops to 130 mEq/L may present with more symptoms than a patient who experiences a gradual drop to 120 mEq/L.

Common Causes in Psychiatric Patients

- *Medication-induced:* Psychotropic drugs, diuretics, antiepileptics, and anticancer medications.
- *Psychogenic polydipsia:* Excessive water intake due to psychiatric conditions.
- *Syndrome of inappropriate antidiuretic hormone secretion (SIADH):* Often related to underlying conditions like lung disease, central nervous system disorders (eg, brain injuries), malignancies, or infections.

Evaluation

Identify symptoms

- *Mild (130–134 mEq/L):* Often asymptomatic, but patients might experience nonspecific signs like nausea, headache, dizziness, muscle cramps, and lethargy.
- *Moderate (120–129 mEq/L):* Vomiting, disorientation, agitation, gait disturbances.
- *Severe (<120 mEq/L):* Seizures, coma. In extreme cases, brain herniation may occur as a result of cerebral edema and increased intracranial pressure.

Review medication history

Look for medications that may cause hyponatremia, such as selective serotonin reuptake inhibitors, antipsychotics, carbamazepine, and thiazide diuretics.

Order labs

- *Serum sodium:* Check if it's less than 135 mEq/L.
- *Serum osmolality:* Helps determine if hyponatremia is due to excess water or other causes like hyperglycemia. (Excess glucose draws water out of cells and creates pseudohyponatremia, where serum osmolality will be high despite low sodium levels.)
- *Urine sodium and osmolality:* Provides clues about the underlying cause, such as SIADH (high urine sodium, high urine osmolality) or fluid overload (low urine sodium, high urine osmolality).

Management Strategies

- Mild cases:
  - Fluid restriction: 1000–1500 mL/day or less.
  - Discontinue or adjust offending medications.
  - Oral salt tablets: eg, 1 g twice daily.
  - Encourage a high-salt diet.
  - Monitor electrolytes daily until serum sodium level returns to normal range (135 mEq/L or greater).
- For psychogenic polydipsia, implement behavioral strategies and educate the patient about the importance of fluid restriction (see the "Psychogenic Polydipsia: Diagnosis and Treatment" fact sheet in the Managing Comorbid Medical Conditions section).

When to Involve the Medical Team

- *Sodium <130 mEq/L:* Patients, especially if symptomatic, may need IV saline (3% sodium chloride). The medical unit will increase serum sodium gradually to avoid osmotic demyelination syndrome, a potentially fatal condition where rapid correction of sodium levels causes severe brain damage.
- *SIADH:* You might suspect SIADH if the patient has a urine sodium >20 mEq/L and urine osmolality >100 mOsm/kg. Involve the medical team for diagnosis and management, which will include treating the underlying condition and prescribing medications like vasopressin receptor antagonists.
- *Severe symptoms:* Transfer patients with severe symptoms like seizures or coma immediately to a medical unit.
- *Complex cases:* Get a medical consultation if your initial interventions are ineffective or if the cause is unclear.

Lice and Scabies

Outbreaks of lice and scabies are unfortunately not unusual in congregate settings like psychiatric units. Given how easily these parasites can spread, swift identification and treatment are critical.

Diagnosis

Lice

- *Visual inspection:* A thorough examination of the hair, particularly around the neck and behind the ears, can reveal adult lice or their eggs, known as nits.

Scabies

- *Physical examination:* Check for a rash and characteristic burrows typically located in skin folds like the wrists, elbows, and between fingers.
- *Skin scraping test:* A more definitive diagnosis involves microscopic examination of a skin scraping, which may reveal scabies mites or their eggs.

Treatment Recommendations

Lice

- *Permethrin 1% shampoo:* Should be applied to damp hair and left on for 10 minutes before rinsing out.
- *Malathion 0.5% lotion or ivermectin 0.5% lotion:* For tougher cases.
- *Oral ivermectin:* For severe cases or for those who can't tolerate topical treatments. The dosage is 200 mcg/kg, taken orally as a single dose, with a possible second dose a week later.
- All clothes, bedding, and personal items must be washed in hot water and dried on a hot cycle to kill remaining lice and nits.

Scabies

- *Permethrin 5% cream:* Should be applied to all skin from the neck down and left on for eight to 14 hours before washing it off.
- *Oral ivermectin:* As for lice, this is reserved for severe cases or for those who can't tolerate topical treatments. The dosage is 200 mcg/kg, taken orally as a single dose, with a possible second dose a week later.
- Prescribe antihistamines like diphenhydramine to alleviate itching.
- Similar to lice treatment, washing and hot-drying all clothing, bedding, and personal items is necessary to kill mites and their eggs.

Preventive Measures

- Patients should avoid sharing personal items like towels, combs, and clothing.
- Isolate affected individuals until they are declared noncontagious:
  - *For lice:* Patients are checked 24 hours after the lice-killing product has been applied; if no live lice are found, the patient is considered noncontagious.
  - *For scabies:* Individuals are considered noncontagious after 24 hours if they have used a prescription scabicidal treatment like permethrin cream.
  - *For both lice and scabies:* For those taking oral medications like ivermectin, check for live lice or new burrows/rashes 24–48 hours after treatment; if none are found, the patient is no longer considered contagious. If lice/scabies are still present, repeat ivermectin dose seven days after the first dose.

Pain Management

When you manage pain in inpatient psychiatric settings, you will face unique challenges, including risk of drug interactions, potential for substance misuse, and worry that inadequately managed pain will exacerbate psychiatric conditions like depression and anxiety. This guide outlines strategies for managing varying degrees of pain in psychiatric inpatients. Collaborate with pain specialists, nurses, and physical therapists for the best outcomes.

Identify the Cause of Pain

- Common causes of pain in psychiatric inpatients: Recent injuries, infections, chronic conditions like arthritis or gout, neurological disorders, GI issues, and headaches. Cancer-related and postoperative pain are also significant concerns.
- Obtain a history of the treatment of the root cause as well as the pain syndrome itself. If there has been no clear treatment, start the process of getting medical consultation and making referrals for outpatient treatment.

Assess Pain Severity

- Use a simple pain scale to assess severity and monitor treatment response, particularly for moderate to severe pain.
  - *1–10 scale:* "Can you tell me how bad your pain feels right now on a scale from 1 to 10? With 1 being very little pain, almost none, and 10 being the worst pain you can imagine, like if you hurt yourself really badly."
  - *FACES scale:* Here is a link to the Wong-Baker FACES Pain Rating scale that you can use: www.tinyurl.com/2afcfys3

Nonpharmacological Interventions

- *Cognitive behavioral therapy:* Can help modify pain perception and is particularly beneficial for chronic pain.
- *Physical therapy:* Customized exercises can alleviate specific types of pain, like back pain.
- *Relaxation techniques:* Meditation, deep breathing, and progressive muscle relaxation can reduce stress and pain sensation (see the "Relaxation and Deep Breathing Exercises" fact sheet in the Psychotherapy on the Inpatient Unit section).

Pharmacological Interventions

Mild pain

- *Acetaminophen (Tylenol):* Safe with most psychiatric medications. Dose at 325–650 mg every four to six hours. Max dose is 4000 mg daily. Monitor for liver toxicity, especially when used with other potentially hepatotoxic medications like valproate.
- *NSAIDs:* Ibuprofen 400–600 mg every six hours as needed. Caution with SSRIs due to increased risk of GI bleeding.

Moderate pain

- *Tramadol:* 50–100 mg every four to six hours as needed. Watch for serotonin syndrome with SSRIs and SNRIs.
- *Codeine:* Often combined with acetaminophen. Start with low doses (eg, codeine 15 mg combined with acetaminophen 300 mg) to minimize the risk of dependence and interactions with CYP2D6-metabolized drugs.
- *Gabapentin:* Particularly useful for neuropathic pain. Starting dose is 100–300 mg at bedtime, with gradual titration up to 1800 mg/day divided into three doses. Also has anxiolytic effects.
- *Pregabalin (Lyrica):* For neuropathic pain and fibromyalgia. Start at 75 mg twice a day or 50 mg three times a day, up to a maximum of 600 mg/day. Also works as an anxiolytic.
- *SNRIs (eg, duloxetine, venlafaxine):* Effective for chronic pain, including neuropathic pain and fibromyalgia. Start with a low dosage and adjust based on pain relief and tolerability. SNRIs are particularly useful in patients with comorbid depressive or anxiety disorders.
- *Nortriptyline:* Another antidepressant that is effective for neuropathic pain. Start at 10–25 mg at night and increase as needed. Monitor for anticholinergic side effects and potential cardiac effects, especially in older adults.

Severe pain

Involve your hospital's pain specialists. Typical recommendations include:

- *Morphine:* Begin with low doses, such as 2.5–5 mg every four hours as needed, and closely monitor for respiratory depression and potential interactions with benzodiazepines.
- *Oxycodone:* Use with caution due to the risk of dependence and overdose. Dose 5–15 mg every four to six hours as needed for pain, with careful monitoring for signs of opioid dependence and respiratory depression.

Additional Medications and Considerations

- *Topical analgesics:* Topical NSAIDs (eg, diclofenac gel) or capsaicin cream have lower systemic absorption and might be preferable for patients at risk of systemic side effects.
- *Muscle relaxants:* In cases of muscle spasms contributing to pain, use muscle relaxants (eg, cyclobenzaprine 5–10 mg TID) on a short-term basis. Watch for their sedative effects.
- *Lidocaine patches:* For neuropathic pain or localized areas of intense pain; minimal systemic effects.

Special Populations

- *Elderly patients:* Use lower starting doses and increase the dose gradually.
- *Patients with substance use history:* Use nonopioid pain alternatives when possible and remain vigilant for discrepancies between reported pain and observed behavior.

Parkinson's Disease

Parkinson's disease (PD) can be a challenge on an inpatient psych unit, given its overlap with other movement disorders and its array of psychiatric complications. Here's a practical guide to help you navigate diagnosis, distinguishing features, common psychiatric complications, and treatment strategies.

Pathophysiology

PD is primarily caused by the degeneration of dopamine-producing neurons in the substantia nigra, a region of the midbrain. The exact cause of this neuronal degeneration remains unclear but likely involves a combination of genetic and environmental factors.

Diagnosis

Step 1: Determine presence of core features

- Bradykinesia (slowness of movement) is required.
- In addition, at least one of the following is required:
  - Rest tremor (4–6 Hz, "pill-rolling" tremor).
  - Rigidity (increased muscle tone felt during passive movement).
  - Postural instability (impaired balance and difficulty maintaining an upright posture—both of which can lead to falls).

Step 2: Rule out other conditions

Conditions that can mimic PD include:

- Atypical parkinsonism, such as dementia with Lewy bodies, progressive supranuclear palsy, and others (requires consultation with neurology).
- Repeated strokes with stepwise progression.
- History of repeated head injury.
- Severe dementia.
- Antipsychotic treatment at symptom onset.

Step 3: Assess supportive criteria

There's no minimum, but the more of these that are present, the more confident you can be in the diagnosis:

- Unilateral onset: Symptoms begin on one side of the body.
- Progressive disorder: Symptoms progressively worsen over time.
- Persistent asymmetry: Symptoms remain more severe on the side of onset.
- Excellent response (70%–100%) to levodopa.

Table 14: **Distinguishing Antipsychotic-Induced Parkinsonism from PD**

	Antipsychotic-Induced Parkinsonism	PD
Onset	Days to weeks after starting/increasing antipsychotic	Gradual onset over months to years
Symmetry	Symmetrical	Unilateral onset
Tremor	Less pronounced or absent resting tremor	Classic "pill-rolling" resting tremor
Progression	Nonprogressive if medication is adjusted	Progressive
Response to Antipsychotic Adjustment	Symptoms improve or resolve	Symptoms persist and progress
Response to Levodopa	Little to no improvement	Significant improvement
Nonmotor Symptoms	Less likely to have typical PD nonmotor symptoms	Often has nonmotor symptoms (REM sleep behavior disorder, constipation, anosmia)

Treatment

Medications

Patients with PD are often on multiple medications to manage their motor symptoms. Unfortunately, many of these medications can cause psychiatric side effects like hallucinations, confusion, and poor impulse control.

- *Levodopa/carbidopa (Sinemet):* The cornerstone of PD treatment; helps replenish dopamine. Can cause side effects such as hallucinations, confusion, and mood changes. Can interact with antipsychotics, potentially reducing their effectiveness.
- *Dopamine agonists (pramipexole, ropinirole):* Mimic dopamine effects. Used as monotherapy in early PD or as adjunct to levodopa in advanced stages. Can cause impulse control disorders (eg, gambling, hypersexuality), and psychosis.
- *Monoamine oxidase-B (MAO-B) inhibitors (selegiline, rasagiline):* Reduce dopamine breakdown. Often used in early PD or as adjunct therapy, these can interact with serotonergic psychiatric medications (such as selective serotonin

reuptake inhibitors [SSRIs] and serotonin/norepinephrine reuptake inhibitors [SNRIs]), increasing the risk of serotonin syndrome.
- *Catechol-O-methyltransferase (COMT) inhibitors (entacapone, tolcapone):* Used with levodopa to prolong its effect. Can increase the risk of hallucinations and confusion.
- *Amantadine:* Helpful for managing involuntary movements (such as jerking or twitching) in advanced PD. Can cause confusion, hallucinations, and agitation.

Surgical option
Deep brain stimulation is used for treatment-resistant PD.

Lifestyle and supportive therapies
- *Physical therapy:* Improves mobility and flexibility.
- *Occupational therapy:* Helps with daily activities.
- *Speech therapy:* Addresses speech and swallowing difficulties.
- *Exercise:* Regular aerobic exercise can improve overall function and well-being.
- *Diet:* Balanced diet, adequate hydration, and fiber intake to manage constipation.

Common Psychiatric Symptoms and Treatment

Depression
Patients with PD often present with apathy and reduced motivation rather than sadness.
- SSRIs are often used; consider mirtazapine for insomnia and weight loss. Both bupropion and pramipexole (Mirapex) can help with apathy and low motivation. Low-dose tricyclic antidepressants can be helpful for depression, and their anticholinergic side effects can help PD symptoms like insomnia, pain, muscle stiffness, and overactive neurogenic bladder.

Psychosis
Hallucinations, especially visual, are common in advanced PD, resulting both from the disease as well as from PD medications.
- Clozapine or quetiapine are preferred (with clozapine usually first-line) due to lower risk of worsening motor symptoms. Low doses (up to 50 mg at bedtime) are often effective. Nuplazid (pimavanserin) is specifically approved for treating PD psychosis and does not worsen motor symptoms—however, it is weaker than standard antipsychotics and may take two weeks to work. It tends to be stimulating, allowing patients to be more alert during the day.

Anxiety
Panic disorder, generalized anxiety disorder, and various other anxiety issues may respond to standard treatment with SSRIs. However, anxiety in PD sometimes reflects inadequate doses of dopaminergic medication. If anxiety is worse in the morning (when PD medication blood levels are at their lowest), it may respond to increasing levodopa or adding ropinirole (Requip) or bupropion.

Cognitive impairment
Presentation can range from mild cognitive impairment to more severe forms such as Parkinson's disease dementia and dementia with Lewy bodies.
- Cholinesterase inhibitors and memantine are somewhat helpful in slowing the progression of dementia.

Poor impulse control
Compulsive gambling, hypersexuality, and binge eating are often associated with dopamine agonist therapy.
- Lower dopamine agonists (in collaboration with the patient's neurologist); however, if this worsens motor symptoms, use antipsychotics such as clozapine or pimavanserin.

Best Practices for Managing PD in the Psychiatric Unit

Interdisciplinary collaboration
- Work closely with neurologists to adjust PD medications to optimize motor symptom control while minimizing psychiatric side effects.
- Involve physical therapists to help patients maintain mobility and balance.
- Ask the unit's occupational therapist to assist with daily living activities.

Emotional and social support
- Encourage participation in support groups and therapeutic activities, like music and art therapy.
- Provide supportive counseling to address the emotional impact of PD.
- Educate patients and families about PD and its management.

Medication management
Coordinate with nursing staff to ensure PD medications are administered on time to prevent "off" periods—times when symptoms reemerge due to low medication levels.

Poststroke Psychiatric Symptoms

Poststroke patients will present with a range of psychiatric symptoms in addition to neurological issues. One of your challenges is to determine whether the psychiatric problems are related to the stroke. For instance, does your patient have preexisting depression aggravated by stroke, a new depression caused by stroke, or a new depression unrelated to the stroke? There are rarely clear answers to these kinds of questions. In this fact sheet, we will go through the major poststroke symptoms you are likely to encounter and provide some tips on diagnosis and treatment.

Diagnosis and Workup

Comprehensive assessment

- *Clinical history:* Determine the stroke's timing, type (hemorrhagic or ischemic), and initial symptoms. What sort of functional recovery did the patient make since the event? Is more recovery of function thought to be likely?
- *Psychosocial history:* Investigate any prestroke psychiatric symptoms and their similarity to current symptoms. Try to identify whether current psychiatric issues started de novo poststroke or were aggravated by it.
- *Current symptoms:* Conduct a detailed mental status exam. Differentiate between mood disturbances and the physical sequelae of the stroke, such as psychomotor retardation.
- *Current stroke treatments:* Coordinate with the patient's medical/neurological provider to ensure they receive gold-standard stroke treatment. Review current stroke medications with specialists and work with them to assess the need for additional neuroimaging while the patient is on your unit.

Neuropsychological evaluation

If available at your hospital, a neuropsychologist evaluation will help differentiate between primary psychiatric conditions and those secondary to the stroke, assess cognitive deficits, and guide individualized rehabilitation plans.

Poststroke psychiatric symptoms

- *Depression:* The most common psychiatric outcome poststroke, depression affects about one-third of stroke survivors, potentially appearing from one month to over a year poststroke.
- *Anxiety disorders:* May present as generalized anxiety, phobias, or panic disorders, often triggered by new physical limitations and the psychological impact of the stroke.
- *Apathy:* Characterized by a lack of initiative; distinct from depression as patients with apathy deny feeling sad and generally enjoy activities initiated by others.
- *Fatigue:* A common condition described as a lack of mental and physical energy that interferes with daily activities.
- *Mania:* Though rare, mania can occur, particularly after right frontal strokes.
- *Personality changes:* Patients may display disinhibition, inappropriate social behavior, and poor judgment; often associated with frontal lobe strokes.
- *Psychosis:* Not common, and usually presents as a single psychotic symptom (eg, visual hallucinations with occipital lobe stroke).
- *Pseudobulbar affect (PBA):* Also known as pathological laughter and crying (PLC) and involuntary emotional expression disorder (IEED). Patients experience uncontrollable episodes of crying or laughing that don't match the situation. Symptoms can be sudden and last from seconds to minutes. PBA can be mistaken for depression or bipolar disorder, but patients will readily tell you their reactions are not connected to their actual feelings.

Treatment

Pharmacotherapy

- *Antidepressants:* Selective serotonin reuptake inhibitors (SSRIs), tricyclic antidepressants, and serotonin/norepinephrine reuptake inhibitors for poststroke depression and anxiety. SSRIs increase bleeding risk, so they're less suitable for patients who have had hemorrhagic strokes.
- *Antipsychotics:* For poststroke psychotic symptoms.
- *Buspirone:* For poststroke anxiety disorders.
- *Dextromethorphan/quinidine (Nuedexta):* FDA approved for treating PBA. Start with one capsule daily for seven days, then increase to one capsule twice daily. Watch for side effects like loose stool, dizziness, cough, weakness, QT prolongation, elevated liver enzymes, and thrombocytopenia.
- *Modafinil:* Helpful for poststroke fatigue and apathy.
- *Mood stabilizers:* For poststroke mania.

Psychotherapy

Cognitive behavioral therapy and supportive therapy are helpful for poststroke depression and anxiety.

Nonpharmacological interventions

- Techniques like yoga, tai chi, mindfulness, and relaxation can benefit poststroke anxiety and emotional lability.

- Behavioral interventions, like group-based approaches to promote activity, are effective for addressing poststroke apathy. Positive reinforcement techniques are useful in managing disinhibition and inappropriate behaviors.
- Graduated exercise programs can help manage poststroke fatigue.
- Skills training programs help patients with poststroke personality changes relearn appropriate social interactions.

Psychogenic Polydipsia: Diagnosis and Treatment

Patients with psychogenic polydipsia (PP) consume excessive amounts of water, making their blood dangerously dilute. This condition is surprisingly common, with a prevalence of 3%–25% in institutionalized patients. You'll see it most often among patients with schizophrenia, but it also occurs in patients with mood and anxiety disorders.

Diagnosis

Clinical manifestations

- Suspect PP in patients who often complain of thirst or who repeatedly request or consume large amounts of water.
- Neuropsychiatric manifestations of hyponatremia (a consequence of water intoxication) include nausea, headache, cramping, dysarthric speech, lethargy, and confusion. Seizures and delirium occur in extreme cases.

Labs

- Obtain a basic metabolic panel. Sodium will be low (<135 mEq/L).
- Obtain a urine sample for urine osmolality and sodium. Both will be low (urine osmolality <100 mOsmol/kg; urine sodium <10 mEq/L).

Differential Diagnosis

- *Diabetes mellitus:* The primary problem is hyperglycemia, which leads to polyuria because excess glucose in the urine draws excess water along with it. The excess thirst is a result of the dehydration caused by the polyuria. Key diagnostic features are hyperglycemia and glucosuria (glucose in the urine)—neither of which occur in PP.
- *Diabetes insipidus:* The primary problem is inadequate production/response to antidiuretic hormone (ADH). Urine is dilute, but unlike PP, serum sodium will be high as the serum is concentrated from free water loss.
- *Syndrome of inappropriate antidiuretic hormone secretion (SIADH):* The primary problem is too much ADH, caused by medications including oxcarbazepine, carbamazepine, and serotonergic antidepressants. The kidneys absorb excessive water, so serum sodium levels will be low, but urine will be concentrated, unlike in PP.

Treatment

- *Water restriction:* The most important treatment strategy for PP is fluid restriction, which is harder than it sounds. Patients with PP are often highly driven to consume water. If you try to limit their water intake, they may find surreptitious ways of drinking water (eg, from the toilet or sink). Limit water to 1000–1500 mL/day; this will quickly resolve hyponatremia. Patients may need 1:1 supervision if you suspect they are drinking water surreptitiously.
- *Sodium supplementation:* Prescribe sodium chloride tablets, 1–3 g daily.
- *Discontinue certain medications:* Some medications exacerbate PP—these are typically anticholinergic antipsychotics that cause dry mouth, such as chlorpromazine, diphenhydramine, and tricyclic antidepressants. In response, patients may drink more water.
- *Transfer to medicine floor:* In severe cases, with serum sodium levels in the low 120s or below, patients will require transfer to a medicine unit for closely monitored sodium repletion using IV saline (a 3% saline solution, rather than the usual 0.9%).
- *Long-term treatment:* There is no established long-term treatment for PP, but naltrexone 50 mg daily may help.

Seizure Disorders

Epilepsy is often comorbid with psychiatric conditions like depression, anxiety, and psychosis, so it is likely that some of your patients will suffer from seizure disorders. Here are practical recommendations for managing these disorders in the inpatient psychiatric unit.

Types of Seizures

Generalized-onset seizures

- *Tonic-clonic seizures (grand mal seizures):* Loss of consciousness, with body stiffening (tonic phase) followed by jerking (clonic phase), typically lasting one to three minutes. Commonly associated with epilepsy.
  - Watch for signs suggesting the patient might instead be experiencing psychogenic nonepileptic seizures, or PNES, which is also called functional neurological disorder (see the "Functional Neurological Disorder" fact sheet in the Common Psychiatric Conditions section, Less Common Syndromes subsection). PNES typically presents with asynchronous shaking, side-to-side head movements, pelvic thrusting, closed eyes, and no postictal confusion. Interestingly, 10%–30% of patients with epilepsy also have PNES.
- *Absence seizures:* Brief lapses in awareness (usually less than 20 seconds), often mistaken for daydreaming. More common in children but can occur in adults.
- *Myoclonic, tonic, atonic, clonic seizures:* Sudden, brief muscle jerks (myoclonic), increased muscle tone (tonic), loss of muscle tone (atonic), or repeated jerking movements (clonic).

Focal-onset seizures

This is the most common type, accounting for approximately 60% of all cases of epilepsy.

- *Focal aware seizures (simple partial seizures):* Consciousness is not impaired. May involve unusual sensations or movements, like tingling, visual disturbances, or jerking movements of a limb.
- *Focal impaired-awareness seizures (complex partial seizures):* Impaired consciousness; may involve repetitive movements or staring.
- *Focal to bilateral tonic-clonic seizures:* Seizures start in one area of the brain and spread to involve both sides, leading to a tonic-clonic seizure.

Status epilepticus

Prolonged or repeated seizures without recovery in between. This is a medical emergency, as patients are at risk of permanent brain damage.

Acute symptomatic seizures (provoked by certain conditions)

- *Alcohol withdrawal seizures:* These typically occur six to 48 hours after the last drink in individuals with chronic alcohol use.
- *Drug-induced seizures:* Seizures caused by the withdrawal of drugs, like benzodiazepines, or from the use of medications or recreational drugs, like stimulants or cocaine.
- *Other causes of seizures:*
  - Metabolic disturbances: Typically due to hypoglycemia, hyponatremia, or hypocalcemia.
  - Head trauma.
  - Severe sleep deprivation, central nervous system infections, eclampsia, high fever (febrile seizures; these mostly occur in young children).

Postictal States

Many types of seizures are followed by a postictal state, which can include confusion, agitation, and sleepiness lasting from minutes to hours.

Initial Assessment

- *Obtain a history:* This should include the seizure type, frequency, triggers (eg, lack of sleep, flashing lights, hormonal changes), and treatments. Find out when the patient had their last seizure to assess their seizure control and frequency.
- *Review the patient's antiepileptic drugs (AEDs):* Ask which drugs the patient is taking, including dosages, and ask about medication adherence and any recent changes.
- *Obtain labs:*
  - Serum levels of AEDs: To ensure therapeutic levels.
  - Routine blood tests: To monitor for AED side effects like elevated liver function tests or depressed platelet counts.
- *Consult with a neurologist:* This is especially important if seizures are poorly controlled, there are sudden changes in seizure patterns, or the patient presents with new neurological symptoms.

Management Tips

- *Adjust AED dosages:* Adjustments should be based on blood levels and in consultation with the neurology team.
- *Choose psychotropic medications with less risk of lowering the seizure threshold:* Try to avoid drugs known to exacerbate seizures, such as the following:
  - Bupropion
  - Clozapine
  - Tricyclic antidepressants (eg, amitriptyline)
  - Chlorpromazine
- *Be mindful of drug interactions:* AEDs can interact with other medications. For example, carbamazepine is notorious for inducing hepatic enzymes. For patients on hormonal contraception, this interaction can render the contraceptive ineffective.
- *Monitor for psychiatric side effects:* Several AEDs have been associated with causing or exacerbating psychosis and agitation, particularly levetiracetam and zonisamide. Some studies have also reported higher rates of depression and even suicidality with certain AEDs, like phenobarbital.
- *Exercise caution with teratogenic AEDs:* Some AEDs, valproate in particular, are known teratogens and should be used with caution in patients of reproductive age.
- *Order seizure precautions:* These will notify nurses to order a bed with padded bed rails and to provide close supervision during activities that pose a risk of injury, such as showering.

What to Do if Your Patient Has a Seizure on the Unit

For an isolated seizure

- Clear the area of any harmful objects, protect the patient's head, position them on their side to prevent aspiration, and wait for the seizure to pass. Most seizures last no more than two minutes.
- Once the seizure is over, assess vital signs and neurological status to identify any immediate complications like respiratory distress or neurologic complications. Look for potential triggers (eg, lack of sleep, missed medications). Consult with the neurology team for next steps.

Status epilepticus

- Administer benzodiazepines as quickly as possible. IV medications take effect more quickly, so use that route whenever feasible.
  - *Lorazepam (Ativan):* 0.1 mg/kg IV or IM, up to 4 mg/dose. Can be repeated once after 10–15 minutes if the seizure persists.
  - *Diazepam (Valium):* 0.2 mg/kg IV or IM, up to 10 mg/dose. Can be repeated once after 10–15 minutes if the seizure persists.
  - *Midazolam:* 0.1–0.2 mg/kg IV, IM, or intranasal, up to 10 mg/dose.
- Arrange immediate transfer to a medical unit as the patient will need continuous EEG monitoring as well as close monitoring for potential complications like recurrent seizures and respiratory depression.

Sexually Transmitted Diseases

You'll sometimes encounter sexually transmitted diseases (STDs) among patients in psychiatric units. Here we review diagnoses and treatments for the most common STDs. Inform patients that their partners should be treated simultaneously to prevent reinfection.

Gonorrhea

- *Symptoms:* Often asymptomatic; pain or burning during urination, yellowish discharge, bleeding outside menstrual cycles, testicular swelling.
- *Diagnosis:* Swabs (throat, rectum, urethra), urine test.
- *Treatment:* Single injection of ceftriaxone 500 mg IM.

Chlamydia

- High rate of co-infection with gonorrhea, so patients are often treated for both simultaneously.
- *Symptoms:* Often asymptomatic; if symptoms occur, they typically include dysuria and abnormal vaginal or penile discharge.
- *Diagnosis:* Swabs, urine tests.
- *Treatment:* Doxycycline 100 mg orally twice daily for seven days or azithromycin 1 g orally in a single dose (recommended for pregnant patients).

Trichomoniasis

- *Symptoms:* Women: Genital itching, burning, discharge with fishy odor, spotting. Men: Often asymptomatic; possible irritation, discharge.
- *Diagnosis:* PCR test, eg, from patient-collected swab of vaginal/penile area. You can treat empirically if other common causes of vaginitis (eg, yeast infection) have been ruled out.
- *Treatment:* Metronidazole (2 g orally once or 500 mg twice daily for seven days) or tinidazole (2 g orally once).

Herpes (HSV)

- *Types:* HSV-1 (oral), HSV-2 (genital).
- *Symptoms:* Flu-like symptoms, blisters, open sores; milder recurrent outbreaks.
- *Diagnosis:* Examination, viral culture, PCR, blood test for antibodies.
- *Treatment:* Acyclovir.
  - Initial outbreak: 200 mg five times daily or 400 mg three times daily for seven to 10 days.
  - Recurrent: 800 mg twice daily for five days or three times daily for two days.
  - Suppressive: 400 mg twice daily.
  - Cold sores can also be treated with acyclovir 5% topical cream Q3 hours for seven days.

Yeast Infection (Candidiasis)

- Not an STD, but sexually transmittable and often mistaken for an STD.
- *Symptoms:* Itching, irritation, swelling, redness. Women: "Cottage cheese-like" discharge. Men: White patches, odor, discharge.
- *Diagnosis:* PCR test, eg, from patient-collected swab. You can treat empirically if the patient presents with classic symptoms.
- *Treatment:* Antifungals like fluconazole (Diflucan) 150 mg orally once, miconazole cream (Monistat) 4% for three days, or clotrimazole cream (Lotrimin) 1% for seven days.

Bacterial Vaginosis (BV)

- Also not an STD, but sexually transmittable and often mistaken for an STD.
- *Symptoms:* Thin white, gray, or green vaginal discharge; fish-like odor.
- *Diagnosis:* PCR test, eg, from patient-collected swab.
- *Treatment:* Metronidazole (500 mg BID for seven days), metronidazole 0.75% vaginal gel (one applicator QHS for five days), or clindamycin 2% cream (one applicator intravaginally QHS for seven days).

Swollen Feet, Ankles, and Calves

Swollen feet, ankles, and calves can be due to various reasons, some incidental and others requiring immediate attention. Psychiatric patients are at higher risk for these symptoms due to medication side effects, prolonged immobility, and underlying medical conditions that can be exacerbated by psychiatric disorders or their treatments. Here's a guide to help identify and manage the underlying causes. Involve the medical team early in the workup, especially for urgent cases like possible deep vein thrombosis (DVT).

Common Causes

Cardiovascular

- *DVT:* Look for unilateral swelling with pain, redness, and warmth.
- *Heart failure:* Bilateral swelling, often associated with shortness of breath and fatigue.
- *Venous insufficiency:* Unilateral or bilateral swelling. Look for varicose veins, skin changes (eg, hyperpigmentation), and ulcers.

Hepatic

- *Liver cirrhosis:* Often accompanied by ascites and jaundice.

Infection

- *Abscess:* Unilateral swelling with localized erythema, warmth.
- *Cellulitis:* Unilateral swelling with redness, warmth, and tenderness.

Lymphatic

- *Lymphedema:* Can be bilateral or unilateral. Look for thickened skin (elephantiasis).

Medications

- *Psychiatric meds (eg, antipsychotics, antidepressants, lithium):* Typically bilateral swelling. Look for recent changes in medication or dosage.
- *Calcium channel blockers, NSAIDs:* Bilateral swelling, often without other systemic symptoms like shortness of breath, fever, or significant pain.

Musculoskeletal

- *Gout:* Unilateral swelling, often affecting the big toe (podagra). Look for redness, warmth, and severe pain, often with a rapid onset.
- *Trauma:* Unilateral swelling with a history of injury, pain, and possible bruising.
- *Tendinitis or bursitis:* Inflammation of the tendons or bursae in the foot, causing localized pain and swelling.

Renal

- *Chronic kidney disease:* Often with generalized edema (anasarca). Look for signs of hypertension and uremia (waste buildup), like fatigue, pruritus, and a metallic taste.
- *Nephrotic syndrome:* Bilateral swelling, especially in the legs and around the eyes (periorbital edema). Look for proteinuria, hypoalbuminemia, and hyperlipidemia.

Other

- *Electrolyte imbalances:* Bilateral swelling. Look for signs of underlying conditions such as muscle cramps, weakness, or cardiac arrhythmias, which may indicate imbalances in sodium, potassium, calcium, or magnesium.
- *Hypoalbuminemia:* Look for signs of malnutrition or underlying chronic disease, such as muscle wasting and fatigue, and check serum albumin levels to confirm hypoalbuminemia.
- *Prolonged immobility:* Bilateral swelling, common in patients who are bedridden or sedentary. Look for dependent edema (worse at the end of the day or after prolonged sitting).

Assessment

History

- *Onset and duration:* When did the swelling start? Is it constant or intermittent?
- *Location and laterality:* Is it one foot or both? What specific areas are affected?
- *Associated symptoms:* Pain, redness, warmth, fever, shortness of breath.
- *Medical history:* Heart disease, kidney disease, liver disease, diabetes, recent infections, trauma.
- *Medication history:* Recent changes in medications, new medications.
- *Lifestyle factors:* Recent immobility, dietary habits (eg, high sodium intake or low protein), fluid intake (too much or too little).

Physical examination

- Look for signs of trauma, erythema, cyanosis, and any visible deformities.
- Check for warmth, tenderness, and pitting edema.
- Assess gait and any limitations in movement.

Vital signs

- Blood pressure, heart rate, respiratory rate, temperature.

Involving Specialists

- *Podiatry:* For cases related to musculoskeletal issues like tendinitis, bursitis, gout, or trauma.
- *Internal medicine:* For cases related to cardiovascular, renal, hepatic, or infection-related etiologies.

Diagnostic Workup

Laboratory tests

- *Complete blood count (CBC):* To check for infection or anemia.
- *Complete metabolic panel (CMP):* To assess kidney function, liver function, and electrolyte imbalances.
- *B-type natriuretic peptide (BNP):* To evaluate for heart failure.
- *D-dimer:* If you suspect a DVT.
- *Urinalysis:* To check for proteinuria and other renal issues.
- *Uric acid:* To assess for gout or hyperuricemia.
- *Erythrocyte sedimentation rate (ESR)/C-reactive protein (CRP):* To evaluate for inflammatory processes.

Imaging studies

- *Ultrasound:* For DVT assessment.
- *X-ray:* To rule out fractures or joint abnormalities.
- *ECG:* If heart failure is suspected.
- *Venous Doppler:* To assess for venous insufficiency or DVT.

Management

Management is based on underlying cause:

- *Heart failure:* Diuretics, angiotensin-converting enzyme (ACE) inhibitors, beta-blockers, and lifestyle modifications (eg, reduced sodium intake, fluid management).
- *Renal issues:* Medication adjustment, fluid balance management, and dietary modifications (eg, low sodium, adequate protein intake).
- *Liver disease:* Dietary modifications, diuretics, and management of underlying liver condition.
- *Infection:* Antibiotics for cellulitis and abscesses; drainage of abscesses if necessary.
- *DVT:* Anticoagulation therapy, compression stockings, and encouraging mobility.
- *Venous insufficiency:* Compression stockings and leg elevation; avoidance of prolonged standing or sitting.
- *Lymphedema:* Compression therapy, manual lymphatic drainage, and leg elevation.
- *Gout:* NSAIDs, colchicine, urate-lowering therapy, and dietary modifications.
- *Arthritis:* Anti-inflammatory medications (NSAIDs) and physical therapy.
- *Trauma:* Rest, ice, compression, and elevation (RICE); pain management.
- *Tendinitis or bursitis:* Rest, ice, anti-inflammatory medications, and physical therapy.

Syphilis

Syphilis, often termed the "great imitator," is a sexually transmitted infection that can present symptoms similar to many other conditions, including psychotic and mood disorders. Here we review its stages, diagnosis, and treatment.

Stages and Symptoms

- *Primary stage*
  - 10–90 days postexposure, patients may exhibit sores or "chancres" on the genitals or in the mouth. These tend to be firm, round, and painless.
- *Secondary stage*
  - Following the disappearance of the chancres, a pink to brown rash may develop all over the body, with about half of cases showing on palms and soles.
  - "Snail trail" mucous patches may be visible in the mouth.
  - Ocular neurosyphilis is common, often presenting as uveitis.
  - Syphilitic meningitis symptoms include stiff neck, headache, and vertigo, and can progress to strokes and seizures if untreated.
  - Other manifestations: Fatigue, fever, swollen lymph glands.
- *Latent stage*
  - If untreated, the infection progresses to a latent phase that can last for years, during which patients are free of any outward symptoms.
  - Many people stay in this stage indefinitely, but if left untreated, about 30% go on to the tertiary stage.
- *Tertiary stage*
  - Involves invasion of the spirochete into the central nervous system and can present with general paresis, which includes memory loss, mood changes, psychosis, seizures, and dementia.

Diagnosis

- Screen all new psychiatric inpatients due to the significant importance of early detection.
- High-risk populations include men who have sex with men, individuals in commercialized sex, and substance users.
- Start with a nontreponemal test (eg, rapid plasma reagin [RPR] or venereal disease research laboratory [VDRL] test). If reactive, confirm with a treponemal test like fluorescent treponemal antibody absorption (FTA-ABS) or *T. pallidum* particle agglutination (TP-PA).
- A combination of clinical symptoms, cerebrospinal fluid abnormalities (pleocytosis, elevated protein, positive VDRL), and brain imaging showing cerebral atrophy can help distinguish neurosyphilis from primary psychiatric illness.
- Neurosyphilis—meaning syphilitic infection of the central nervous system—can occur at any stage of the illness.

Treatment

- *Primary to early latent stages:* A single dose of intramuscular penicillin G benzathine 2.4 million units.
  - Early latent syphilis refers to the stage of infection occurring within the first year after the initial infection, during which the person is asymptomatic but still infectious.
- *Late latent stage:* Three doses of weekly intramuscular penicillin G benzathine 2.4 million units.
- *Penicillin allergy:* Doxycycline 100 mg BID for 14 days—but not for pregnant women.
- *Neurosyphilis:* IV penicillin G or ceftriaxone for 10–14 days.
- *Jarisch-Herxheimer reaction:* Posttreatment fever and flu-like symptoms within 24 hours. It's not a penicillin allergy, and supportive treatment suffices.
- *Mood and psychotic symptoms in tertiary stage:* Second-generation antipsychotics like olanzapine, aripiprazole, and quetiapine can help, but once patients progress to general paresis, their response to treatment is poor.

Systemic Lupus Erythematosus

Lupus, or systemic lupus erythematosus (SLE), is an autoimmune disease where the immune system attacks its own tissues, causing widespread inflammation and tissue damage. It presents with a range of symptoms, including psychiatric manifestations. In rare cases, psychosis is the presenting sign, but most of the time you'll encounter psychiatric symptoms in patients with preexisting SLE. Lupus is more common in women, particularly those of childbearing age, and has a higher prevalence in certain ethnic groups, including Blacks, Hispanics, and Asians.

Common Symptoms

- *Fatigue:* Almost everyone with lupus experiences this, and it can be debilitating.
- *Joint pain and swelling:* Particularly in the hands, wrists, and knees.
- *Skin rashes:* The classic "butterfly" rash across the cheeks and nose is a hallmark.
- *Photosensitivity:* Sensitivity to sunlight, which can exacerbate skin rashes.
- *Fever:* Low-grade fever is common and can signal a flare-up.
- *Mouth or nose ulcers:* Usually painless.
- *Raynaud's phenomenon* (fingers turning white/blue in the cold).

Systemic Symptoms

- *Kidney issues:* Lupus nephritis, which can lead to proteinuria and, if untreated, kidney failure.
- *Cardiovascular problems:* Increased risk of heart disease and stroke.
- *Pulmonary issues:* Pleuritis or pleurisy, which can cause chest pain and shortness of breath.
- *Neurological problems:* Seizures, headaches, and cognitive dysfunction can occur.

Psychiatric Manifestations

- *Cognitive dysfunction:* "Lupus fog" affects memory, concentration, and problem solving.
- *Mood disorders:* Depression and anxiety are common conditions in patients with SLE.
- *Psychosis:* Some patients experience delusions or hallucinations.
- *Behavioral changes:* Including irritability and personality changes.

Diagnosing Lupus

Clinical criteria

The diagnosis requires at least four criteria, including rashes (malar or butterfly rash; discoid rash), oral ulcers, arthritis, photosensitivity, kidney disease, seizures, psychosis, and abnormal labs.

Lab Findings

Note that not all of these findings need to be present for a positive diagnosis.

- Antinuclear antibody (ANA).
- Presence of specific antibodies (anti-dsDNA, anti-Smith, anti-phospholipid antibodies).
- Low counts of red blood cells, white blood cells, or platelets.

Treatment

Medications

- *NSAIDs:* For mild pain and inflammation.
- *Antimalarials:* Hydroxychloroquine is often used for skin and joint symptoms.
- *Corticosteroids:* To reduce inflammation and immune response.
- *Immunosuppressants:* Drugs like azathioprine, methotrexate, or mycophenolate for more severe cases.
- *Biologics:* Belimumab for refractory lupus.

Lifestyle

- Balanced diet, regular exercise, and stress management.
- Sun protection to prevent flare-ups.
- Smoking cessation.

Psychiatric Aspects

Psychiatric management is crucial, as lupus can significantly impact mental health.

- *Depression and anxiety:* Common due to chronic pain, fatigue, and the stress of living with a chronic illness. Use antidepressants, antipsychotics, or anxiolytics as needed.
- *Cognitive dysfunction:* Lupus fog can involve memory problems, difficulty concentrating, and confusion. Cognitive behavioral strategies and occupational therapy can help.
- *Psychotropic medications:* Be cautious with prescribing these, as lupus patients may have impaired renal or hepatic function. Monitor closely for side effects and drug interactions with lupus medications.
- *Steroid-induced psychiatric symptoms:* Long-term corticosteroid use can lead to mood swings, depression, mania, and psychosis. Monitor closely and adjust medications as necessary.

Thyroid Disease

Thyroid diseases encompass a range of disorders affecting the thyroid gland, which regulates metabolism, energy, and overall hormonal balance. The two most common thyroid conditions are hypothyroidism (underactive thyroid) and hyperthyroidism (overactive thyroid). These conditions can have significant implications for psychiatric illness. You'll often order thyroid function tests as part of your standard screening for newly admitted patients, as well as for patients taking lithium.

Thyroid Hormone Basics

- The butterfly-shaped thyroid gland wraps around the trachea and plays a crucial role in regulating (mainly boosting) metabolism.
- Thyroxine (T4) is the main hormone released by the thyroid, and it is converted into the more potent triiodothyronine (T3) in other tissues and organs, like in the liver, kidneys, and muscles.
- Thyroid-stimulating hormone (TSH) is produced by the pituitary gland and stimulates the thyroid to release T4 and T3. In a feedback loop, high levels of thyroid hormone suppress TSH production, while low levels of thyroid hormone stimulate it.
- Hypothyroidism symptoms: Fatigue, weight gain, cold intolerance, constipation, dry skin, hair loss, and depression.
- Hyperthyroidism symptoms: Weight loss, heat intolerance, palpitations, increased appetite, tremors, anxiety, and excessive sweating.
- Subclinical hypo- or hyperthyroidism: This refers to situations where the TSH is high or low, but T4/T3 levels are normal. This means mild or early-stage thyroid disease and is often followed conservatively by periodic testing.

Pathophysiology

Hypothyroidism

Often caused by Hashimoto's thyroiditis, an autoimmune condition where the immune system attacks the thyroid. Other causes include iodine deficiency, thyroid surgery, radiation therapy, and lithium use.

Hyperthyroidism

Frequently caused by Graves' disease, another autoimmune disorder. Other causes include thyroid nodules, thyroiditis, and excessive iodine intake.

When to Order Thyroid Testing

- *Evaluating psychiatric symptoms:* Consider thyroid testing for symptoms like unresponsive depressive symptoms or unexpected anxiety/agitation, which may indicate thyroid dysfunction.
- *Medication monitoring:* Some psychiatric medications, like lithium, can affect thyroid function.
- *Use of thyroid hormone in psychopharmacology:* T3 is sometimes prescribed for refractory mood disorders and requires monitoring of thyroid hormone levels and patient response.

What Tests to Order

Thyroid-stimulating hormone

This is the primary test for thyroid screening. Normal range: 0.4–4.5 mIU/L.

- *Normal TSH:* Typically, no need for further testing.
- *Elevated TSH:* Suggests hypothyroidism.
  - Order free T4 (normal range 0.8–1.8 ng/dL). If low, it confirms hypothyroidism; refer to endocrinology. If normal, consider rechecking TSH in six weeks for possible subclinical hypothyroidism.
- *Decreased TSH:* Suggests hyperthyroidism.
  - Order both free T3 (normal range 2.3–4.2 pg/mL) and free T4. High levels confirm hyperthyroidism; normal levels suggest subclinical hyperthyroidism.

Thyroid antibodies

Anti-thyroid peroxidase (TPO) antibodies for hypothyroidism; TSH receptor antibodies (TRAb) for hyperthyroidism.

Treatment

Work with medicine or endocrinology to evaluate and manage thyroid disorders.

Hypothyroidism

- *Medications:* Levothyroxine (synthetic T4) to normalize thyroid hormone levels.
- *Monitoring:* Regular blood tests to adjust medication dosage.

Hyperthyroidism

- *Medications:* Antithyroid drugs (methimazole, propylthiouracil) to reduce thyroid hormone production; beta-blockers to manage symptoms.

- *Radioactive iodine therapy:* To destroy overactive thyroid cells.
- *Surgery:* Thyroidectomy in severe or refractory cases.
- *Lifestyle:* Avoidance of iodine-rich foods and managing stress.

Psychiatric Aspects

Hypothyroidism

- *Depression:* The treatment of hypothyroidism often alleviates depressive symptoms. However, if depression persists, antidepressants and psychotherapy can be effective adjuncts.
- *Cognitive dysfunction:* Cognitive impairments, like slowed thinking and poor memory, are likely to get better with normalization of thyroid function, although improvement might occur gradually over several weeks to months. To support this recovery, your hospital's occupational therapists and neuropsychologists can provide cognitive rehabilitation exercises to improve memory and attention.
- *Psychotropic medications:* Be cautious with dosing as hypothyroidism can slow drug metabolism, potentially increasing the risk of side effects and toxicity.
- *Lithium-induced:* Lithium can induce hypothyroidism in about 10% of patients. Order screening TSH at baseline, at three months, then annually. In cases of lithium-induced hypothyroidism, consider adjusting the lithium dosage or switching to an alternate mood stabilizer.

Hyperthyroidism

- *Anxiety and agitation:* These symptoms can be severe and may require the use of anxiolytics or beta-blockers.
- *Mania and psychosis:* Can occur, especially in untreated cases. Antipsychotics may be necessary.
- *Psychotropic medications:* Adjust dosages carefully due to accelerated drug metabolism in hyperthyroid states.

Upper Respiratory Infections

Upper respiratory infections (URIs) are common in psychiatric units due to close living quarters and shared spaces. When patients complain of cough, congestion, or feeling "sick," your primary goal is to distinguish between a simple viral illness (a common cold), which is self-limiting, and conditions that require specific interventions.

Evaluate Symptoms and History

Start with asking about symptom onset, associated symptoms (like body aches, fever, and sore throat), and if they've been around anyone sick. Here are the typical clinical pictures of the most common illnesses you will encounter.

Viral URI (common cold)

- *Symptoms:* Gradual onset of cough, runny nose, mild sore throat, and sneezing. Typically lacks high fever and severe body aches.
- *History:* Often no specific exposure; community prevalence common.
- *Onset and progression:* Symptoms develop over one to two days; usually improve with supportive care within a week.

Influenza

- *Symptoms:* Sudden onset of high fever, severe body aches, profound fatigue, and cough. May have headaches and chills.
- *History:* Recent exposure to known flu cases or unvaccinated status. Seasonal occurrence typically in fall and winter.
- *Onset and progression:* Rapid symptom onset and more intense severity compared to a common cold. Can lead to serious complications, especially in high-risk groups (eg, the elderly, young children, and those with certain health conditions), such as pneumonia, bronchitis, sinus infections, and worsening of chronic medical conditions.

Bacterial infections (eg, strep throat)

- *Symptoms:* Severe sore throat, pain on swallowing, white patches on tonsils, and swollen lymph nodes. Generally lacks cough.
- *History:* Exposure to known cases may be relevant; more common in children and adolescents.
- *Onset and progression:* Symptoms are localized and severe from the onset.

COVID-19

- *Symptoms:* Can vary but often include fever, dry cough, fatigue, and loss of taste or smell. Symptoms can range from mild to severe and may include breathing difficulties.
- *History:* Recent travel to affected areas or contact with confirmed cases. Relevant during ongoing pandemic periods.
- *Onset and progression:* Symptoms can appear two to 14 days after exposure, with a wide range of severity.

Physical Exam and Diagnostic Testing

Perform a basic physical exam focused on ENT (ear, nose, throat) and respiratory systems. Look for signs of infection (eg, redness, swelling, discharge). Assess breathing quality and listen for wheezing or abnormal lung sounds.

If you suspect the common cold, no testing is necessary. For more severe symptoms, your hospital probably offers multiplex PCR testing, which simultaneously checks for multiple pathogens including respiratory syncytial virus, influenza, and COVID-19. For suspected strep throat, a rapid strep test can be useful. Coordinate with medical consultants about who should order these tests based on your unit's protocols.

Management

Symptomatic treatment for presumed viral URI

- *Fever and pain:* Primarily use acetaminophen since it's safe to use with most psychiatric medications. Monitor lithium levels if you use NSAIDs, as they can increase lithium retention.
- *Cough:* Administer expectorants like guaifenesin to loosen mucus if the cough is productive. For a dry cough, prescribe cough suppressants like dextromethorphan to reduce coughing.
- *Congestion:* Saline nasal sprays are helpful. If patients need additional interventions, consider decongestants, but avoid pseudoephedrine or phenylephrine in patients taking monoamine oxidase inhibitors due to the risk of hypertensive crisis. For a runny nose, opt for second-generation antihistamines like loratadine or cetirizine, which are less sedating than first-generation ones like diphenhydramine.
- *Sore throat:* Lozenges and saline throat sprays will alleviate throat discomfort.

Treatment for other illnesses

Usually ordered by medical consultants, though the specific agent will vary:

- *Influenza:* Antiviral medications like oseltamivir (Tamiflu) within 48 hours of symptom onset.
- *Strep throat:* Antibiotic therapy (eg, penicillin or amoxicillin).
- *COVID-19:* The most common antiviral treatment is nirmatrelvir/ritonavir (Paxlovid). Infectious disease consultants might recommend other treatments, including other antivirals and monoclonal antibodies.

Urinary Tract Infections

Urinary tract infections (UTIs) are common, especially among female patients. In younger patients, an uncomplicated UTI doesn't normally affect psychiatric symptoms, and you will typically order a urinalysis and initiate antibiotic treatment. In geriatric patients, however, UTIs can cause a variety of psychiatric symptoms, including confusion and agitation. Here we review strategies to diagnose and manage UTIs.

Symptoms

- Typical symptoms: Dysuria (pain or burning during urination), urgency, frequency, and abdominal pain.
- Elderly psychiatric patients, especially those with dementia, might present with atypical symptoms like unexplained agitation and confusion. They may not have the capacity to describe their urinary symptoms, making diagnosis more challenging.
- Fever may or may not be present.

Urinalysis

- Typical urinalysis findings include:
  - Cloudy or odorous urine.
  - Positive leukocyte esterase, an enzyme found in white blood cells (WBCs); it's a surrogate marker suggesting the presence of pyuria (WBCs in urine).
  - Positive nitrites: Bacterial conversion of nitrate, which is normally found in urine, to nitrite is a strong indicator of bacterial UTI.
  - Increased WBCs.
  - Hematuria (presence of red blood cells).
  - Visible bacteria on microscopic exam.
- Large numbers of squamous cells and common skin flora (eg, *Staphylococcus epidermidis* or *Staphylococcus aureus*) suggest contamination. Order a "clean catch" repeat test if necessary.

Urine Culture

- This is used to identify the causative organism and guide the choice of antibiotic.
- You don't normally need a urine culture for uncomplicated UTIs as they can be treated empirically based on symptoms and urinalysis findings.
- Do obtain urine cultures in these cases: recurrent UTIs, UTIs during pregnancy, and complicated UTIs (eg, patients with kidney stones or using a urinary catheter).
- Consult medicine to review the findings and initiate treatment if you order a culture.

When Is Treatment Necessary?

- As a psychiatric practitioner, you can generally prescribe antibiotics in uncomplicated UTIs. It's best to consult medicine in the following situations:
  - Underlying complex medical conditions.
  - Recurrent UTIs.
  - When initial treatment fails.
- Don't prescribe antibiotics for asymptomatic cases as they don't improve outcomes and may contribute to antibiotic resistance.
- Exceptions include pregnant individuals and confused elderly patients who may not report symptoms accurately.

Management Strategies

- *Nitrofurantoin (Macrobid):* 100 mg twice daily for five days. Avoid in patients with severe renal impairment.
- *Trimethoprim/sulfamethoxazole (Bactrim/Septra):* One double-strength tablet twice daily for three days.
- *Fosfomycin (Monurol):* A single 3 g dose. Helpful for patients who might have problems with medication adherence.
- *Cephalexin (Keflex):* 500 mg twice daily for seven days. Good for patients with sulfa allergies.
- *Symptomatic relief:* Phenazopyridine (Pyridium) can be used for dysuria relief but isn't a substitute for antibiotic therapy.
- *Monitoring and follow-up:* Reassess symptoms after 48–72 hours of antibiotic therapy. Consider a posttreatment urine culture in cases of complicated UTIs or persistent symptoms.

Viral Hepatitis

Hepatitis B and C are prevalent among psychiatric inpatients, often transmitted through shared needles and sexual contact. This fact sheet serves as a concise guide on the pathophysiology, diagnosis, and treatment of these conditions, tailored for the psychiatric setting.

Hepatitis A (HAV)

- *Transmission:* Through contaminated food or water.
- *Nature of infection:* Acute, presenting with fever, malaise, jaundice, nausea, and abdominal discomfort. Does not progress to chronic liver disease. Not commonly seen in psychiatric units but presented here for context, as many patients will not know the differences among the various types of hepatitis.

Hepatitis B (HBV)

- *Transmission:* Via infected blood and semen, through needle sharing and sexual contact.
- *Symptoms:* The acute illness typically occurs within two weeks of exposure and causes flu-like symptoms, including fever, joint pain, fatigue, and sometimes jaundice. While most patients eventually clear the virus and develop lifelong immunity, about 5% of patients develop chronic HBV. Of these, about 10% will develop liver cancer or cirrhosis, which will often be fatal.
- *Labs:*
  - *Hepatitis B surface antigen (HBsAg):* This is a protein on the surface of the virus. If present, the virus is in the blood and the person is contagious.
  - *Anti-HBs:* This antibody against HBsAg signifies immunity to HBV, either from previous infection or vaccination. It indicates that the person is not currently infected.
  - *Immunoglobulin M (IgM):* Indicates a recent infection, generally within the last six months.
- *Treatment:*
  - *Vaccine:* There is a vaccine to prevent HBV.
  - *Active infections:* There is no specific treatment for active infections other than supportive care.
  - *Chronic infections:* Unlike hepatitis C, there is no cure for chronic HBV, but daily use of oral antiviral medications significantly reduces liver damage and the risk of liver cancer. These medications must be taken daily for about a year (or sometimes for longer, depending on response to treatment) and include tenofovir disoproxil, tenofovir alafenamide, and entecavir. In some cases, pegylated interferon (weekly injections for six months to one year) is used for younger patients with good liver function.

Hepatitis C (HCV)

- *Transmission:* Primarily through needle-sharing among IV drug users, but also through sexual contact and perinatal transmission.
- *Symptoms:* Acute infection is mild and usually without symptoms, but it is much more likely to convert to a chronic infection than HBV, with 75% of patients developing chronic HCV. HCV has historically been a major cause of liver cirrhosis, cancer, and eventual need for liver transplantation.
- *Labs:*
  - *Anti-HCV antibodies:* Indicate past or current exposure to the virus.
  - *HCV RNA:* Detects the presence of the virus in the blood, indicating an active infection.
- *Treatment:*
  - No vaccine is available for HCV.
  - *Direct-acting antivirals (DAAs):* These medications, including combination pills like Harvoni and Zepatier, offer a cure rate of approximately 90%, with treatment durations of 12–24 weeks.

Psychiatric Implications of HBV and HCV

- *Screening:* Consider routine screening for viral hepatitis in patients with a history of IV drug use, high-risk sexual behaviors, or known exposure to the viruses. Include HIV screening due to overlapping transmission routes.
- *Stigma:* Address and combat the stigma associated with HBV and HCV, particularly for infections acquired through needle sharing or unprotected sex. Supportive, nonjudgmental care encourages treatment adherence and disclosure.
- *Substance use:* Educate substance-using patients about the high risk of transmitting viruses through needle sharing and unprotected sexual encounters. Encourage moderation of alcohol use to avoid further liver damage.
- *Medication management:* Obtain liver function tests to assess whether you will need to decrease dosages of psychiatric medications.

Specific Populations

Management of Agitation in Children and Adolescents in Hospital Settings

When managing agitation in children and adolescents in hospital settings, you're not just focusing on their immediate safety and that of those around them; you're also trying to minimize the trauma that can occur in such high-stress environments. In this guide, we'll walk through the core principles for handling these sensitive situations.

Treatment Principles

- Begin by reducing excessive stimulation. If possible, move kids to a quiet, uncrowded space.
- Speak at the patient's eye level, using clear, simple language.
- Encourage family members to bring comforting items from home.
- Don't underestimate the use of snacks (eg, Goldfish crackers) and other rewards in de-escalation efforts.
- Target the underlying cause of agitation, whether it's due to a psychiatric illness, substance use or withdrawal, developmental delay/autism, or delirium.
- Utilize sitters like ED techs and nursing assistants to engage kids in activities like playing games, which can be calming.
- Communicate regularly with family members and caregivers for a comprehensive understanding of the child's needs, including triggers and calming techniques.
- Set firm limits for unacceptable behaviors and praise appropriate behaviors.
- Keep kids' developmental stages in mind. The younger the kids are, the harder it will be for them to manage their agitation.
- Establish a routine quickly. Use visual schedules, or at least tell the kids what their day is going to look like. Cards with "if-then" statements are helpful (eg, "If you take your medicine, then you get your iPad").
- Start treatment promptly, even in the ED. You might be able to get the child well enough to go home instead of waiting for an inpatient bed.
- Use physical restraint only as a last resort when there is an imminent risk of harm, for the shortest duration necessary, and with continuous monitoring. After removal, conduct a debriefing with the child and family.

Medication Principles

- Whenever possible, use monotherapy—but combinations of medications may be necessary in some cases, like for severe agitation.
- Check for existing home medications before introducing new ones to avoid additional side effects and drug interactions.
- Diphenhydramine and benzodiazepines are good choices for younger children and those with anxiety or agitation without a clear psychiatric history—but be careful about using these meds in kids with delirium or developmental delays/autism as they can cause disinhibition.
- Antipsychotics like chlorpromazine, haloperidol, olanzapine, quetiapine, and risperidone are helpful for severe agitation due to their sedating effects. Ziprasidone is problematic since it can prolong QT intervals and needs to be taken with food.
- Remember, children are more prone to side effects like dystonia.

Table 15: **ED Dosing Recommendations for Children and Adolescents**

Medication	Dose	Peak Effect	Max Daily Dose	Notes
Chlorpromazine	PO/IM: 12.5–60 mg (IM should be half PO dose) or 0.55 mg/kg/dose	PO: 30–60 minutes IM: 15 minutes	• Child <5 years: 40 mg/day • Child >5 years: 75 mg/day	• Monitor for hypotension and QT prolongation
Clonidine	PO: 0.05–0.1 mg	30–60 minutes	• 27–40.5 kg: 0.2 mg/day • 40–45 kg: 0.3 mg/day • >45 kg: 0.4 mg/day	• Monitor for hypotension and bradycardia • Avoid giving with benzodiazepines or antipsychotics due to hypotension risk
Diphenhydramine	PO/IM: 12.5–50 mg or 1 mg/kg/dose	2 hours	• Child: 50–100 mg • Adolescent: 100–200 mg	• Avoid in delirium • Can be combined with haloperidol or chlorpromazine if concerns for EPS • Can cause disinhibition or delirium in younger or developmentally disabled youth
Haloperidol	PO/IM: 0.5–5 mg (IM should be half PO dose)	PO: 2 hours IM: 20 minutes	• 15–40 kg: 6 mg • >40 kg: 15 mg • Dependent on prior antipsychotic exposure	• Consider ECG or cardiac monitoring for QT prolongation, especially if given IV • Monitor hypotension • Note EPS risk with MDD >3 mg/day, with IV dosing having very high EPS risk • Consider AIMS testing
Lorazepam	PO/IM/IV/NGT: 0.5–2 mg or 0.05–0.1 mg/kg/dose	PO/IM: 1–2 hours IV: 10 minutes	• Child: 4 mg • Adolescent: 6–8 mg • Dependent on weight and prior exposure	• Can cause disinhibition or delirium in younger or developmentally disabled youth • Can be given with haloperidol, chlorpromazine, or risperidone • Do not give with olanzapine (especially IM due to risk of respiratory suppression)
Olanzapine	PO/ODT/IM: 2.5–10 mg (IM should be 1/4–1/2 PO dose)	PO: 5 hours (range 1–8 hours) IM: 15–45 minutes	• 10–20 mg • Dependent on prior antipsychotic exposure	• Do not give within one hour of benzodiazepine
Quetiapine	PO: 25–50 mg or 1–1.5 mg/kg/dose (or divided)	PO: 30 minutes–2 hours	• >10 years: 600 mg • Dependent on prior antipsychotic exposure	• More sedating at lower doses • Monitor for hypotension
Risperidone	PO/ODT: 0.25–1 mg or 0.005–0.01 mg/kg/dose	PO: 1 hour	• Child: 1–2 mg • Adolescent: 2–3 mg • Dependent on prior antipsychotic exposure	• Can cause akathisia at higher doses • FDA approved for autism-related irritability

Source: Gerson R et al, *West J Emerg Med* 2019;20(2):409–418.

Management of Suicidality and Self-Harm in Children and Adolescents

If you work with children and adolescents in a psychiatric inpatient unit, you're likely to encounter kids experiencing suicidal and self-injurious thoughts. Over the past decade, there's been a significant increase in the number of kids showing up to hospitals for thoughts or incidents of self-harm. Here's a guide to help you navigate these challenging situations.

Safety Planning

- Start by sitting down with your patient and working together to develop a safety plan. Ask them, "What helps you feel safe when you're having these thoughts?" Involving them in identifying coping strategies and supportive contacts can empower them and help them feel more understood.
- Implement continuous or frequent monitoring based on the level of risk (see the "Assessing Suicide Risk" fact sheet in the Suicide and Self-Injurious Behaviors section). Use a standardized risk assessment tool upon admission, such as the Columbia Suicide Severity Rating Scale (C-SSRS): www.tinyurl.com/mu2964kp
- Ensure that no means of self-harm are accessible, like phone charging cords, shoelaces, mirrors, or pencils. Say, "Let's make sure your environment is safe. What items might we need to remove or secure?"

Treatment

Therapy

- Cognitive behavioral therapy (CBT)
  - *Introduction:* "CBT helps us understand how our thoughts, feelings, and actions are connected. Let's find some of your negative thoughts and see how they make you feel and act."
  - *Activity:* "We'll work on spotting and challenging these negative thoughts. For example, if you think, 'I'm worthless,' let's look at the evidence for and against this thought. Then we'll practice replacing it with a more balanced thought."
  - *Homework:* "Between our sessions, keep a thought diary. Write down any negative thoughts you have, what triggered them, and how you challenged those thoughts."
- Dialectical behavior therapy (DBT)
  - *Introduction:* "DBT teaches skills to handle emotions and improve relationships. We'll focus on mindfulness, dealing with stress, controlling emotions, and getting along with others."
  - *Activity:* "Let's start with mindfulness. Close your eyes and take deep breaths. Focus on the feeling of your breath. If your mind wanders, gently bring it back to your breath."
  - *Distress tolerance:* "Next time you feel overwhelmed, try the 'TIPP' skills: **T**emperature (splash cold water on your face), **I**ntense exercise (do jumping jacks), **P**aced breathing, and **P**rogressive muscle relaxation."
  - *Emotion regulation:* "Keep an emotion diary to track your feelings and what triggers them. We'll use this to find patterns and develop coping strategies."
  - *Interpersonal effectiveness:* "Let's role-play a situation where you need to stand up for yourself. For example, if a friend is pressuring you to do something you're uncomfortable with, how can you do a better job of handling it?"
  - *Group therapy:* "Joining a group can provide support from people your age who understand what you're going through."
  - *Family therapy:* Address systemic issues and enhance the patient's support system.

Pharmacotherapy

- *Antidepressants:* Selective serotonin reuptake inhibitors like fluoxetine (Prozac) are commonly used but require close monitoring for any increase in suicidal ideation, especially during the initial stages.
- *Mood stabilizers:* Medications like lithium or lamotrigine can be effective, particularly in cases of comorbid bipolar disorder.
- *Antipsychotics:* Second-generation antipsychotics like aripiprazole or risperidone may be considered for severe mood dysregulation or psychotic features.

Psychoeducation

- Educate the patient about their condition, treatment options, and strategies for managing symptoms. Say, "Knowledge is power. Let's talk about what you're experiencing and how we can manage it together."
- Provide the family with information on how to support their loved one, recognize warning signs, and access crisis resources.

Discharge Planning

- Once the patient has shown consistent improvement and stability, work with the team social worker and discharge planner to arrange a follow-up appointment soon after discharge, ideally within a week.
- Prior to discharge, sit with the patient to develop a detailed safety plan that includes warning signs and coping strategies (see the "Creating a Patient Safety Plan" fact sheet in the Suicide and Self-Injurious Behaviors section).
- Make sure the patient and their family know about crisis hotlines and emergency services, including local mental health crisis teams, national hotlines like the National Suicide Prevention Lifeline (1-800-273-8255), 988, and text services like the Crisis Text Line (text HOME to 741741).

Working with Pregnant Patients

It's not uncommon to encounter pregnant patients in a general adult psychiatric unit. Providing comprehensive care to these patients requires a solid understanding of the obstetric care needed at different stages of pregnancy, along with vigilance for potential complications. Here we review the basics of prenatal care, with emphasis on aspects that are particularly relevant in psychiatric settings.

Initial Assessment

Upon confirming a pregnancy, reach out to the OB-GYN team. Depending on the stage of pregnancy at which the patient presents, the following assessments will be initiated or updated:

- *Laboratory tests:* Blood type; Rh factor; complete blood count; urinalysis; tests for HIV, hepatitis B, and syphilis; immunity to rubella; and a Pap smear.
- *Ultrasound:* To confirm the pregnancy's viability and establish gestational age.

Informed Consent and Capacity

- *Capacity assessment:* The OB-GYN team will seek your input to evaluate the patient's ability to make informed decisions, especially regarding invasive procedures like cesarean sections. This involves assessing whether the patient understands the treatment's nature and purpose, whether they know the benefits and risks involved, and whether they can communicate their decision.
- *Surrogate decision making:* If the patient is deemed incapable of making informed decisions:
  - *Primary surrogates:* Typically, a next of kin, such as a spouse or adult child, will make health care decisions on the patient's behalf.
  - *Appointed guardian/conservator:* If no next of kin is available or suitable, a court-appointed guardian or conservator may need to be designated.
- *Bioethics team involvement:* For urgent decisions where a surrogate decision maker is not immediately available, the hospital's bioethics team may act temporarily to ensure the patient's best interests.
- *Emergency exception rule:* In life-threatening situations where there is no time to secure informed consent and no surrogate is available, health care providers may proceed under the emergency exception rule.
- Continuously reassess the patient's capacity to make informed decisions and care for the infant throughout pregnancy and delivery. A lack of capacity at one stage does not necessarily imply a lack at another.

Ongoing Prenatal Care

Ensure regular OB-GYN visits are scheduled:

- Monthly until 28 weeks.
- Biweekly from 28 to 36 weeks.
- Weekly from 36 weeks to delivery.

Common Pregnancy Complications

- *Gestational diabetes:* The OB-GYN team will perform an oral glucose tolerance test between 24 and 28 weeks of gestation, or possibly earlier for high-risk patients (eg, patients with a history of gestational diabetes, obese patients, or patients on antipsychotic medications like olanzapine or quetiapine).
- *Preeclampsia:* Characterized by high blood pressure and proteinuria. The OB-GYN team will assess blood pressure and urine protein levels at each prenatal visit. Alert the OB-GYN team if the patient develops high blood pressure between visits. Preeclampsia can lead to serious complications, including acute renal failure, seizures, placental abruption, and preterm birth.
- *Vaginal bleeding:* Light spotting is common and generally not a concern. In cases of moderate to heavy bleeding, immediately reach out to the OB-GYN team.

Labor

- Signs of labor include:
  - Regular contractions that increase in intensity and frequency.
  - Pain in the lower back radiating to the abdomen.
  - Leakage of amniotic fluid.
- Ensure that all nursing and staff members know how to contact the labor and delivery team after hours.

Postpartum Care

- *Monitoring for complications:* The OB-GYN team will keep a close watch for potential complications such as postpartum hemorrhage and infection. Although patients typically return to the psychiatric unit within a day of delivery, the OB-GYN team will continue to oversee the patient's health during this transition period.
- *Psychiatric relapse:* Monitor closely for signs of postpartum depression or psychosis. Early detection and intervention are critical to managing these relapses effectively.

- *Breastfeeding support:* Provide access to breast pumps and related supplies to facilitate breastfeeding. Regular milk expression is necessary to prevent complications (eg, painful breast engorgement, mastitis) and to maintain milk production, particularly for those planning to continue breastfeeding after discharge.

Newborn Care and Coordination

- *Immediate postnatal care:* After delivery, the pediatric and neonatology teams will ensure the newborn is healthy and stable. This includes assessing the Apgar score at one minute and again at five minutes after birth. This score evaluates the newborn's heart rate, breathing, muscle tone, reflex response, and skin color. Each of these five criteria is scored from 0 to 2, with total scores ranging from 0 to 10. A score of 7–10 is considered normal.
- *Psychosocial care:* Continue to work with the patient's family, social services, and Child Protective Services if there are concerns about the mother's ability to safely care for the baby due to severe mental illness or active substance abuse, to determine the best course of action for the infant's living arrangements.

Treatment of Bipolar Disorder in Pregnant and Postpartum Women

Preconception Management

Begin preparation at least six months before conception to ensure stability, switch to safer medications, and manage psychosocial stressors.

Course of Bipolar Disorder During Pregnancy and Postpartum

- *Pregnancy:* Low risk; only about 5% relapse rate.
- *Postpartum:* High risk; about one in three women with bipolar disorder relapse.

Predictors of Relapse

Early onset of illness, rapid cycling, history of multiple recurrences, and abrupt discontinuation of medications are significant red flags.

Impact on Pregnancy Outcomes

Increased risks of substance use, low birth weight, preterm birth, and inadequate prenatal care.

Lithium and Pregnancy

- *Risks:* Mainly cardiac anomalies, including Epstein's anomaly. Risk is dose dependent: No significant increase in risk with a daily dose of 600 mg or less, but risk increases three-fold with a daily dose of over 900 mg.
- Developmental outcomes in children exposed to lithium in utero appear normal.
- *Management:* Use the lowest effective dose, obtain a fetal ECG at week 18–24, and adjust doses carefully throughout pregnancy and postpartum.
  - Obtain lithium levels at least monthly.
  - Lithium levels drop as much as 34% by third trimester.
  - Reduce lithium back to pre-pregnancy dose at delivery to avoid lithium toxicity in the mother.

Other Mood Stabilizers

- *Valproate and carbamazepine:* High risk of neural tube defects (NTD); avoid in pregnancy.
  - Risk is linked to these medications' antifolate properties, but even high doses of supplemental folate during pregnancy don't reliably prevent the risk of NTD.
  - Prenatal valproate is also associated with poor school performance, lower IQ, and even autism.
- *Lamotrigine:* No significant risk of birth defects, but clearance can increase by 250% during pregnancy, requiring dose increases as necessary for symptom control.

Antipsychotics During Pregnancy

- There's some evidence of increased rate of birth defects among antipsychotic-exposed infants, but no specific patterns, suggesting that the underlying illness or unidentified confounds might explain this excess risk of birth defects.
- Keep antipsychotic doses at the lowest effective dose during pregnancy to minimize potential adverse sequelae in newborns like sleepiness, jitteriness, and extrapyramidal symptoms.
- Most data are with haloperidol, olanzapine, risperidone, and quetiapine.
- Minimize use of medications for which there are few pregnancy data, like asenapine, paliperidone, lurasidone, and clozapine.

Electroconvulsive Therapy

- Safe, rapid, and effective for patients with bipolar disorder.
- Main complications are preterm labor and transient fetal arrhythmias, but these are rare.
- Produces minimal fetal medication exposure and rapid symptom resolution.

FDA Use in Pregnancy Ratings

- These have been recently revised and the A, B, C, D, X categories are being phased out.
- Don't base your choice of medication solely on FDA ratings; information from large numbers of human exposures is far more meaningful.

Prophylactic Treatment for Postpartum Psychosis

- Patients with bipolar disorder should begin prophylactic treatment immediately upon delivery to prevent relapse if they're not already on a mood stabilizer.
- Lamotrigine and lithium are good options, but careful monitoring and dose adjustments are crucial.

Breastfeeding Considerations

- *Lithium:* Generally not recommended due to the potential for high serum levels in nursing infants, especially if the infant experiences dehydration from conditions like diarrhea or fever.
- *Carbamazepine and valproate:* Generally okay to use in breastfeeding due to their high protein binding.
- *Lamotrigine:* Generally okay to use in breastfeeding, although infant blood levels have been reported to vary widely. Monitor the baby for side effects, especially rash.
- *Antipsychotics:* Generally considered safe; monitor for dose-dependent exposure risks, like sedation in the baby.
- *Pharmacokinetics:* Highly protein-bound medications with short half-lives tend to produce the least infant exposure through breast milk.

Summary

- *Preconception:* Begin management early, with a focus on switching to safer medications and stabilizing the patient.
- *Pregnancy:* Monitor closely for signs of relapse, adjust medication doses as needed, and avoid high-risk medications like valproate and carbamazepine. Lithium and lamotrigine levels vary widely as pregnancy progresses. First-trimester exposure to lithium increases the risk of cardiac defects in a dose-dependent manner.
- *Postpartum:* Implement prophylactic treatment to prevent relapse for patients who are not already on a mood stabilizer.
- *Breastfeeding:* Many medications can be safely taken during breastfeeding, although lithium is best avoided.
- *Documentation:* Carefully document discussions about the risks and benefits of treatment and the patient's capacity to consent. Also, document that you've informed the patient of the 2%–4% baseline risk of birth defects, regardless of medication exposures. Indicate whether the patient's symptoms are improving with the medication. If they are not improving, document that you will discontinue an ineffective medication rather than continue to expose the fetus to the medication.

Depression in Pregnancy: Diagnosis and Treatment

Prenatal depression is common, affecting 10%–15% of pregnant patients. Make sure to screen for this condition as it's linked with negative birth outcomes like low birth weight and preterm birth. Early detection and intervention are key to protecting both maternal and fetal health.

Diagnosis

You'll diagnose depression in pregnancy in the same way as any other time, but be careful about over-relying on neurovegetative symptoms like poor sleep, fatigue, and changes in weight and appetite, as these are common in pregnancy. Focus instead on cognitive, emotional, and behavioral aspects of depression, like persistent feelings of sadness or worthlessness, poor concentration, loss of interest or pleasure in activities (anhedonia), and/or suicidal thoughts.

Treatment of Depression During Pregnancy

Therapy

Several forms of therapy are helpful during pregnancy, including supportive therapy, couples counseling, and cognitive behavioral therapy.

Antidepressants

Most studies show no increased risk for major malformations or developmental disorders following prenatal antidepressant use, except for paroxetine, which has been linked with fetal cardiovascular anomalies.

- Citalopram, fluoxetine, and sertraline are most often used.
- Minimize the use of tricyclic antidepressants as they can exacerbate pregnancy symptoms like weight gain, constipation, and dizziness.
- Infants exposed to selective serotonin reuptake inhibitors or serotonin/norepinephrine reuptake inhibitors during pregnancy, especially in the third trimester, may experience transient neonatal distress, including restlessness and poor feeding. Symptoms resolve spontaneously after one to four days.

Electroconvulsive therapy (ECT)

ECT is a relatively safe and effective option, but it requires close monitoring of the mother and fetus during the procedure.

Management of Preexisting Depression

It's generally advised to continue antidepressants during pregnancy. Discontinuation is associated with higher rates of relapse.

Risk/Benefit Discussions

- Engage in joint decision making with the patient, ideally also involving the baby's other parent. Discuss previous medication discontinuations and their outcomes.
- Document the discussion of risks, including those of untreated depression and medication use during pregnancy.

Support and Educational Resources

- MotherToBaby: Provides expert consultation and free second opinions with teratology specialists (www.mothertobaby.org, 866-626-6847).
- Massachusetts General Hospital Center for Women's Mental Health: Provides information on perinatal mental health (www.womensmentalhealth.org).

How to Recognize and Treat Postpartum Depression

Postpartum depression (PPD) is surprisingly common, affecting 10%–20% of new mothers in the first year after giving birth. Severe cases may require inpatient psychiatric hospitalization. Here we review key principles in the diagnosis and treatment of PPD.

Diagnosis

The diagnosis of PPD follows criteria similar to those for major depression, with the specification that onset occurs within the first four weeks after childbirth. However, clinical practice recognizes that symptoms can emerge any time within the first year postpartum. The key symptoms include:

- Persistent sadness or low mood.
- Marked loss of interest or pleasure in activities previously enjoyed.
- Significant weight loss when not dieting, weight gain, or decrease or increase in appetite.
- Insomnia or excessive sleep.
- Psychomotor agitation or retardation.
- Fatigue or loss of energy.
- Feelings of worthlessness or excessive or inappropriate guilt.
- Diminished ability to think or concentrate, or indecisiveness.
- Recurrent thoughts of death, suicidal ideation, or a suicide attempt or plan.

Screen for bipolar disorder also since many cases of PPD reflect bipolar depression.

Differentiating from Baby Blues

Don't confuse PPD with the "baby blues," a transient state of emotional disturbance occurring in up to 80% of mothers during the first two weeks postpartum. Unlike PPD, the baby blues are characterized by mild mood swings, irritability, and tearfulness, resolving without medical intervention. In contrast, PPD presents with more severe, persistent symptoms that can impair a mother's ability to care for the child and themselves.

Use of Screening Tools

To aid in diagnosis, use the Edinburgh Postnatal Depression Scale, an easy-to-use, 10-item questionnaire (see: www.thecarlatreport.com/AdministeringEPDS).

Treatment Considerations

- If the patient was breastfeeding before being admitted to the hospital, ensure they have access to a breast pump. This will prevent breast engorgement and help maintain their milk supply. The patient may wish to collect the milk so it can be picked up and given to the infant during the patient's hospitalization.
- Make use of perinatal psychiatry-focused partial hospitalization programs or inpatient units in your area if they're available (www.tinyurl.com/mrxk7dnh).

Treatment Options

Nonpharmacologic approaches

- Encourage patients to participate in individual and group psychotherapy and peer support groups if available on the unit.
- Postpartum Support International offers a wide array of free, virtual, facilitator-led peer support groups that patients may be able to access while on the unit and after discharge (1-800-944-4773; www.postpartum.net).

Pharmacologic approaches

- Select antidepressant medications based on past response, side effects, cost, etc.
- Breastfeeding is not a contraindication for starting or continuing an antidepressant, as adverse events in the infant are extremely rare.
- Sertraline is often favored due to undetectably low levels in breastfeeding infants, but don't switch from an effective regimen to sertraline to prevent destabilizing the parent's mental health.
- Sometimes patients want to know when antidepressant levels peak in breast milk so they can "pump and dump" to minimize the baby's exposure, but since exposure to antidepressants in breast milk does not adversely affect the baby, all this does is waste milk.
- Intravenous brexanolone is FDA approved for PPD and works quickly, but it requires a 60-hour infusion in a health care setting and enrollment in a federal Risk Evaluation and Mitigation Strategy (REMS) program due to safety concerns of excessive sedation and hypoxia. Its high cost also limits its use.
- Zuranolone, a neurosteroid like brexanolone, recently received FDA approval for PPD. It's costly but seems to work faster than traditional antidepressants. It's prescribed in a 50 mg evening dose, taken with a fatty meal, for 14 days. Its main side effects are drowsiness and dizziness.

Postpartum Psychosis: Diagnosis and Treatment

Once you see a case of postpartum psychosis, you'll never forget it. New mothers who appear stable one day can become severely impaired almost overnight. These mothers are in no condition to care for their newborns, and in extreme cases, they might even pose a danger to the child. Here we dive into the key points in identifying and managing this challenging condition.

Symptoms and Presentation

- Develops within the four weeks following childbirth.
- Watch for delirium-like symptoms (eg, confusion, fluctuating consciousness).
- Patients also experience delusions, hallucinations, and manic or depressive symptoms.
- Delusions often involve the infant, like beliefs that the baby is possessed. In extreme cases, the mother might believe it's necessary to harm or even kill the baby.
- Obsessive thoughts about the newborn are common.

Differential Diagnosis

- Rule out substance use; obtain a urine toxicology screen.
- Postpartum depression and anxiety disorders are in the differential, but these don't present with delusions or hallucinations.
- Schizophrenia—but new-onset schizophrenia is rare in the first four weeks postpartum.
- Postpartum obsessive-compulsive disorder (OCD) is probably the most likely syndrome to be confused with postpartum psychosis. The risk of new onset or exacerbation of OCD rises after childbirth, and patients' intrusive thoughts (eg, thoughts that the baby might fall out an open window) can be so extreme as to seem delusional. But obsessive thoughts are highly distressing, in contrast to the delusions of postpartum psychosis.
- Work with OB-GYN to exclude medical conditions that mimic psychiatric symptoms. These include delirium, thyroiditis, lupus, autoimmune encephalitis, medication side effects (eg, steroid-induced mania), and Sheehan's syndrome (postpartum pituitary necrosis).

Risk Factors

- The primary risk factor is a history of bipolar disorder, implicated in 20%–30% of cases.
- Other factors include previous episodes of postpartum psychosis, family history of bipolar disorder, sleep deprivation, and first childbirth.

Treatment

- Immediate inpatient admission.
- Treat as psychotic mania: Antipsychotic, mood stabilizer, benzodiazepine for agitation.
- Lithium is often the most effective mood stabilizer in these cases.
- Educate the family on the importance of sleep, medication adherence, and keeping the mother supervised until fully recovered.
- After remission, taper the antipsychotic and benzodiazepine, but continue lithium for at least nine months, longer if you suspect underlying bipolar disorder.
- Consider electroconvulsive therapy for nonresponders or severe cases.

Prophylactic Treatment

For patients with a history of postpartum psychosis, consider prophylactic treatment with antipsychotic meds and/or mood stabilizers in late pregnancy or immediately postpartum.

Use of Psychiatric Medications in Breastfeeding Patients

When new mothers are admitted to the inpatient psychiatric unit, they might ask about the safety of taking psychiatric medications while breastfeeding. If they were nursing an infant prior to admission, provide them with a breast pump so they can continue producing milk. The milk should be refrigerated until a family member or designated person can pick it up. Most psychiatric medications pose little risk to breastfeeding infants. Here's a guide to the safety of psychiatric medications during breastfeeding.

Antidepressants

- Most antidepressants are safe to use in breastfeeding. These include paroxetine and sertraline (for which we have the most data). Bupropion, citalopram, mirtazapine, and venlafaxine have less data but are also considered safe.
- Antidepressants that are not recommended include fluoxetine, due to long half-life and risk of causing jitteriness in the baby; tricyclics, which can cause excess sedation in the baby (especially doxepin); and vilazodone, vortioxetine, and monoamine oxidase inhibitors (as we have little data on these meds).

Antipsychotics

- Most antipsychotics are considered safe, including haloperidol, olanzapine, and quetiapine (which have the most safety data). Aripiprazole, risperidone, and ziprasidone are also considered safe.
- Antipsychotics that are not recommended include brexpiprazole, cariprazine, iloperidone, lumateperone, and lurasidone, as we know little about their safety in breastfeeding.
- Clozapine is contraindicated in nursing.
- Monitor infants for side effects like extrapyramidal symptoms (these are rare) and sedation.

Anxiolytics/Hypnotics

- Anxiolytics/hypnotics that are safe to use in breastfeeding include lorazepam, diphenhydramine, and melatonin, but monitor for signs of infant sedation. Buspirone, gabapentin, and trazodone are probably okay to use at low doses, but breastfeeding data are sparse.
- Anxiolytics/hypnotics that are not recommended include clonazepam, diazepam, and chlordiazepoxide due to their long half-lives and risk of sedation in the baby. Alprazolam, temazepam, ramelteon, suvorexant, zaleplon, and zolpidem are also not recommended due to lack of data.

Mood Stabilizers

- Lithium can lead to relatively high blood levels in infants, so it's best to avoid or minimize its use during breastfeeding. Some clinicians prescribe it to new mothers, though. If you do, monitor the baby closely for potential side effects (eg, lethargy, feeding difficulties) and follow these guidelines:
  - Regular lab tests for the infant (lithium level, thyroid-stimulating hormone [TSH], blood urea nitrogen [BUN], creatinine), eg, at two and 10 days postpartum and then at 30 and 60 days postpartum.
  - If the infant's lithium level is greater than 0.2 mEq/L, or if there are increases in TSH, BUN, or creatinine, recommend that the mother reduce breastfeeding and supplement with formula, or discontinue breastfeeding entirely.
  - Advise mothers to hold off on breastfeeding, or to combine it with formula, during periods when the baby may be dehydrated, such as if the baby has diarrhea or fever.
- Valproate, lamotrigine, and carbamazepine are generally okay to use in breastfeeding. Monitor the infant for sedation. Mothers on lamotrigine should stop nursing if the baby develops a rash.

Additional Considerations

For medication safety information during breastfeeding, refer to the Drugs and Lactation Database (LactMed; www.tinyurl.com/atnyr6xd).

Table 16: **Psychiatric Medications in Pregnancy and Lactation**

Medication	Pregnancy	Breastfeeding	Recommendations
Anxiolytics/Hypnotics			
Benzodiazepines (various agents)	Possible increased incidence of cleft lip or palate (with first trimester exposure); floppy infant syndrome (with exposure just before delivery); neonatal withdrawal syndrome; lower Apgar scores	Excretion less than 10%. Excessive sedation in infant, lethargy with consequent feeding difficulty and weight loss reported.	• Try to avoid in first trimester and late in pregnancy (although intermittent use less likely to induce withdrawal symptoms in neonate) • Lorazepam (Ativan) may be best in class to use due to lack of active metabolites and relatively shorter half-life • Monitor sedation in breastfed infants; use of shorter-acting agents preferred
Buspirone (BuSpar)	Minimal data; difficult to determine risks	Low to undetectable infant levels reported	• Avoid in pregnancy due to limited data • Likely safe in breastfeeding
Diphenhydramine (Benadryl)	Fairly consistent data show lack of associated malformations	Larger doses or more prolonged use may cause adverse effects in the infant	• Considered to be the safest hypnotic in pregnancy and breastfeeding
Nonbenzodiazepines: Eszopiclone (Lunesta) Zaleplon (Sonata) Zolpidem (Ambien)	No increased risk of malformations, but data fairly sparse	Relatively low levels in breast milk. Most data are with zolpidem. Zolpidem is relatively hydrophilic and excreted rapidly; therefore, may be favored.	• Reserve for second-line use due to paucity of data • Zolpidem at low dose is the best option when nonbenzos are needed
Daridorexant (Quviviq), lemborexant (Dayvigo), suvorexant (Belsomra)	No data	No data	• Use other agents with more data and longer record of experience
Trazodone	Fewer data show no increased risk of malformations	<1% excretion; not expected to cause adverse effects in breastfed infants	• Probably safe in pregnancy and breastfeeding
Mood Stabilizers			
Carbamazepine (Tegretol)	Rate of major malformation 2.2%–7.9%. Neural tube defects (0.5%–1%), craniofacial defects, cardiovascular malformations, and hypospadias reported.	Relatively high levels in breast milk but with few adverse effects reported. Sedation, poor sucking, withdrawal reactions, and three cases of hepatic dysfunction have been reported.	• Avoid if possible • If use unavoidable, add high-dose (4 mg) folic acid supplementation
Lamotrigine (Lamictal)	Rate of major malformations 1%–5.6%. Increased risk of oral clefts (0.4%).	Based on limited data, thought to be safe; however, infant exposure can be high and can vary widely (reports of 18%–60% of maternal concentrations); monitor infant. Relatively high infant exposure (22.7%); avoid or exercise caution.	• Safest of the anticonvulsants in pregnancy, though good safety data are sparse. Serum levels should be monitored; levels usually decrease over course of pregnancy.
Lithium (Eskalith, Lithobid)	Rate of major malformations 4%–12%. Risk of Ebstein's anomaly (cardiac problem) is lower than previously thought (0.05%–0.1%). Increased maternal risk of diabetes, polyhydramnios, thyroid dysfunction during pregnancy.	30%–50% excretion; not recommended due to high risk of toxicity	• Try to avoid, particularly in first trimester • If first trimester use required, fetal echocardiogram recommended • Check serum levels and thyroid function frequently during pregnancy, since changes in metabolism and total body water require dose adjustments, particularly in third trimester • Avoid in breastfeeding if possible
Oxcarbazepine (Trileptal)	Danish study showed no increased risk of major malformation. However, data are limited.	Possible adverse effects in breastfed infants; monitor infant for drowsiness, adequate weight gain, and developmental milestones	• Relatively safe, though more data are needed

Medication	Pregnancy	Breastfeeding	Recommendations
Valproate (Depakote)	Most teratogenic of all mood stabilizers, with a 6.2%–20.3% rate of congenital malformations, with neural tube defects most prominent. Teratogenic effects are dose-related with greatest risk at doses >1000 mg per day. Recently, exposure linked to autism.	Relatively low excretion (0.68%); considered compatible with breastfeeding	• Avoid in pregnancy unless absolutely required • If use unavoidable, add high-dose (4 mg) folic acid supplementation • Safe in breastfeeding
Antipsychotics			
First-generation	No increased risk of malformations seen with high-potency agents. Small increased risk with low-potency agents such as chlorpromazine (Thorazine). Transient extrapyramidal side effects; sedation; withdrawal symptoms in neonates.	Relatively low excretion reported although little data available. Sedation and parkinsonism effects possible in breastfed infants.	• Haloperidol (Haldol), fluphenazine (Prolixin) favored during pregnancy because of long history of safe use • Relatively safe in breastfeeding
Second-generation	Fewer data available, most showing no increased risk of malformations. Maternal hyperglycemia, impaired glucose tolerance, and weight gain may lead to maternal complications. Large-for-gestational-age infants reported. Floppy infant syndrome reported in clozapine exposure; monitor neutrophils in neonate for six months.	Excretion low, usually <3%, with exception of clozapine (Clozaril), which is seen in relatively high concentrations in breast milk	• Overall, relatively safe in pregnancy; not treating serious mental illness in pregnancy poses greater risk. Most data with risperidone, olanzapine, quetiapine. • Avoid clozapine in breastfeeding if possible.
Antidepressants			
Bupropion (Wellbutrin)	No increased risk of malformation	<1% excretion with no adverse outcomes reported	• Safe for use in pregnancy and breastfeeding
Duloxetine (Cymbalta)	Little data	No published data, though exposure is low	• Not enough data to recommend
Levomilnacipran (Fetzima)	No data	No published data	• Not enough data to recommend
Mirtazapine (Remeron)	Sparse data, but one small study suggests no increased rate of major malformation	Low excretion; compatible with breastfeeding	• Likely safe in pregnancy and breastfeeding
SSRIs	Controversial data regarding cardiovascular malformation with first-trimester paroxetine (Paxil) exposure. Larger and more recent studies show no overall increased risk for malformations with SSRIs. Conflicting reports, with some showing decreased gestational age, low birth weight, poor neonatal adaptation, low Apgar scores (some of which could be due to underlying depression or anxiety). Conflicting reports regarding SSRI use in later pregnancy and persistent pulmonary hypertension (PPHN). Neonatal toxicity reported as transient jitteriness, tremulousness, and tachypnea. No problems detected in behavioral or cognitive development—greatest data with fluoxetine (Prozac).	Relatively low excretion, varies by agent: Citalopram (Celexa): 5%–10% Fluoxetine: 3%–9% Fluvoxamine (Luvox): <2% Paroxetine: <4% Sertraline (Zoloft): <2%	• SSRIs are relatively safe in pregnancy; avoid paroxetine if possible • Sertraline is safest in breastfeeding • Avoid fluoxetine in breastfeeding due to long half-life and active metabolite

Medication	Pregnancy	Breastfeeding	Recommendations
Tricyclics	Relatively large database; recent meta-analysis of 300,000 live births revealed no increased risk of malformations. Some data indicate clomipramine may increase risk for congenital heart malformations. Neonatal anticholinergic effects. Transient neonatal withdrawal symptoms reported.	<1%–5% excretion; appear relatively safe during breastfeeding, with possible exception of doxepin	• Safe in pregnancy; desipramine and nortriptyline preferred due to lower anticholinergic and orthostatic hypotension risks • Relatively safe in breastfeeding; monitor infant for sedation
Venlafaxine (Effexor)/ desvenlafaxine (Pristiq)	Earlier data regarding major malformations reassuring, but one more recent study suggested a possible association with birth defects; additional studies needed. Increased maternal blood pressure may be a concern during pregnancy, particularly at higher doses.	2%–9.2% excretion; no adverse outcomes reported	• Less recommended than other antidepressants
Vilazodone (Viibryd)	No data	No published data	• Not enough data to recommend
Vortioxetine (Trintellix)	No data	No published data	• Not enough data to recommend
Stimulants			
Amphetamines and methylphenidates	No apparent congenital malformations; may constrict blood flow to placenta, which reduces oxygen flow to developing fetus. May cause premature delivery, small for gestational age and low-birth-weight babies; however, data inconclusive. Neonatal withdrawal possible.	0.2% excreted into breast milk; adverse effects usually not observed	• Not recommended in pregnancy due to possibility of vasoconstriction and ability to disrupt blood flow to the fetus • Likely safe in breastfeeding

Cross-Cultural Issues on the Inpatient Psychiatric Unit

Cross-cultural factors can shape how patients express symptoms, convey needs, and adhere to treatment. Here we review common cross-cultural issues and tips to keep in mind when you work with patients of diverse backgrounds. At the same time, beware of stereotyping cultural groups; each patient has a unique cultural and personal perspective.

Communication and Decision Making

- Limited English proficiency can mimic paucity of thought and thought disorganization. Use professional interpreter services whenever possible; avoid asking family members to translate.
- Patients, especially from Latinx and Asian backgrounds, may consent to treatments out of respect, even without full comprehension. Foster open dialogue with statements like, "Many patients have concerns about new medications. What are your thoughts?"

Cultural Expressions and Manifestation of Illness

- Watch for somatic symptoms such as GI distress and headaches, as these might indicate mental distress in patients from Asian, Latinx, and Middle Eastern backgrounds.
- In some cultures, phenomena such as seeing spirits or hearing deceased loved ones are normative. Evaluate such experiences within their cultural context before deeming them pathological.
- Be mindful of culture-specific syndromes when arriving at your diagnoses. For instance, ataque de nervios (seen mainly among Hispanic individuals, especially those from Puerto Rico) involves uncontrollable shaking, crying, and even seizure-like activity after a stressful event.

Trust in Health Care

- Past discrimination experiences can foster mistrust toward health care, leading to inconsistent treatment adherence. Empower patients by providing options and involving them in health care decisions.
- Patients might be reluctant to attend outpatient appointments after discharge due to deportation fears if they are living in the US illegally. Reassure them that their information is confidential and used strictly for clinical purposes.

Sociocultural and Environmental Stressors

- Experiences like the trauma from immigration or adjusting to a new culture can profoundly impact a patient's mental well-being. Delve deeper into the motives behind the patient's migration, whether escaping political turmoil or seeking better employment opportunities, to better grasp their potential emotional implications.
- In various cultures, mental health topics are taboo, so patients may conceal or downplay their symptoms. Educate and reassure patients about the privacy of their diagnosis and treatment and emphasize that your goal is to support their well-being.
- Erratic health care follow-up may be due to unstable living situations and frequent moves. Consider arranging for telehealth follow-up post-discharge.

Family and Community Dynamics

- In Latinx and Asian cultures, many value family participation in decision making. Ask, "How would you like your family to be involved in your treatment?"
- Explore traditional healing practices that are often rooted in community practices or beliefs. Ask, "Besides medications, have you tried other treatments like home remedies or acupuncture?"

Potential Biases and Discrepancies

Be mindful of implicit bias. Black patients, for instance, are more likely than White patients to be given a more severe diagnosis for comparable symptoms, such as receiving a diagnosis of schizophrenia instead of a mood disorder.

Traditions, Religion, and Spirituality

- For Muslim patients observing the month-long Ramadan fast, consider adjusting medication schedules. Since observants abstain from eating or drinking from sunrise to sunset, a once- or twice-daily dosing regimen—preferably early morning and at bedtime—might enhance adherence compared to a thrice-daily schedule.
- Certain religious beliefs, like those in Orthodox Judaism and some Islamic traditions, prohibit touching by members of the opposite sex. When physical examinations are necessary, clinicians should ideally be of the same gender as the patient to respect these beliefs.

Pharmacogenomic Differences

- Medication metabolism varies considerably across ethnic groups due to genetic differences. For instance, less than 1% of individuals from China and Japan are poor metabolizers of the P450 enzyme 2D6. In contrast, this percentage is around 10% for those of Central and Northern European descent and rises to 19% for individuals from South Africa.
- Poor 2D6 metabolizers might experience more side effects at standard doses of specific drugs, including olanzapine, risperidone, paroxetine, fluoxetine, and venlafaxine.
- Ultrarapid metabolizers are infrequent in the general population but constitute up to 30% of the population in the Middle East and Northeastern Africa. These individuals may require higher than usual doses to achieve therapeutic benefits.

Providing Gender-Affirming Care to LGBTQIA+ Patients in Hospital Units

You'll often work with patients who are part of the LGBTQIA+ community. To make sure your care is informed and supportive, keep these points in mind.

Cultural Sensitivity

- Always ask for and use patients' preferred pronouns and names. You can say, "I want to ensure I address you correctly. What name and pronouns do you prefer to use?"
- Stay up to date with LGBTQIA+ terminologies:
  - *Cisgender:* Gender that is aligned with a person's sex recorded at birth.
  - *Gender-expansive:* A term that emphasizes the fluidity and individuality of gender.
  - *Genderqueer:* Not adhering to the gender binary. Can also indicate sexual attraction.
  - *Nonbinary/nonconforming:* Does not identify strictly as masculine or feminine.
  - *Queer:* An umbrella term that can be used to describe a sexual orientation, gender identity, or gender expression that does not conform to dominant societal norms.
  - *Transgender:* A discrepancy between a person's sex recorded at birth and their gender.
- Strive to maintain an environment where LGBTQIA+ patients feel supported by promptly addressing any forms of bias or prejudicial conduct.

History Taking

- Make sure electronic health records reflect the patient's preferred name and pronouns.
- Use gender-neutral language, such as "partner" or "relationship status."
- Ask about a history of discrimination, violence, or other trauma: "Sometimes experiences of discrimination or trauma can have a big impact on our mental health. Have you had any experiences like this that you feel comfortable sharing with me?"
- Include questions about past or future gender-affirming treatments: "Can we talk about any medical treatments or procedures that you've undergone or are considering, such as hormone therapy or surgeries? Only share what you feel comfortable with."
- Pay extra attention to LGBTQIA+ youth, who may be dealing with family rejection or homelessness. You can ask, "How has your experience been with your family regarding your gender identity or sexual orientation?"
- Be cautious about privacy. Some patients may not be "out" to family or friends. You can say, "Your privacy is very important. Is there anyone in your life who is unaware of your gender identity or sexual orientation that I should be mindful of when discussing your care?"

Environmental Accommodations

Talk to nonbinary patients about their room preferences, without making assumptions based on their sex at birth. Offer private or unisex bathroom facilities when possible.

Health Care Management in Gender Transitioning

- Continue hormonal treatments for transgender patients during their hospital stay unless there's a medical concern (eg, a heightened risk for thromboembolism in a bed-bound patient).
- Watch for interactions with other medications, like lithium with spironolactone or carbamazepine with estrogen.
- You might be asked to provide a letter of support for a patient's gender-affirming treatments.
- Familiarize yourself with resources for patients seeking or undergoing gender transition, such as therapists, endocrinologists, and support groups.

Appendices

Appendix A: National Mental Health Resources

Providing patients with resources as they transition from inpatient psychiatric units to outpatient care is vital for their continued support and recovery. Here are several valuable national resources.

General Mental Health Resources

National Alliance on Mental Illness (NAMI)

- **Website:** www.nami.org
- **Phone:** 1-800-950-NAMI (1-800-950-6264)
- **Description:** Offers support groups, education programs, and advocacy for individuals with mental illness and their families.

Mental Health America (MHA)

- **Website:** www.mhanational.org
- **Description:** Provides resources for mental health awareness, including screening tools and information on various mental health conditions.

National Institute of Mental Health (NIMH)

- **Website:** www.nimh.nih.gov
- **Description:** Offers extensive information on mental disorders, current research, and educational materials.

Crisis and Suicide Prevention Resources

988 Suicide and Crisis Lifeline

- **Website:** www.suicidepreventionlifeline.org
- **Phone:** 988
- **Description:** Offers free and confidential support 24/7 for individuals in distress, along with suicide prevention and crisis resources.

American Foundation for Suicide Prevention (AFSP)

- **Website:** www.afsp.org
- **Description:** Provides resources for suicide prevention, including education, advocacy, and support for those affected by suicide.

Substance Use Resources

Substance Abuse and Mental Health Services Administration (SAMHSA)

- **Website:** www.samhsa.gov
- **National Helpline:** 1-800-662-HELP (1-800-662-4357)
- **Description:** Offers comprehensive information and support for substance use disorders, including treatment referrals and support services.

Anxiety and Depression Resources

Anxiety and Depression Association of America (ADAA)

- **Website:** www.adaa.org
- **Description:** Provides information on prevention, treatment, and symptoms of anxiety, depression, and related conditions.

Depression and Bipolar Support Alliance (DBSA)

- **Website:** www.dbsalliance.org
- **Description:** Offers peer-led support groups and resources for individuals living with depression and bipolar disorder.

Veteran Services

Veterans Crisis Line

- **Website:** www.veteranscrisisline.net
- **Phone:** 988, then press 1
- **Description:** Provides 24/7 confidential support for veterans and their loved ones experiencing mental health crises or suicidal thoughts.

LGBTQIA+ Resources

The Trevor Project

- **Website:** www.thetrevorproject.org
- **Phone:** 1-866-488-7386

- **Description:** Offers crisis intervention and suicide prevention services specifically for LGBTQIA+ youth under 25 years old.

LGBT National Help Center

- **Website:** www.lgbthotline.org
- **Description:** Provides free and confidential peer-support and local resources for LGBTQIA+ individuals through hotlines and online chat services.

Maternal Mental Health Resources

Postpartum Support International (PSI)

- **Website:** www.postpartum.net
- **Phone:** 1-800-944-4773
- **Description:** Dedicated to supporting families dealing with postpartum depression, anxiety, and distress through helplines, support groups, and informational resources. Services available in English and Spanish.

National Maternal Mental Health Hotline

- **Phone:** 1-833-TLC-MAMA (1-833-852-6262)
- **Description:** Provides free and confidential support and resources 24/7 to pregnant and postpartum individuals experiencing mental health challenges. Assistance available in English and Spanish via call or text.

Culturally Specific Resources

Asian Mental Health Collective

- **Website:** www.asianmhc.org/apisaa
- **Description:** Provides mental health support and resources tailored for the Asian American and Pacific Islander communities, including directories for culturally competent therapists.

Latino Behavioral Health Services

- **Website:** www.latinobehavioral.org
- **Description:** Offers culturally relevant mental health services, including online therapy and support programs for the Latino community.

Black Men Heal

- **Website:** www.blackmenheal.org
- **Description:** Provides free mental health services and resources to men of color, aiming to reduce the stigma and barriers associated with seeking mental health support.

Therapy for Black Girls

- **Website:** https://providers.therapyforblackgirls.com
- **Description:** Offers a directory of Black female therapists and resources dedicated to the mental wellness of Black women and girls.

Appendix B: SMART Goals and Interventions in Psychiatric Care

CMS and The Joint Commission require that you participate in regular interdisciplinary treatment plan meetings. While meeting with other staff about your patients is always a good idea, these agencies require certain types of documentation that are confusing and often of debatable usefulness. Nonetheless, hospitals are required to produce these documents, and you should be a good team player and do your part. One of the most confusing aspects of these plans are the long-term goals and short-term goals. They are supposed to be "SMART" goals—**S**pecific, **M**easurable, **A**chievable, **R**elevant, and **T**ime-bound. Here, to make your job easier, we provide a goal bank and an interventions bank with examples of long-term/short-term goals (LTGs/STGs) and interventions (LTIs/STIs) you can customize for your interdisciplinary treatment plans. (AEB in these example statements stands for "as evidenced by.")

Goal Bank

Target Symptom	Goals
Depression	**LTG:** Demonstrate stabilized mood AEB participation in group programs at least ___ times weekly for ___ consecutive weeks. **STG:** Actively participate and attend at least ___ groups per day for ___ consecutive days within ___ days. **STG:** Increase PO intake AEB eating at least ___% of meals for ___ consecutive days within ___ days. **STG:** Increase socialization AEB initiating conversation with at least ___ staff members or peers per day for ___ consecutive days.
Mania	**LTG:** Demonstrate stabilized mood AEB maintaining consistent participation in structured activities and group therapy at least ___ times per week for ___ consecutive weeks. **STG:** Demonstrate a ___% decrease in grandiose delusions AEB by verbalizing less than ___ grandiose statements per shift within ___ days. **STG:** Display a ___% decrease in intrusive behavior AEB tolerating ___ groups per day within ___ days.
Psychosis	**LTG:** Demonstrate reduced psychotic symptoms AEB reporting no auditory hallucinations for ___ consecutive weeks. **STG:** Demonstrate a decrease in delusional thinking AEB verbalizing reality-based thoughts at least ___ times per day for ___ consecutive days. **STG:** Increase reality orientation AEB participating in reality orientation groups at least ___ times per week for ___ consecutive weeks.
Suicidal ideation	**LTG:** Demonstrate increased self-awareness AEB no reported suicidal ideation or attempts for ___ consecutive weeks. **STG:** Decrease in suicidal ideation AEB denying active intent to harm self for ___ consecutive days over ___ days. **STG:** Demonstrate improved impulse control AEB no impulsive actions for ___ consecutive days.
Anxiety	**LTG:** Demonstrate a decrease in anxiety AEB reporting anxiety levels of ___ or below on a 10-point scale for ___ consecutive weeks. **STG:** Demonstrate a decrease in anxiety AEB reporting ___ or less panic episodes per day for ___ consecutive days. **STG:** Demonstrate a decrease in anxiety AEB reporting anxiety levels of ___ or below on a 10-point scale for ___ consecutive days.
Agitation/combativeness	**LTG:** Demonstrate improved behavioral control AEB no incidents of physical aggression for ___ consecutive weeks. **STG:** Demonstrate improved impulse control AEB having less than ___ episodes of verbal aggression per shift for ___ days within ___ days. **STG:** Demonstrate improved self-control AEB initiating use of ___ coping skills per shift for ___ consecutive days.
PO intake	**LTG:** Demonstrate improved ability to care for self AEB by eating at least ___% of meals for ___ consecutive weeks. **STG:** Demonstrate improved oral intake AEB eating at least ___ meals per day in the dining room for ___ consecutive days over ___ days. **STG:** Demonstrate improved insight into nutrition status AEB by identifying ___ negative effects of poor PO intake within ___ days.
Medication compliance/ hospital relapse	**LTG:** Develop a safe discharge plan AEB identifying ___ outpatient supports over ___ days. **STG:** Demonstrate medication adherence AEB identifying at least ___ consequences of nonadherence within ___ days. **STG:** Demonstrate improved medication adherence AEB by accepting all medications with no more than ___ prompts per shift over ___ consecutive days.
Sleep	**LTG:** Demonstrate improved sleep AEB sleeping ___ hours per night for ___ consecutive weeks. **STG:** Demonstrate increased sleep AEB sleeping more than ___ hours per night for ___ consecutive days. **STG:** Demonstrate improved sleep hygiene AEB spending less than ___ hours per day in bed for ___ consecutive days over ___ days.
Falls	**LTG:** Demonstrate improved safety awareness AEB consistently complying with fall prevention interventions for ___ consecutive weeks. **STG:** Demonstrate decreased risk of falls AEB use of fall prevention interventions with minimal staff prompting for ___ consecutive days over __ days.

Interventions Bank

Target Symptom	Interventions
Depression	**LTI:** Encourage participation in weekly therapy sessions and adjust pharmacotherapy as needed over the next ___ weeks. **STI:** Educate the patient on the nature of depression and available treatment options at least ___ times per week over the next ___ days. **STI:** Encourage participation in group activities to enhance socialization and reduce isolation at least ___ times daily over the next ___ days.
Mania	**LTI:** Identify and manage factors that trigger manic episodes, such as stress and sleep disruptions, while continuing mood stabilizer therapy at least ___ per week for the next ___ weeks. **STI:** Monitor behavior and set clear, consistent limits to manage symptoms at least ___ times daily over the next ___ days. **STI:** Offer structured activities to channel excess energy positively at least ___ times daily over the next ___ days. **STI:** Reassure and validate patient's feelings to reduce paranoia and intrusive thoughts at least ___ times daily over the next ___ days.
Psychosis	**LTI:** Engage in antipsychotic medication management and regular assessment of symptoms at least ___ times weekly over the next ___ weeks. **STI:** Use reality orientation techniques during daily interactions at least ___ times daily over the next ___ days. **STI:** Encourage participation in reality orientation groups at least ___ times per week over the next ___ days. **STI:** Provide a calm and structured environment to reduce sensory overload and stressors at least ___ times daily over the next ___ days.
Suicidal ideation	**LTI:** Engage in cognitive behavioral therapy and safety planning at least ___ times weekly over the next ___ weeks. **STI:** Collaborate with the patient at least ___ times daily to create a detailed safety plan within the next ___ days. **STI:** Increase observation levels at least ___ times per shift as needed to ensure safety over the next ___ days. **STI:** Engage in therapeutic communication to explore underlying issues and provide support at least ___ times daily over the next ___ days.
Anxiety	**LTI:** Educate on relaxation techniques at least ___ times weekly for the next ___ weeks. **STI:** Teach and encourage the use of relaxation techniques, such as deep breathing or progressive muscle relaxation, at least ___ times daily over the next ___ days. **STI:** Help the patient establish a daily routine to reduce anxiety triggers, reviewed at least every ___ days for the next ___ days. **STI:** Utilize cognitive behavioral techniques to challenge and reframe anxious thoughts during therapy sessions at least ___ times weekly over the next ___ days.
Agitation/combativeness	**LTI:** Encourage participation in weekly anger management sessions and regular physical activity over the next ___ weeks. **STI:** Use de-escalation techniques to manage aggressive behavior as needed, reviewed at each incident, for the next ___ days. **STI:** Encourage physical activities to help release pent-up energy at least ___ times daily over the next ___ days. **STI:** Teach and reinforce the use of coping skills to manage anger and agitation during daily sessions for the next ___ days.
PO intake	**LTI:** Work with a nutritionist to develop and follow a balanced meal plan daily over the next ___ weeks. **STI:** Provide education on the importance of nutrition and its impact on mental health at least ___ times in the next ___ days. **STI:** Use positive reinforcement to encourage increased food intake at ___% of meals over the next ___ days. **STI:** Supervise meals to ensure adequate intake and address any issues at ___% of meals over the next ___ days.
Medication compliance/ hospital relapse	**LTI:** Educate the patient about the importance of medication adherence at least ___ times weekly over the next ___ weeks. **STI:** Supervise medication administration at least ___ times daily to ensure compliance over the next ___ days. **STI:** Address any concerns about side effects to improve adherence at least every ___ days over the next ___ days.
Sleep	**LTI:** Encourage the use of a structured sleep hygiene plan at least ___ times weekly over the next ___ weeks. **STI:** Educate the patient on good sleep hygiene practices at least every ___ days over the next ___ days. **STI:** Help the patient establish a consistent nightly bedtime routine by reviewing and reinforcing it at least ___ times in the next ___ days.
Falls	**LTI:** Attend multidisciplinary meetings to review fall prevention strategies at least ___ times over the next ___ weeks. **STI:** Educate the patient on fall prevention strategies at least ___ times over the next ___ days. **STI:** Ensure the environment is safe and free of fall hazards, checked at least ___ times a day over the next ___ days. **STI:** Provide supervision and assistance as needed to prevent falls, reviewed at least ___ times a day over the next ___ days.

Appendix C: Clinical Scales

We've included essential clinical scales to help you accurately assess and monitor your patients. These tools are invaluable for understanding patient conditions and tailoring effective treatment plans.

Table 17: **Commonly Used Clinical Scales**

Scale	Link
Administering the Abnormal Involuntary Movement Scale (AIMS)	www.thecarlatreport.com/AdministeringAIMS
Aid to Capacity Evaluation (ACE) – Administration	www.thecarlatreport.com/AdministeringACE
How to Administer the Bush-Francis Catatonia Rating Scale	www.thecarlatreport.com/BushFrancisCatatoniaRatingScale
Clinical Institute Withdrawal Assessment for Alcohol Scale, Revised (CIWA-Ar)	www.thecarlatreport.com/CIWA-Ar
Clinical Opiate Withdrawal Scale (COWS)	www.thecarlatreport.com/AdministeringCOWS
How to Administer the Montreal Cognitive Assessment (MoCA)	www.thecarlatreport.com/AdministeringMoCA
Edinburgh Postnatal Depression Scale (EPDS)	www.thecarlatreport.com/AdministeringEPDS
Short Form of the Informant Questionnaire on Cognitive Decline in the Elderly (Short IQCODE)	www.thecarlatreport.com/shortIQCODE
Yale-Brown Obsessive-Compulsive Scale (Y-BOCS)	www.thecarlatreport.com/Y-BOCS

Index

Index

A

Abdominal pain, 226
Acute stress disorder, DSM-5 criteria, 87
ADHD in adults, 108
Adolescents
- dosing recommendations, 267
- management of agitation, 266–267
- suicidality and self-harm, 268

Agitation, 63–69
- medication, 66–67
- nonpharmacological interventions, 67
- physical restraint and seclusion, 68
- restraints, 67
- verbal de-escalation, 64–65

Agranulocytosis, 198
- clozapine and, 142

Akathisia, 174
Alcohol withdrawal, 149
Alpha-1 adrenergic blockers, trauma-related disorders, 87
Alpha-2 agonists, trauma-related disorders, 88
Alzheimer's disease, 119
Anger management, 168
Anorexia nervosa, 111–112
- forced refeeding, 113

Anticonvulsants, dementia, 123
Antidepressants
- anorexia nervosa, 111
- breastfeeding patients, 276
- dementia, 123
- depression in pregnancy, 273
- insomnia, 117
- major depressive disorder, 101
- postpartum women, 274
- prolonged grief disorder, 102
- schizoaffective disorder, 136
- schizophrenia, 135
- suicidality and self-harm in children and adolescents, 268
- TBI, 125

Antihistamines, 66
- insomnia, 117

Anti-NMDA receptor encephalitis, 228
Antipsychotics, 66
- anorexia nervosa, 111
- bipolar depression, 96
- breastfeeding patients, 276
- brief psychotic disorder, 138
- delusional disorder, 137
- dementia, 123
- effect on lab tests, 197
- fast facts for, 139–141
- insomnia, 117
- long-acting injectable, 143–146
- manic episodes, 94
- personality disorders, 127
- pregnant patients, 271
- schizoaffective disorder, 136
- schizophrenia, 135
- second generation (SGAs)
  - effect on lab tests, 197
  - long-acting injectable, 143–145
  - schizophrenia, 135
- suicidality and self-harm in children and adolescents, 268

Antisocial personality disorder (ASPD), 127
Anxiety disorders, screening for, 83–91
Anxiolytics, prolonged grief disorder, 102
Anxiolytics/hypnotics, breastfeeding patients, 276
Aripiprazole (Abilify), 139
Armodafinil (Nuvigil), bipolar depression, 96
Asenapine (Saphris), 141
Assault precautions, 58
Atypical depression, differential diagnosis, 98
Autism spectrum disorder (ASD)
- DSM-5 criteria, 109
- medications, 109

Avoidant personality disorder (AvPD), 127

B

Baby blues, 274
Bacterial vaginosis (BV), 255
Basic metabolic panel, 201–202
Behavioral management
- nurses, 10
- plan, 169

Benzodiazepines, 66
- catatonia, 155
- choosing and managing, 90–91
- comparative table of, 91
- dementia, 123
- insomnia, 117
- manic episodes, 94
- panic disorder, 86
- schizophrenia, 135

Beta-blockers, anxiety management, 89
Billing, 52–53
Bipolar depression, 96
- differential diagnosis, 98

Bipolar disorder, 92–96
- DSM-5 criteria, 93
- pregnant and postpartum patients, 271–272
- psychoeducation, 96
- psychosis and, 132

Bone marrow suppression, 198
Borderline personality disorder (BPD), 127
- defense mechanisms, 128–129
- DSM-5 criteria, 128
- four key domains of, 128
- overview, 128
- psychopharmacology, 129
- psychotherapy, 129

Breastfeeding considerations
- medications in postpartum women, 272
- psychiatric medications in, 276–279

Brexpiprazole (Rexulti), 140
Brief psychotic disorder, 132, 138
Bruxism, 175
Bulimia nervosa, 114
Buprenorphine, opioid withdrawal, 150
Buspirone, anxiety management, 89

C

Capacity evaluation, 44
- anorexia nervosa, 113
- pregnant patients, 269

Carbamazepine, effect on lab tests, 197
Cariprazine (Vraylar), 141
- bipolar depression, 96

Case managers, 12
Catatonia, 155
Chemical restraint, use in agitated patients, 68
Chest pain, 229–230
Children
- dosing recommendations, 267
- management of agitation, 266–267
- suicidality and self-harm, 268

Chlamydia, 255
Chlorpromazine (Thorazine), 66, 141
Cholinesterase inhibitors, dementia, 123
Chronic obstructive pulmonary disease (COPD), 231–232
Citalopram, effect on diagnostic tests, 197
Clinical scales, 288
Clonazepam (Klonopin)
- dementia, 123
- insomnia, 117

Clozapine, 139, 142
- agranulocytosis and, 142
- effect on lab tests, 197
- neutropenia and, 142
- schizophrenia, 135

Coding and billing, 52–53
Cognitive behavioral therapy (CBT)
- delusional disorder, 137
- insomnia, 116
- OCD, 85
- panic disorder, 86
- psychotherapy and, 160
- psychotic disorders (CBTp), 166
- schizoaffective disorder, 136
- suicidality and self-harm in children and adolescents, 268
- TBI, 125
- techniques, 162

Cognitive rehabilitation therapy, TBI, 125
Columbia Suicide Severity Rating Scale (C-SSRS), 74
Commitment of patients, 41
Comorbid conditions, 223–264. see also specific condition
Complete blood count (CBC), 198–200
Compliance, 62
- in health care administration, 12
- legal, 46

Confidentiality, 45–46
Confusion, 122
Constipation, 176
Conversion disorder. see Functional neurological disorder
Court order, involuntary medications, 43
CPR, 233–234
Cross-cultural issues, inpatient psych unit, 280
Cyproheptadine, anorexia nervosa, 112

D

Danger to others, 79–81
Daridorexant (Quviviq), insomnia, 117
Deep breathing exercises, 167
De-escalation strategies, 60, 64
Deliberate foreign body ingestion (DFBI), 78
Delirium, 122
Delusional disorder, 132, 137
- common types of, 137
- DSM-5 criteria, 137
- prognosis, 137

Delusions, in psychosis, 132
Dementia
- behavioral and psychological symptoms, 123
- clinical evaluation, 119–120
- medication treatment, 121

Dementia with Lewy bodies, 119
Depakote, dementia, 123
Dependent personality disorder (DPD), 127
Depression, 97–105. see also specific type
- postpartum, 274
- in pregnancy, 273

Depression with mixed manic features, differential diagnosis, 98
Depression with psychotic features, 100
Desipramine, bulimia nervosa, 114
Desvenlafaxine, effect on diagnostic tests, 197
Diabetes, 235–236
Dialectical behavior therapy (DBT), 160
- suicidality and self-harm in children and adolescents, 268

Diarrhea, 177
Digestive issues, 221
Diphenhydramine (Benadryl), insomnia, 117

Discharge planning
  children and adolescents, 268
  notes for coding and billing, 53
  social workers and case managers, 12
  summaries, 26–27
Disclosure without consent, 46
Dissociative identity disorder (DID), 156
Documentation
  ED, 19
  legal compliance and, 46
  requirements for coding and billing, 52
  steps to follow after suicide, 77
  suicide risk, 74
  Tarasoff obligations, 81
Donepezil (Aricept), dementia, 121, 123
Dosing recommendations in ED, children and adolescents, 267
Doxepin (Silenor), insomnia, 117
Doxylamine (Unisom), insomnia, 117
Dronabinol, anorexia nervosa, 112
Drug interactions, 214–215
Dry mouth (xerostomia), 178
Dual orexin receptor antagonists (DORAs), insomnia, 117
Duty to protect, 81
Duty to warn, 81
Dystonia, 179

E

Eating disorders, 110–114
ECG, 211
Edinburgh Postnatal Depression Scale, 274
Electroconvulsive therapy (ECT), 103–104
  depression in pregnant patients, 273
  pregnant patients, 271
Electronic health record (EHR), hospital pharmacy and, 16
Elopement precautions, 58
Emergency department (psychiatric ED), 18–19
Escitalopram, dementia, 123
Eszopiclone (Lunesta), insomnia, 117

F

Factitious disorder, 157
Fall precautions, 58
Family and caregiver liaison, social workers and case managers, 12, 13
Family-focused therapy (FFT), 166
Family psychiatric history, 21
Fatigue, 181
Fluoxetine (Prozac)
  anorexia nervosa, 111
  bulimia nervosa, 114
Fluphenazine (Prolixin), 140
Forced refeeding, anorexia nervosa, 113
Formulary, pharmacists and, 15
Frontotemporal dementia, 119
Functional neurological disorder, 158

G

Gabapentin, dementia, 123
Galantamine (Razadyne, Razadyne ER), dementia, 121, 123
Gastroesophageal reflux disease (GERD), 237
Gender-affirming care, inpatient psych unit, 281
Gonorrhea, 255
Group programs, 164–165
Guardianship, anorexia nervosa and refeeding, 113

H

Hallucinations, in psychosis, 132
Haloperidol (Haldol), 66, 139
Headaches, 238–239
Health care proxy (HCP), 42
  anorexia nervosa and refeeding, 113
Herpes (HSV), 255
HIPAA, 45
Histrionic personality disorder (HPD), 127
HIV, 240–241
Homicide risk, 80
Hospital-Based Inpatient Psychiatric Services (HBIPS), 55
Hospital pharmacy, 16
Hospital safety protocols, 57–62
Huntington's disease, 242
Hydroxyzine, anxiety management, 89
Hyperhidrosis. see Sweating
Hyperlipidemia, 224
Hyperprolactinemia, 182
Hypersexual precautions, 58
Hypersalivation. see Sialorrhea
Hypertension, 243–244
Hyponatremia, 245

I

Iloperidone (Fanapt), 139
Informant Questionnaire on Cognitive Decline in the Elerly (IQCODE), 120
Informed consent, 40
  involuntary medications, 43
  pregnant patients, 269
Ingesting harmful substances, 73
Inpatient Psychiatric Facility Quality Reporting (IPFQR), 55
Insomnia, 115–117
  medication management, 117
Insulin sliding scale protocol, 236
Intellectual disabilities
  DSM-5 criteria, 107
  medications, 107
Interpersonal therapy (IPT), 160
Involuntary medications, 43
Isolation precautions, 58

K

Kidney function testing, 203
Kidney impairment, psychiatric medications in, 218

L

Laboratory data, 22
Lab tests
  guidelines, 196–197
  recommended tests for medications, 216–217
Lamotrigine (Lamictal), bipolar depression, 96
Legal and ethical considerations, 39–46
Lemborexant (Belsomra), insomnia, 117
Leukopenia, 198
Levomilnacipran, effect on lab tests, 197
LGBTQIA+ patients, 281
Lice and scabies, 246
Licensed Clinical Social Worker (LCSW), 12
Licensed Practical Nurse (LPN), 10
Lipid panel, 224
Lithium
  bipolar depression, 96
  dementia, 123
  effect on lab tests, 197
  manic episodes, 94
  pregnancy and, 271
Liver function tests, 204
Liver impairment, psychiatric medications in, 219–220
Locked-door seclusion, use in agitated patients, 68
Lorazepam (Ativan)
  catatonia, 155
  dementia, 123
  insomnia, 117
  manic episodes, 94
Lumateperone (Caplyta), 139
Lurasidone (Latuda), 140

M

Major depression
  differential diagnosis, 98
  how to diagnose, 99
  psychosis and, 132
Major neurocognitive disorders
  DSM-5 criteria, 119
  medication, 121
Manic episodes, 94–95
Mechanical restraint, use in agitated patients, 68
Medicaid, 49
Medicare, 48
Medication errors, 62
Medication reconciliation, hospital pharmacy and, 16
Melancholic depression, differential diagnosis, 98
Melatonin, insomnia, 117
Melatonin receptor agonists, insomnia, 117
Memantine IR and XR (Namenda), dementia, 121
Mental status examination (MSE), 23–24, 32–33
Metabolic syndrome, 173
Methadone, opioid withdrawal, 150
Methamphetamine, 151
Mindfulness and relaxation techniques, panic disorder, 86
Mindfulness-based cognitive therapy, 160
Mirtazapine (Remeron)
  anorexia nervosa, 111–112
  dementia, 123
  effect on lab tests, 197
  insomnia, 117
Monoamine oxidase inhibitors (MAOIs), bulimia nervosa, 114
Montreal Cognitive Assessment (MoCA), 120
Mood stabilizers
  bipolar depression, 96
  breastfeeding patients, 276
  dementia, 123
  manic episodes, 94
  personality disorders, 127
  pregnant patients, 271
  schizoaffective disorder, 136
  schizophrenia, 135
  suicidality and self-harm in children and adolescents, 268
  TBI, 125
Motivational interviewing (MI), 161
Multidisciplinary teams, 9–16
Multiple personality disorder. see Dissociative identity disorder
Munchausen disorder. see Factitious disorder

N

Naltrexone, effect on lab tests, 197
Naltrexone plus bupropion, stimulant use disorder, 151
Narcissistic personality disorder (NPD), 127
National mental health resources, 284–285
Nausea, 183
Negative symptoms, in psychosis, 132
Neurocognitive disorders, 118–125
Neuroimaging, 209
Neuroleptic malignant syndrome, 184
Neurological exam, 37
Neutropenia, 198
  clozapine and, 142
Newborn care, pregnant inpatients, 270
N-methyl-D-aspartate (NMDA), catatonia, 155
Nonviolent physical restraints, use in agitated patients, 69
Nurses, 10–11
Nutritional rehabilitation, anorexia nervosa and forced refeeding, 113

O

Obsessive-compulsive disorder (OCD), 85
Obsessive-compulsive personality disorder (OCPD), 127
Occupational therapists (OTs), 13
Olanzapine, anorexia nervosa, 111
Olanzapine (Zyprexa), 66, 141

Index

Olanzapine/fluoxetine combination (Symbyax), 96
Opioid withdrawal, 150
Orthostatic hypotension, 185
Oxcarbazepine, effect on lab tests, 197

P

Pain management, inpatient setting, 247
Paliperidone (Invega), 140
    effect on lab tests, 197
Pancytopenia, 198
Panic disorder, 86
Parenteral nutrition, forced refeeding, 113
Parkinsonism, 186
Parkinson's disease, 248–249
Patient competency and consent, 45
Patient safety incidents, 62
Patients' rights, involuntary medications, 43
Peer reviewer, 50
Peer-to-peer calls, 51
Perphenazine (Trilafon), 141
Personality disorders (PDs), 126–129
Pharmacists (PharmDs), 15
Pharmacogenetic testing, 210
Physical exams, 22, 36
Physical restraint, use in agitated patients, 68
Pimavanserin (Nuplazid), 140
Platelets, 198
Positive psychology interventions, 160
Postpartum women
    antidepressants in, 274
    bipolar disorder treatment, 271–272
    breastfeeding considerations, 272
    depression in, 274
    psychosis, 275
Poststroke psychiatric symptoms, 250–251
Posttraumatic stress disorder (PTSD), 87–88
    adjunctive and alternative medications, 88
    DSM-5 criteria, 87
    workplace trauma, 61
Power of attorney (POA), 42
    access to health information and, 45
Pramipexole (Mirapex), bipolar depression, 96
Precaution orders, 58
Pregabalin, anxiety management, 89
Pregnant patients, 269–270
    bipolar disorder treatment, 271–272
    common complications, 269
    depression in, 273
Prescription Drug Monitoring Program (PDMP), 19
Privacy breaches, 62
Progress notes, 25
Prolonged grief disorder (PGD), 102
Psychiatric admission notes, 20–24
Psychiatric interview techniques, 28
Psychiatric review of symptoms, 29–31
Psychiatric technicians, 14
Psychogenic polydipsia, 252
Psychosis
    differential diagnosis, 132
    DSM-5 criteria, 132
    interviewing patients, 131
    postpartum, 271–272
    with a major mood component, 132
Psychosocial assessments, social workers and case managers, 12
Psychotherapy, 159–170
    borderline personality disorder, 129
    psychotic disorders, 166
    nurses, 10
Psychotic depression, differential diagnosis, 98
Psychotic disorders, psychotherapy, 166

Q

QT interval prolongation, 187–188
Quality measures, 55–56
Quetiapine (Seroquel), 141
    bipolar depression, 96
    insomnia, 117

R

Ramelteon (Rozerem), insomnia, 117
Recreation therapists, 13
Red blood cells (RBC), 198
Relaxation, 167
Release of information (ROI) forms, 45
Remeron (mirtazapine), insomnia, 117
Reportable events, 62
Respiratory symptoms, 221–222
Restraints
    psychiatric technicians, 14
    use in agitated patients, 67–69
Risperidone (Risperdal), 140–141
Rivastigmine and patch (Exelon, Exelon patch), dementia, 121, 123
Ruminative depression, differential diagnosis, 98

S

SAFE-T (Suicide Assessment Five-step Evaluation and Triage), 74
Safety plan, 76
Schizoaffective disorder, 132
    diagnosis and treatment, 136
Schizophrenia, 130–147
    adjunctive medications, 135
    comorbid depression, 132
    differential diagnosis, 133
    DSM-5 criteria, 132
    key symptoms, 133
    medication, 135
    post-discharge treatment, 134
    prognosis, 133
    psychosis and, 132
    resources for patients, 134

risk factors, 133
Schizophreniform disorder, 132
Schizotypal personality disorder (STPD), 127
Screening for metabolic disorders (SMD), 56
Seclusion, use in agitated patients, 68
Seizure disorders, 253–254
Seizure precautions, 58
Selective serotonin reuptake inhibitors (SSRIs)
anorexia nervosa, 111
bulimia nervosa, 114
dementia, 123
OCD, 85
panic disorder, 86
personality disorders, 127
trauma-related disorders, 87
Self-harm, children and adolescents, 268
Self-hitting, 73
Self-injurious behaviors, 71–78
medication management, 73
Serotonin/norepinephrine reuptake inhibitors (SNRIs)
panic disorder, 86, 89
trauma-related disorders, 87
Serotonin syndrome, 189
Sertraline, dementia, 123
Sexual activity, inpatient unit, 59
Sexual dysfunction, 190
Sexually transmitted diseases (STDs), 255
Sialorrhea (hypersalivation), 191
Side effects, 171–194
Skin and eye care, 222
Sleep disturbances, inpatient psych unit, 116
Sleep hygiene enhancements, 116
SMART goals and interventions, 286–287
Smoking cessation, 222
Social history, collateral contact information, 21
Social workers (MSWs), 12
Stimulants, ADHD, 108
Stimulant use disorders, 151–152
Stroke symptoms, 227
Substance use disorders, 148–153
Substance use history, 21
Suicidality, children and adolescents, 268
Suicide, 71–78
assessing risk, 74–75
precautions, 58
steps to follow after, 77
Supportive therapy, 163
Sweating, excessive (hyperhidrosis), 180
Swollen feet, ankles, and calves, 256–257
Symptom-Triggered Withdrawal Protocol (CIWA protocol), 149
Syphilis, 258
Systemic lupus erythematosus (SLE), 259

T

Tarasoff obligations, 81
Tardive dyskinesia (TD), 192
Temazepam (Restoril), insomnia, 117
The Joint Commission, 54
Therapeutic drug monitoring, 206
Therapeutic groups, psychiatric technicians and, 14
Thiamine, 153
Thyroid disease, 260–261
Token economy, 170
Topiramate
bulimia nervosa, 114
stimulant use disorder, 151
Transcranial magnetic stimulation (TMS), 105
OCD, 85
Traumatic brain injury (TBI), 124–125
DSM-5 criteria, 124
Trazodone (Desyrel)
bulimia nervosa, 114
insomnia, 117
Tremor, 193
Trichomoniasis, 255
Tricyclic antidepressants (TCAs)
bulimia nervosa, 114
panic disorder, 86

U

Upper respiratory conditions, 262
Urinalysis, 205
Urinary tract infections, 263
Urine drug screening (UDS), 207–208
Utilization review (UR), 50–51
social workers and case managers, 12

V

Valproic acid, manic episodes, 94
Vascular neurocognitive disorder, 119
Verbal de-escalation, 64–65
Viral hepatitis, 264

W

Weight gain, 194
Wernicke's encephalopathy (WE), 153
White blood cells (WBCs), 198
Workplace violence, prevention and safety, 60

X

Xerostomia. see Dry mouth

Y

Yale-Brown Obsessive-Compulsive Scale (Y-BOCS), 85
Yeast infection (Candidiasis), 255

Z

Zaleplon (Sonata), insomnia, 117
Ziprasidone (Geodon), 66, 139
Zolpidem CR (Ambien), insomnia, 117
Zolpidem SL (Intermezzo), insomnia, 117

Index

www.ingramcontent.com/pod-product-compliance
Lightning Source LLC
LaVergne TN
LVHW070850210926
848482LV00016B/907
9798989326426